Orthopedic Rehabilitation Science

Principles for Clinical Management of Nonmineralized Connective Tissue

Orthopedic Rehabilitation Science

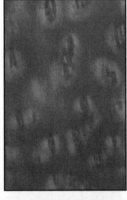

Principles for
Clinical
Management of
Nonmineralized
Connective
Tissue

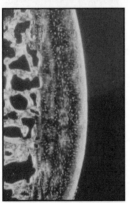

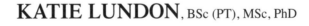

KATIE LUNDON, BSc (PT), MSc, PhD

Assistant Professor, Department of Physical Therapy
and Graduate Department of Rehabilitation Science,
Faculty of Medicine, University of Toronto,
Toronto, Ontario

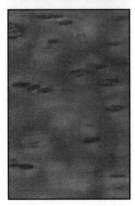

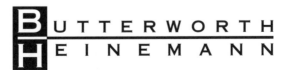

BUTTERWORTH
HEINEMANN

An Imprint of Elsevier Science
Amsterdam   Boston   London   New York   Oxford   Paris
San Diego   San Francisco   Singapore   Sydney   Tokyo

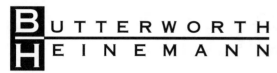

An Imprint of Elsevier Science

11830 Westline Industrial Drive
St. Louis, Missouri 63146

NOTICE

Orthopedics is an ever-changing field. Standard safety precautions must be followed, but as new research and clinical experience broaden our knowledge, changes in treatment and drug therapy may become necessary or appropriate. Readers are advised to check the most current product information provided by the manufacturer of each drug to be administered to verify the recommended dose, the method and duration of administration, and contraindications. It is the responsibility of the licensed prescriber, relying on experience and knowledge of the patient, to determine dosages and the best treatment for each individual patient. Neither the publisher nor the author assumes any liability for any injury and/or damage to persons or property arising from this publication.

International Standard Book Number 0-7506-7347-8
Acquisitions Editor: Andrew Allen
Developmental Editor: Rebecca Swisher
Publishing Services Manager: Linda McKinley
Project Manager: Jim Rygelski
Designer: Julia Dummitt

KI/MVY

Printed in the United States

Last digit is the print number: 9 8 7 6 5 4 3 2 1

Contributors

Harpal K. Gahunia, BSc, MSc, PhD
Senior Scientist
Orthobiologic Department
DePuy Orthopedics, Inc. (A Johnson and Johnson Company)
Warsaw, Indiana

Pamela Houghton, BSc(PT), PhD
Associate Professor
Chair, Undergraduate Program
School of Physical Therapy
Elborn College
University of Western Ontario
London, Ontario
Canada

This book is dedicated to my children: Sophie, Sam, and Robyn.
May they share a lifelong love of learning.

Preface

This text provides information about the basic science underpinnings of select dense nonmineralized connective tissues as they relate to the clinical science of orthopaedic rehabilitation. The nature of this work resembles and is closely associated with material found in its companion volume, *Orthopedic Rehabilitation Science: Principles for Clinical Management of Bone*.

The fundamentals of development, morphology, and function of nonmineralized dense connective tissue-based structures are presented. A thorough understanding of some basic pathophysiologic events common to these structures across the lifespan, in both health and disease, is essential knowledge for clinicians involved in orthōpaedic physical therapy practice. The premise upon which this material is compiled is that sound clinical judgement in orthopaedic physical therapy practice results from the judicious use of this knowledge.

Extensive knowledge of connective tissue dynamics in response to injury and repair is important to the physical therapist for two reasons. First, the selection of the appropriate strategy for management of dense connective tissues should be guided by evidence-based studies of how these tissues respond to physical intervention in health, injury, and disease. Secondly, physical methods, including manual therapy and electrophysical agents, should appropriately aim to promote the optimal repair of injured connective tissues and endeavor to improve function of the replacement tissue after injury.

This book is designed to help clinicians do the following:

1. Gain a basic understanding of the biology of dense nonmineralized connective tissues in terms of normal structure, function, growth, and repair processes in the adult skeleton

2. Obtain a basic level of knowledge of pathophysiologic processes inherent to dense nonmineralized connective tissue in response to injury and disease

3. Understand the rationale for physical intervention in the orthopaedic management of structures comprised of nonmineralized connective tissues in health and disease

4. Be cognizant of both the results of and direction for future research studies involving nonmineralized connective tissues that would have an impact on the advancement of orthopaedic rehabilitation and establishment of best practices within this field.

The goals of this book are the following:

1. To effectively present the current basic science background underlying nonmineralized dense connective tissue dynamics in health and selected conditions commonly encountered in physical rehabilitation practice

2. To serve as a practical reference for students of professional physical therapy programs and practicing clinicians alike by offering a comprehensive and integrated text on nonmineralized connective tissue metabolism, selected clinical disorders, and pertinent applications to clinical practice in physical rehabilitation

3. To facilitate the clinician's understanding of the basic science mechanisms of skeletal pathophysiology that underlie clinical decision making in the physical assessment and

treatment of selected nonmineralized connective tissue disorders

Therefore the knowledge objectives are as follows:

1. To describe the normal structure and function of the dense nonmineralized connective tissues
2. To describe the normal repair processes of the dense nonmineralized connective tissues in response to injury
3. To differentiate acute versus chronic repair processes after injury in dense nonmineralized connective tissue
4. To understand the principles underlying select physical therapy interventions, including manual and electrophysical therapies in determining the healing, repair, and subsequent behavior of these tissues

This book is organized into seven chapters. Chapters 1 and 2 introduce the general structure, function, and metabolic properties inherent to the dense nonmineralized connective tissues. Chapters 3, 4, and 5 address the morphology and general physiology of tendon and ligaments, articular cartilage and meniscus, and the intervertebral disc, respectively. Chapter 6 reflects the physical behavior of these structures as well as their response to physical stresses encompassing issues such as immobilization and principles for (re)mobilization

of these tissues. Finally, Chapter 7 addresses the rationale for and effect of select electrotherapeutic modalities on the healing and repair of injured dense connective tissues.

The intent of this book is to effectively present the basic science principles underlying the nonmineralized connective tissues and select pathologic states affecting them that are important to orthopaedic rehabilitation practice. The rationale for physical intervention strategies in the management of the nonmineralized connective tissues in both health and disease is examined.

There is a clear need for a unified presentation of the scientific underpinnings of clinical care of dense nonmineralized connective tissues in physical therapy practice. The physical management of these tissues, including tendon, ligament, intervertebral disc, and articular cartilage should incorporate and be constantly guided by the knowledge of the dynamics of their metabolism in health and disease as well as the changes that affect them across the lifespan. Advanced practice in orthopaedic physical therapy continues to develop with an inherent dependency for fluency in the basic and clinical sciences. This text, along with its companion text, *Orthopedic Rehabilitation Science: Principles for Clinical Management of Bone* is critical information for the contemporary practitioner actively involved in the musculoskeletal field of practice.

Acknowledgments

I would like to thank the members of the team at Elsevier Sciences who worked with such thoroughness, efficiency, and enthusiasm on the editing and overall production of this book. A special note of appreciation is extended to Laurie Anello, Rebecca Swisher, Jim Rygelski, and Leslie Forman (previously with Butterworth-Heinemann). I would like to express my sincere gratitude to my two contributing authors, Dr. Harpal (Polly) Gahunia and Dr. Pamela Houghton, for their outstanding work on this project. Finally, I would like to extend my heartfelt appreciation to my students, both undergraduate and graduate, who over the past decade have shown ceaseless curiosity and eagerness to learn.

Contents

CHAPTER 1

Connective Tissues: Structure, Function, and Metabolic Properties, 1

CHAPTER 2

Structure, Function, and Metabolic Properties of Nonmineralized Connective Tissues, 5

    Composition of Connective Tissue, 5
    Components of Connective Tissue:
      Overview, 5
    Constituents of the Nonmineralized
      Connective Tissues: Specific Cellular
      Components, 7
    Regular Dense Connective Tissue: The
      Extracellular Matrix, 8
    The Molecular Structure of Collagen, 12
    Stabilization of Fibrillar Collagens, 15
    Collagen Biosynthesis, 17
    Summary, 29

CHAPTER 3

The Nature of the Dense Connective Tissues of the Musculoskeletal System: Structure, Function, and Biomechanics of Tendon, Ligament, and the Joint Capsule, 33

    Tendon and Ligament: General
      Characteristics, 33
    Tendon: Specific Characteristics, 34
    Tendon Structure and Structures that
      Surround Tendon, 38

    Organization of Tendon: Paratenon,
      Epitenon, Endotenon, 38
    Healing and Repair in Tendon Injury, 41
    Ligament: Specific Characteristics, 48
    Summary, 57

CHAPTER 4

The Nature of the Dense Connective Tissues of the Musculoskeletal System: Structure, Function, and Biomechanics of Articular Cartilage and Meniscus, 63
Harpal K. Gahunia

    Articular Cartilage Structure and
      Biochemistry, 63
    Articular Cartilage Heterogeneity, 67
    Articular Cartilage Function and
      Biomechanics, 68
    Articular Cartilage Formation, Growth, and
      Remodeling, 69
    Age-Related Changes in Articular
      Cartilage, 71
    Articular Cartilage Degradation and
      Related Diseases, 71
    Articular Cartilage Visualization in Health
      and Disease, 74
    Articular Cartilage Repair, 77
    Meniscal Anatomy, 81
    Meniscal Structure, 82
    Meniscal Function and Biomechanics, 83
    Meniscal Degradation, 84
    Meniscal Repair, 84
    Summary, 86

CHAPTER 5

The Nature of the Dense Connective Tissues of the Musculoskeletal System: Structure, Function, and Biomechanics of the Intervertebral Disc, 97

The Nonimpaired Intervertebral Disc, 97

General Morphology of the Intervertebral Disc, 100

Biomechanics of the Intervertebral Disc, 101

Intervertebral Disc: Common Pathologies, 107

Lesions of the IVD: Morphological Characteristics, 109

Summary, 111

CHAPTER 6

Dynamics of the Nonmineralized Connective Tissues of the Musculoskeletal System, 117

Connective Tissue Biomechanics, 117

Connective Tissue Response to Immobilization, 127

Joint Hypomobility, 132

Joint Hypermobility, 134

Pharmacologic Management of Soft Tissue Injuries, 135

Summary, 135

CHAPTER 7

Therapeutic Modalities for the Treatment of Orthopaedic Conditions, 139

Pamela Houghton

Superficial Hot and Cold, 139

Electrical Stimulation, 143

Electromagnetic Fields, 147

Laser, 147

Ultrasound, 150

Ankle Sprains, 153

Periarticular Inflammatory Conditions, 158

Shoulder Tendonitis, 165

Acute and Chronic Low Back and Neck Pain, 167

Summary, 175

Chapter 1

Connective Tissues: Structure, Function, and Metabolic Properties

Impairments of the musculoskeletal system often stem from changes in structures composed of non-mineralized connective tissues such as ligaments and tendons, articular cartilage, intervertebral discs, and joint capsules. The impairments caused by affliction or change in these tissues because of disease or age-related processes are largely represented in orthopaedic physical therapy practice and result in weakness, pain with movement, and restriction of motion (Jette 1990). Musculoskeletal impairments constitute the most prevalent and symptomatic group of problems affecting the health of middle-aged and older individuals (Brock et al. 1990; Jette et al. 1990). This cohort is demographically prominent in both the United States, where between 1990 and 2010 the number of people older than 45 years is projected to have increased from 82,000,000 to 124,000,000 (U.S. Bureau of the Census 1992) and in Canada, where the projected increase during that same time period is from 11,000,000 to 14,500,000 (Statistics Canada, CANSIM 2001).

Connective tissues present as tremendously diverse forms within the human musculoskeletal system. One has only to reflect on the toughness and characteristic ability of tendon and ligament to sustain significant stress, or the resilience and viscoelastic properties inherent to articular cartilage and the intervertebral disc to respect this variance. The design of load-bearing collagenous-based tissues reflects different mechanical principles. For instance, tendon is a fiber-reinforced composite material, whereas the mechanical properties of cartilage depend on osmotic pressure developed within an aqueous proteoglycan gel and resisted by tension in a collagenous network (Ker 1999).

Connective tissues bind cells together and are therefore critical elements to multicellular animals. The common link among all of the connective tissues in the human body is that the composition of their extracellular matrices is largely collagen-based.

The physical therapist must be familiar with numerous structures within the musculoskeletal system in terms of their biologic behavior across the lifespan and the factors that influence their integrity in health and disease, as well as processes that underlie the healing and restoration of these tissues after injury and during rehabilitation. Principles for providing the most appropriate physical management for these tissues are derived from such knowledge. The structures composed of dense nonmineralized connective tissue, whose qualities in terms of their form and function will be addressed in subsequent chapters, include tendon, ligament, and joint capsule (Chapter 3), articular cartilage (Chapter 4) and the intervertebral disc (Chapter 5). The basic science underpinnings of the dense nonmineralized connective tissue-based structures in the musculoskeletal system will be highlighted in terms of their relationship to, and implications for, clinical orthopaedic physical therapy practice.

Connective tissues serve to support and connect as well as protect tissues and organs throughout the body. In addition, connective tissues have other specialized functions (Table 1-1). The interstitial tissue of the musculoskeletal system is composed of various forms of specialized connective tissues. Common to all forms of connective tissue found in the musculoskeletal system is the presence of connective tissue cells embedded in an abundant

Table 1-1. Main Types of Connective Tissues and Their Function

Type	Presentation	Function
Ordinary connective tissue	Loose	Tissue/organ protection
	Dense	
	Irregular (e.g., capsule, dermis)	Connecting functions
	Regular	
	Cartilage	Connects, supports, bears weight
	Bone	Connects, protects, supports, bears weight
	Ligament, tendon	Connects, supports, stabilizes, and imparts tensile strength
Specialized connective tissue	Adipose (fat) tissue	Space occupying and has cushioning effects
	Blood cells and blood-forming tissue	

From Lundon K. Orthopedic Rehabilitation Science Principles for Clinical Management of Bone. Boston: Butterworth-Heinemann, 2000.

extracellular matrix that the cells produce. The extracellular matrix from different connective tissues comprises many substances, of which only collagen fibers and proteoglycans are ubiquitous components. This interstitial or extracellular matrix is composed of both protein-based structures and complex polysaccharides, the presence and distribution of which determine the metabolic and biomechanical characteristics of each form and contribute to its specialized functions. The biomechanical conditions to which the various connective tissues are subject support a strong relationship between their ultrastructure and function. In health, the connective tissues are not inert structures but are quite metabolically active and achieve a continuous balance of degradation and replacement of their components.

The term *connective tissue* often is used to describe the extracellular matrix plus resident cells such as fibroblasts, macrophages, and mast cells. The amount of connective tissue in organs varies greatly: skin and bone are composed mainly of connective tissue, whereas the brain and spinal cord contain minimal amounts. The relative amounts of the different types of matrix macromolecules and the way in which they are organized within the extracellular matrix vary to a great extent, allowing a large diversity of forms, each specific to the functional requirements of the particular tissue. The extracellular matrix can, for example, calcify to form bone or teeth, or it may assume the ropelike organization of the collagen fibers in tendons, imparting tensile strength. The

ligaments, fasciae, tendons, sclera, and cornea of the eye are all examples of "soft" connective tissues. "Hard" connective tissues, such as bone, dentine, and cementum, are mineralized through the deposition of calcium phosphate in the form of hydroxyapatite $[Ca_{10}(PO_4)_6OH_2]$ crystals. Cartilage, which can be mineralized but usually is not, also is considered a hard connective tissue (Box 1-1).

Connective tissue exists diversely and is integral to systems that perform particular functions. For example, the joints that have bone, cartilage, ligaments, and synovial fluid function to allow movement between long bones. The heart, blood vessels, and blood cells are all formed from cells that develop in the mesenchyme, the embryonic germ layer responsible for connective tissue development. In this way, the blood circulating in vessels that are confined to connective tissue is considered a specialized connective tissue similar to synovial fluid that is confined to the joint.

An appreciation of the morphology, cell biology, biochemistry, and biomechanics inherent to the connective tissues is essential to understand the behavior of normal connective tissues, the response of these tissues to injury, and the potential of these tissues to repair themselves once injured. The study of the repair of connective tissues in the musculoskeletal system is fascinating in that the majority of connective tissues display significant regenerative potential, as can be witnessed by the cellular proliferation and biosynthetic events that occur most notably in response

Box 1-1. Forms of Connective Tissue: Hard Versus Soft

Soft
Ligament
Fasciae
Tendon
Sclera
Cornea of the eye
Hard
Bone*
Dentine*
Cementum*
Cartilage†

*Mineralized
†Nonmineralized
From Lundon K. Orthopedic Rehabilitation Science Principles for Clinical Management of Bone. Boston: Butterworth-Heinemann, 2000.

to injury. Although each tissue has unique intrinsic and extrinsic qualities that influence its response to injury and repair, several common events and processes apply to the musculoskeletal connective tissues.

Because the properties of ordinary connective tissues can differ markedly, two main groups of connective tissue can be described histologically. Depending on the relative amount of fibers, ordinary connective tissue can be distinguished as being loose or dense in nature. Loose connective tissue is also known as *areolar* (*small space*) *tissue*. It is ubiquitous throughout the body and forms a protective covering for many tissues and organs. Loose connective tissue is cellular, compliant, and endowed with many vessels and nerves. Fibers are loosely woven and randomly oriented. Loose connective tissue characteristically has a considerable amount of extracellular matrix containing much the same components as found in dense connective tissues but at lower concentrations. It is also

typically high in tissue fluid, which is important for the supply of nutrients and removal of waste products from the dependent tissues.

The dense connective tissues may be further classified as *regular* or *irregular*, depending on their internal spatial organization. Dense irregular connective tissue (e.g., dermis, joint capsules) has a three-dimensional framework often accompanied by elastic fibers. Dense regular connective tissue (e.g., tendon) displays highly ordered fibers arranged parallel to one another, reflecting the mechanical demands of the tissues.

The intent of this text is to address the structure and functional behavior of specific forms of connective tissue that are the substrate of orthopaedic physical therapy practice. The following six chapters deal exclusively with the basic and clinical science related to form and function of these dense nonmineralized connective tissues across the adult lifespan. This text will not endeavor to cover the rheumatic diseases but rather will use select conditions from a wide spectrum of disorders commonly encountered in orthopaedic physical therapy practice to exemplify the pathobiology of connective tissues.

References

Brock DB, et al. Demography and Epidemiology of Aging in the United States. In EL Schneider, JW Rowe (eds), Handbook of the Biology of Aging (3rd ed). San Diego: Academic Press, 1990;3-23.

Jette A, et al. Musculoskeletal impairments and physical disablement among the aged. J Gerontol 1990;45:M203-M208.

Ker RF. The design of soft collagenous load-bearing tissues. J of Exper Biol 1999;202:3315-3324.

Statistics Canada. CANSIM, Matrix, 2001;6900.

U.S. Bureau of the Census. Projections of the Population of the United States by Age, Sex, and Race 1990–2040. In JW Wright (ed), The Universal Almanac. Kansas City: Andrews and McMeel, 1992;285-286.

Chapter 2

Structure, Function, and Metabolic Properties of Nonmineralized Connective Tissues

Composition of Connective Tissue

Connective tissue is a general term that encompasses a diverse group of tissues with a variety of functions. In general, connective tissue is composed of cells, the macromolecular elements they have synthesized (i.e., extracellular fibers embedded in a matrix of "ground substance"), and the interstitial fluid in which they reside. The environment that the cells (e.g., fibroblast/cyte, chondroblast/cyte, and endothelial cells) have created and in which they may be subsequently embedded is known as the *extracellular matrix (ECM)*. The macromolecular component of connective tissues consists of either protein or complex polysaccharides. The extracellular matrix can be further described in terms of the fibrous or nonfibrous components with which proteins or complex polysaccharides may be associated.

The nonmineralized connective tissue-based structures of the musculoskeletal system that will be discussed in the following chapters include ligaments, tendons, joint capsules, articular cartilage, and the intervertebral disc. Common to each of these structures is their specialized role in providing mechanical support within the body. Each form of regular dense connective tissue is highly specialized and associated with an important function. For instance, articular cartilage is important in bearing compressive loads in joints; its destruction manifests variably in joint diseases such as rheumatoid arthritis and osteoarthritis. The study of cartilage and its role as the precursor for some types of bone tissue during development allows closer investigation into mechanisms of skeletal development and joint diseases. The uniqueness of each form of regular dense

connective tissue also is attributable to the ECM components. For instance, aggrecan is one of the major components of cartilage and binds to hyaluronan (HA) and link protein to form huge aggregates, which in turn lead to the hydrated gel-like structure of cartilage and its resistance to compression and deformation in joints (Watanabe et al. 1998).

Components of Connective Tissue: Overview

Connective tissue proper is derived from mesenchyme, the embryonic form of connective tissue. Mesenchyme has its origin from mesoderm and neural crest ectoderm. The factors that regulate the growth and development of mesenchymal precursor cells toward development of specific forms of connective tissue such as processes underlying chondrogenesis (formation of cartilage) are not well identified (Quarto et al. 1997). The molecular basis of the progression from undifferentiated stem cell to hypertrophic chondrocytes, for instance, involves both the genomic potential of the cells (homeo and controlling genes) and their local microenvironment created by the ECM, systemic factors, and other signaling molecules (hormones, growth factors, and cytokines) that can modulate the cellular metabolism in an autocrine/paracrine manner (Cancedda et al. 1995).

Cells

The cells of connective tissues are all mesenchymally derived and include fibroblasts (chondroblasts, osteoblasts, cementoblasts), which are responsible for the synthesis of the ECM, as well as endothelial cells, pericytes, smooth muscle cells, adipocytes (fat cells), plasma cells (lymphocytes), mast cells, and macrophages.

Extracellular Matrix

The ECM of dense regular connective tissues consists of nonfibrous (e.g., ground substance) and fibrous (e.g., collagen, elastin) components. The ECM encompasses all material outside cells and inside the epithelial and endothelial boundaries of multicellular organisms. Other matrix components include proteins and other macromolecules that are associated with specific and nonspecific components of the cell surface. The macromolecular components that form the ECM are produced by connective tissue cells, and other molecules may also become incorporated into the matrix. The ECM often is described as fibrous proteins embedded within a hydrated polysaccharide gel. Loose connective tissue and dense connective tissue are distinguished according to the relative amount of fibers. The dense irregular connective tissues display a dense three-dimensional collagen fiber arrangement (e.g., capsule) compared with the dense regular connective tissues in which the collagen fibers run more or less parallel to each other (e.g., tendon, ligament). The nature of the fibrous components and the components of the "gel" and the interaction between these macromolecules together with other molecules such as water, calcium, and phosphate provide the basis of the various biophysical properties of the different connective tissue matrices. The relationship between the inner structure of collagen fibrils, their diameter and spatial layout, and the functional requirements they must withstand suggests that collagen fibrils may belong to two different forms, indicated as *T-type* and *C-type*. The T-type consists of large, heterogeneous fibrils tightly packed in a roughly parallel fashion and is represented largely in tendons, ligaments, and bone, where these fibrils are subject to tensile stress along their axes. The C-type form consists of small, homogenous fibrils, helically arranged and designed to resist multidirectional stresses, which prevail in highly compliant tissues such as blood vessel walls, skin and nerve sheaths (Box 2-1).

Box 2-1. Model for Architecture of Collagen Fibrils in Relation to Their Function

T-Type Fibers: These fibrils, of large and heterogeneous diameter are almost exclusively found in highly tensile structures such as tendon, ligaments and flat aponeuroses where they are tightly packed in thick, stiff, and roughly parallel bundles aligned with the direction of the force, appearing where high tensile stresses must be withstood with minimum strain. *C-Type Fibers*: The second architectural type of collagen fibrils appears to be represented by fibrils whose molecules run helically with a winding angle (set to 17 degrees) and are widespread across organs such as cornea, skin, nerves, blood vessels, parenchymous organs, and elastic ligaments. They run in loose, thin wavy bundles forming three-dimensional networks that are tough but compliant and are capable of recovery without change from large, cyclical deformation.

From Ottani V et al. Collagen Structure and Functional Implications. Micron 2001; 32(3):251-260. 2001.

The properties of the extracellular components account for the functional characteristics of the various tissue types. Although fibers are the elements of tensile strength and elasticity and thus are useful for imparting mechanical strength and support, the water and other macromolecular components of the matrix ground substance are important for transport between tissue cells and blood. The nature of the components of the extracellular matrices of various connective tissue structures should be understood clearly in terms of its structure, molecular organization, and contribution to overall tissue function and integrity. The extracellular matrix plays an integral part in directing development, tissue repair, and metastasis by regulating the proliferation, differentiation, adhesion, and migration of cells (Hocking et al. 1998). In its most primitive form, the ECM can be thought of as an isotropic network of tangled collagen fibrils of indefinite length, trapping and restraining an unstructured interfibrillar matrix of highly hydrated proteoglycans (PGs) (Ottani et al. 2001). The current interest in the extracellular matrix has evolved from the appreciation that cell biology extends beyond the cell itself and that the plasma membrane of the cell is not so much a boundary but a structure that mediates a continuum of biochemical events that are directed between the cell nucleus and the extracellular matrix. Cells in animal tissues are in contact with a set of well-defined proteins that make up the extracellular matrix. Among these proteins, collagens are ubiquitous in distribution, whereas laminins are found only in basement membranes. In addition to their structural role, collagens and laminins convey messages (signal transduction) to cells via cell receptors (integrins and nonintegrins) (Rousselle and Garrone 1998). Connections attained and mediated through cellular events serve primarily a mechanical purpose but most importantly play a biologically interactive role in growth and development, tissue homeostasis, and development of pathological states.

Constituents of the Nonmineralized Connective Tissues: Specific Cellular Components

The cellular component and activity in regular dense connective tissues varies depending on the nature of the tissue being manufactured or the environment (matrix) in which the cells are embedded. The numerous cell types may be identified as either fixed (resident) cells or wandering (nonresident). Fixed cells may include fibroblasts and fat cells, whereas wandering cells may include macrophages, lymphocytes, plasma cells, and mast cells. Bone marrow contains a small subset of cells that are progenitors of osteoblasts, chondroblasts, and several other types of non-hematopoietic cells. These cells have been referred to as *colony-forming units, fibroblasts,* and *mesenchymal stem cells* but more recently as *marrow stromal cells* (Prockop 1998). They are detailed as follows:

- *Fibroblasts (fibro,* fiber; *blastos,* germ)*:* The fibroblast is the cell that produces the extracellular matrix of connective tissue (Figure 2-1). These cells are fiber-forming cells that also present in specialized forms such as chondroblasts, osteoblasts, odontoblasts, and cementoblasts. Fibroblasts are important in collagen and elastin synthesis and in the manufacturing of the nonfibrous substance of the ECM. The production of collagen fibers involves a series of both intra- and extracellular events. The myofibroblast is a connective tissue cell that displays

properties of both the fibroblast and the smooth muscle cell (i.e., it contains large bundles of myofilaments). This cell plays a special role in facilitating wound contraction during repair of dense connective tissue after injury.

- *Adipocytes:* The function of adipose tissue is the storage of lipid. Adipocytes are found as fixed cells in loose connective tissue. Adipose tissue is a specialized form of connective tissue that consists of fat-storing cells called *adipocytes.* Adipose tissue is responsible for the acute regulation of fuel metabolism, influences steroid hormone conversion and sexual maturation. Adipose tissue is an active endocrine organ, influencing many aspects of fuel metabolism through a network of local and systemic signals, which interact with neuroendocrine regulators of adipose tissue. The network of adipose tissue signaling pathways, arranged in a hierarchical fashion, appears to constitute a metabolic repertoire that enables the organism to adapt to a range of different metabolic challenges, including starvation, reproduction, times of physical activity, stress, infection, and short periods of gross energy excess (Mohamedali et al. 1998).

- *Plasma cells/lymphocytes:* These cells are key players in the immunologic defense of the body.

- *Mast cells:* Mast cells are actively motile and are abundant around small blood vessels. Heparin, a potent anticoagulant, is stored in granules in the mast cell. Mast cells also release

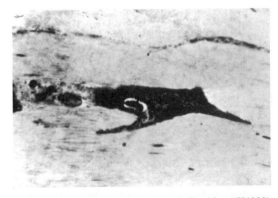

Figure 2-1. Electron micrograph of fibroblast (X4000). (From Woo SL-Y et al. Anatomy, Biology, and Biomechanics of Tendon, Ligament and Meniscus. In SR Simon (ed), Orthopaedic Basic Science. Rosemont, Ill.: American Academy of Orthopaedic Surgeons, 1994;48.)

histamine that binds to heparin in the mast cell granules and causes vasodilation. The mast cell is an ovoid connective tissue cell with a sphere-shaped nucleus.

- *Monocytes/macrophages:* These cells are important in the defense against foreign microorganisms. Macrophages are mostly non-motile cells until they become activated during an inflammatory reaction. The movement of macrophages into an area of inflammation is by chemotaxis. They can phagocytose foreign matter by invagination and formation of vacuoles or phagosomes. The "scavenger" cell behavior of the macrophages is integral to the first line of defense of an organism, since they are highly motile once activated and because of their phagocytic behavior. Monocytes are considered to be the precursors to macrophages.
- *Endothelial cells, pericytes, smooth muscle cells:* These cells are important components in certain vascular tissues.

Regular Dense Connective Tissue: The Extracellular Matrix

Many recent advances have occurred in the identifying, isolating, characterizing, and cloning of molecules important to connective tissue structure and function and also determination of important interactions between matrix proteins and between cellular receptors and connective tissue (Sakai et al. 1996).

Nonfibrous Component of the Extracellular Matrix

Ground substance is the hydrated polysaccharide gel component of the ECM of dense connective tissues in which the cells and fibers are embedded. The matrix proteins, PGs, and polysaccharides are thought to interact and assemble in a large variety of different three-dimensional structures, ordered in part by the cells secreting the matrix. The non-collagenous component of the extracellular matrix contains two large groups of soluble proteins: matrix proteins that bind cell-surface adhesion receptors and PGs that incorporate numerous macromolecules and are composed of core protein

with multiple polysaccharide chains attached. The large polysaccharide HA forms a highly hydrated gel and imparts resilience to compression to the matrix. The amount of PG and hyaluronic acid (HA) contained in ground substance is responsible for its viscous nature. For instance, the high viscosity of HA is important for synovial fluid to act as a joint lubricant. The movement of collagen fibers relative to one another (as in tendon) may be an important result of the lubricating nature of the hydrated ground substance. Additionally, the viscosity imparted by the PGs and HA contributes to the qualities of elasticity and resistance to compression in loose connective tissue, whereas the mechanical integrity of the ECM (Box 2-2) in cartilage is a direct result of PG aggregate interaction with collagen.

Multiadhesive matrix proteins

Although the main role of these matrix proteins is to attach cells to the extracellular matrix, an additional role in initiating cellular responses through classic signal-transduction pathways is now appreciated. Each of these roles is regarded as important for organizing other matrix components and regulating cell attachment to the matrix, cell migration, and cell shape. The multiadhesive matrix proteins are long molecules within which domains bind certain collagen types, other matrix proteins, polysaccharides, cell-surface proteins, and signaling molecules such as growth factors and hormones. Laminin is a large multiadhesive matrix protein and the most prevalent constituent of all basal laminae after type IV collagen. Laminins comprise a family of trimeric extracellular matrix proteins expressed in the basement membranes of many tissues, appearing first during the early stages of embryonic development and later in a wide variety of tissue-specific isoforms (Engvall 1993). For example, one isoform of laminin exists in the myotendinous junction (Ryan and Christiano 1996). The laminins possess a repertoire of biolog-

Box 2-2.

> ECM = fibrous (insoluble fibers of collagen) + nonfibrous (soluble multiadhesive matrix proteins + proteoglycans + hyaluronan)

ical functions including directing cell growth and migration, tissue regeneration, cell differentiation, and cell adhesion (Ryan and Christiano 1996). Laminin binds heparan sulfate and with type IV collagen binds to integrins, which are an important class of specific cell-surface receptor proteins present in the plasma membrane. In turn, these interactions act to attach the basal lamina to adjacent cells. Entactin is a small multiadhesive matrix protein that interacts with laminin and type IV collagen. Fibronectins are another class of soluble multiadhesive matrix proteins that assist cells to link with fibrous collagens (types I, II, III, and V), other matrix components, or other matrix proteins to integrins in the plasma membrane, acting to attach cells to the matrix. Through these attachments, the fibronectins regulate the shape of cells and the organization of the cytoskeleton. Fibronectins are critical for wound healing because they facilitate migration of macrophages and other immune cells into the affected area.

Proteoglycans

PGs are macromolecules of complex structure and composition that consist of a protein backbone to which glycosaminoglycans (GAG) chains are covalently attached. PGs are large molecules with 90% to 95% carbohydrate content by weight in the form of many long, unbranched glycosaminoglycan chains that branch from a linear protein core. PGs are large (molecular weight of 10^6 Da negatively charged hydrophilic molecules that are able to entrap water 50 times their weight. They are found mostly within and between collagen fibrils and fibers (Karpakka 1991). The polysaccharide chains in PGs are long, repeating, linear polymers of 20 to 100 sulfated disaccharides referred to as *glycosaminoglycans* (*glycan*, polysaccharide). They are highly negatively charged as a result of the presence of sulfate groups, carboxyl groups, or both on many of the sugar residues. PGs are typically named according to the structure of their principal repeating disaccharide in the attached GAGs. Some common disaccharides are chondroitin sulfate, dermatan sulfate, heparin sulfate and heparin, and keratin sulfate. PGs are diverse macromolecules that are present both in the extracellular matrix as well as may be attached to the surface of many cells. An important role of PGs is to allow,

via highly charged sidechains, water to be imbibed reversibly into the tissue occupying a solution volume many times its dry weight: in cartilage, for example this swelling is limited by the network of collagen fibrils (Poole 1986). Cartilage matrix may be considered a network of collagen fibers in which compressed aggregates of large PGs are meshed: while the fibers resist high tensile stress, the PG-water gel, as a result of high osmotic swelling pressure and low hydraulic permeability, resists compressive load. The volume of the ECM can be attributed to these hydrated PGs that swell, which in turn allows diffusion of small molecules between tissues and cells. Aggrecan is one of the most important extracellular PGs and the predominant PG in cartilage. The PG aggrecan binds at regular intervals to a centrally based HA molecule to form a very large aggregate. These aggregates impart cartilage, a unique gel-like property, and resistance to deformation. The aggregating PGs thus make significant contributions to the mechanical properties and biological behavior of cartilaginous tissues, including the structural cartilages, articular cartilages of synovial joints, and intervertebral discs (Buckwalter et al. 1994). Age-related changes in PG composition, structure, and organization is believed to alter critical biological and mechanical properties and contribute to the appearance of age-related disorders like osteoarthritis of synovial joints and degeneration of intervertebral discs (Buckwalter et al. 1994). The effect of the PG decorin on collagen fibrillogenesis appears to be to reduce the rate of fibril growth and ultimately increase the diameters of fibrils formed. This suggests that decorin found in fibrous connective tissues may increase type I collagen fibril diameters, resulting in tissues that are better able to withstand tensile forces (Kuc and Scott 1998). In addition to their role as structural components of the ECM and in anchoring cells to matrix, both extracellular and cell-surface PGs also bind many protein growth factors; these smaller PGs may be attached to cell surfaces and assist in cell-matrix interactions and the presentation of certain hormones to their cell-surface receptors. For example, a common PG found on the plasma membrane is syndecan. PGs are thus integral to the normal physiology of connective tissues and their resident cells. This becomes apparent as a disturbance in either their metabolism or their presentation manifests in a variety of pathologic states of connective tissue.

Hyaluronan

The role of HA is to resist compression and facilitate cell migration. HA also is referred to as *hyaluronate* and is major component of the ECM that surrounds migrating and proliferating cells. HA imparts qualities of stiffness and resilience in addition to its lubricating role to many connective tissue structures such as joint complexes. HA is not covalently linked to a protein and is not a long rigid rod; it binds water easily because of the extensive anionic residues on its surface. HA may also be bound to specific receptors (CD44 or homologous protein in the CD44 family) on cells that act to inhibit cell-cell adhesion and facilitate cell migration.

Fibrous Component of the Extracellular Matrix

Collagen is a major component of ECM that holds together the tissues and organs of most complex organisms. Elastin is an example of another non-collagenous, fibrous component of the ECM.

Structure and Function of the Collagens

General

Collagens are the major macromolecules of most connective tissues and are the most abundant (30%) structural proteins in the body. Collagen is a tough, fibrous material that holds complex organisms together. Collagens are a large and diverse family of proteins, found in the extracellular matrix, that play a dominant role in maintaining the structural integrity of various tissues and have numerous other important functions. The collagen superfamily now includes more than 20 collagen types with at least 38 distinct polypeptide classes and more than 15 additional proteins that have collagen-like domains (Myllyharju and Kivirikko 2001). Most collagens assemble into polymers as represented in fibrils, networks, and filaments. Tissues especially rich in collagens are bone, skin, tendon, cartilage, ligaments and vascular walls, but they are found in almost all tissues and have an important role in maintaining the structural integrity of numerous tissues and organs. Collagen fibers are flexible and in general have high tensile strength. Collagens also are recognized as more than elements contributing structure to connective tissue in that they play an important role in normal growth and development and organogenesis, cell attachment, chemotaxis, platelet aggregation, and filtration through basement membranes (Kivirikko 1993). Collagen fibers are the principal and most abundant fibers of connective tissue with a simple main structural presentation and with a periodic amino acid sequence in which every third amino acid is glycine (Gly). The biosynthesis of collagen displays several unique features, including the spontaneous self-assembly observed in the formation of crystals. The three polypeptide chains of the collagen protein fold into a triple-helical conformation by a process that begins with the formation of a small nucleus of triple helix at the C-terminus end

---

Clinical Note

Once hydrated, a hyaluronan (HA) molecule can occupy a volume of about 1000 times the size of the molecule itself. As a result of the pressure created by the waterbound HA molecules, connective tissues have the ability to resist compression forces that are so important to load-bearing tissues such as articular cartilage. In contrast, collagen fibers impart the ability of connective tissues to resist stretching or tensile forces. Since the ultimate strength of tension-bearing elements depends on the substance of which they are made and their cross-sectional area, collagen fibrils are designed exceptionally well to withstand tensile stresses. Collagen inherently has excellent elastic resilience and very high tensile strength; its design as a single element divided into multiple, roughly parallel threads gives the extracellular matrix of connective tissues such as tendon and ligament a high compliance and high safety factor against occasional injuries while not affecting its ultimate tensile strength (Ottani et al. 2001).

of the molecule and propagates itself in a zipper-like fashion (Prockop 1998). This process of self-assembly of the collagen monomers into fibrils is an entropy driven, crystallization-like process (Prockop, 1998) (Figure 2-2).

A number of distinct collagens have been discovered that are clearly related but differ genetically, chemically, and immunologically. In common with one another, the known collagen types have triple-helical domains of variable length, but they differ with respect to their overall size and the nature and location of their globular domains (Dalgleish 1998). In general, a protein can be defined as a *collagen* by the presence of a triple-helical, collagenous domain containing peptide chains with repeating -Gly-X-Y triplets, and by the presence of the amino acids hydroxyproline (Hyp) and hydroxylysine, which are relatively specific to collagen. The variety in structure of different collagen and related proteins supports their diversity in biological functioning (Prockop and Kivirikko 1995). In some collagens, the three alpha chains are identical whereas in other types the molecule contains two or even three different alpha chains.

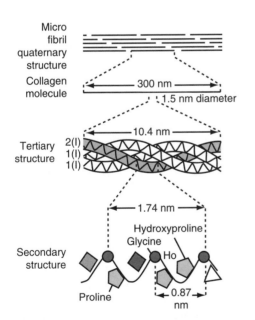

Therefore the current definition of fibrillar collagens is that they are proteins that contain several repeats of an amino acid sequence in which every third amino acid is Gly. The sequence of an alpha chain of a collagen domain in a protein is thus expressed as $(Gly-X-Y)_n$ where X and Y represent amino acids other than Gly. The X position often is occupied by proline (Pro) and the Y position by 4-Hyp (both are amino acids that provide stability for the triple helix), where n varies according to the collagen type and domain (Prockop and Kivirikko 1995). Glycine is the smallest amino acid and its place at every third position is critical as large amino acids are unable to fit into the restricted space in the center of the triple helix where the three chains come together (Myllyharju and Kivirikko 2001). In addition, the term encompasses, to a degree, those molecules able to form supramolecular structures in the extracellular spaces. In collagen-like peptides that form triple helices, the substitution of Hyp for Pro in the Y position of repeating –Gly-X-Y triplets increases the thermal stability of the triple helices by as much as 15°C (Prockop and Kivirikko 1995) and provides additional sites for hydrogen bonding of water molecules in crystals of the peptides. In humans, the hydroxylation of proline residues during biosynthesis of collagen and other fibril forming collagen highlights a mechanism for adjusting the flexibility of the collagen monomer to body temperature (Prockop and Kivirikko 1995).

Much is known about collagen because of its ubiquitous nature, since it exists in various forms tailored to impart structural integrity to various tissues and organs. In fact, the biomechanical properties of connective tissues are regulated by the specific macromolecular organization of their extracellular matrix, the main constituent which is collagen. The collagen molecules, after being secreted by the cells, assemble into characteristic fibers responsible for the functional integrity of tissues such as bone, cartilage, skin, ligaments and tendon. In addition, collagens contribute a structural framework to blood vessels and most organs. The emphasis of this section will be placed on the unique types of collagen present in the skeletal tissues encountered within and influenced by orthopaedic physical therapy practice. These tissues include tendon, ligaments, capsules, articular cartilage and the intervertebral disc.

Figure 2-2. Schematic drawing of structural organization of collagen into the microfibril. (Modified from Woo SL-Y et al. Anatomy, Biology, and Biomechanics of Tendon, Ligament and Meniscus. In SR Simon (ed), Orthopaedic Basic Science. Rosemont, Ill.: American Academy of Orthopaedic Surgeons, 1994;48.)

Clinical Note

Extracellular Matrix Alterations in Chondromalacia of the Patella

In one study of the nature of collagen in chondromalacia of the patella, polarized light microscopy showed decreased biorefringence in the superficial cartilage of these lesions, indicating disorganization or even disappearance of collagen fibers in this zone. The collagen network of chondromalacia lesions of the patella showed gradual disorganization associated with severity of the condition without changes in the concentration or cross-links of collagen (Vaatainen et al. 1998).

The Molecular Structure of Collagen

The Different Collagen Types

The most abundant collagens form extracellular fibrils or network-like structures, but the others fulfill a variety of biological functions (Prockop and Kivirikko 1995). Most of the collagenous proteins are structural elements and help tissues withstand stretching. Some types of collagens are abundant and ubiquitous though the majority are minor components with limited tissue distribution and have specialized functions (Dalgleish 1998). Collagens are secreted by fibroblasts and numerous epithelial cells. Their diversity may be demonstrated in that the different molecules form unique structures that include fibers (collagens I to III, which represent 80% to 90% of the collagen in the body), sheets (type IV), and short insertional straps. Type IV collagen and laminin together form the largest contributing components to the two-dimensional sheetlike reticulum of the basal lamina; most epithelial and endothelial cells rest on a basal lamina linked to specific plasma-membrane receptor proteins and to fibrous collagens and other components of the underlying loose connective tissue. Not only do collagens form distinct structures, but some collagens are produced by and associate themselves with specific cells such as types II, IX, and X with chondrocytes, and, as mentioned before, type IV collagen with epithelial cells.

All collagens encompass noncollagenous components in addition to their collagenous domains. The collagen superfamily can be divided into the following families on the basis of such polymeric structures or other features (Myllyharju and Kivirikko 2001): (1) collagens that form fibrils (types I, II, III, V and XI); (2) collagens located on the surfaces of fibrils and are called *fibril-associated collagens with interrupted triple helices* (FACIT), and structurally related collagens such as types IX, XII, XIV, XVI and XIX); (3) collagens that form hexagonal networks (types VIII and X); (4) the family of type IV collagens found in basement membranes; (5) type VI collagen that forms beaded filaments; (6) type VII collagen that forms anchoring fibrils for basement membranes; (7) collagens with transmembrane domains (types XIII and XVII); and (8) the family of type XV and XVIII collagens. The collagen fibrils found in tissues are often heterogeneous and thus contain more than one collagen type. All collagen molecules form supramolecular aggregates that are stabilized in part by interactions between the triple-helical domains. (An example of supramolecular aggregates is the sheet constituting basement membranes in the case of type IV collagen, and laterally aggregated antiparallel dimers, which are the main constituents of anchoring fibrils typical of type VII collagen.) The collagen triple helix is formed from these polypeptide chains that are coiled into a left-handed helix. Types I, II, III, V and XI collagen form fibrils and are referred to as *fibrillar collagens*. While many types of collagen are evident and at least 25 different types have been classified (Cohen 2000), the collagens most extensively considered in this text are the fibrillar or interstitial collagens (types I to III). Type I collagen, the main constituent of skin, tendon, dentin, bone and vessel walls is synthesized by fibroblasts, smooth-muscle cells, and osteoblasts. Whereas osteoblasts only synthesize type I collagen, smooth-muscle cells also produce type III collagen, which is therefore often found together with type I collagen. Type II collagen, the main collagen constituent of hyaline cartilage, is produced by the chondrocytes. Type X collagen is also a major product of cultured chondrocytes and the calcifying regions of endochondral cartilage.

The Fiber-Forming Collagens: Types I, II, III, V, and XI

The best characterized collagens are the fibril-forming collagens: types I, II, III, V and XI. Types V and XI (Erlebacher et al. 1995) are quantitatively minor tissue constituents, the former co-distributing with type I collagen and the latter with type II collagen (Eyre et al., 1991). In the case of type XI collagen, the proportions of types XI collagen relative to type II collagen decreases with increasing cartilage maturity (Eyre et al., 1991). The unique but common properties of the fibrous collagens I, II, III, V and XI result from the ability of the rodlike triple helices to form side-by-side interactions, their similar size, and their large triple-helical domains with about 1000 amino acids or 330 (Gly-X-Y) repeats per chain. Furthermore, they are first manufactured as larger precursors that are processed via cleavage of N-propeptides and C-propeptides by specific proteinases. In addition, the fibril-forming collagens all assemble into cross-striated fibrils in which each molecule is displaced about one quarter of its length relative to its nearest neighbor above the axis of the fibril (see Figure 2-2).

Type I Collagen

Type I collagen is the most abundant collagen and is found in a variety of connective tissues, including skin, bone, tendon, dentin, fascia, ligament, arteries, and cornea. It is composed of two identical polypeptide chains $\alpha 1(I)$ and one $\alpha 2(I)$ chain. Type I collagen fibrils have tremendous tensile strength in that such collagen can withstand the application of much force without being broken. Type I collagen fibrils are packed side by side in parallel bundles called *collagen fibers* (Figure 2-3). Type I collagen comprises between 80% and 90% of the total body collagen. Bone matrix is primarily type I collagen. The proportion of type I collagen in a particular tissue can vary at different sites during development and with age and pathology. The effect of insertions, deletions, and single amino acid substitutions in the alpha-1 and alpha-2 genes has identified the importance of type I collagen within the musculoskeletal system. The majority of these defects manifest in phenotypic changes in bone development characteristic of diseases such as osteogenesis imperfecta (OI).

NOTE: The type I collagen molecule may not be as uniform a structure as once thought; evidence exists that different domains within the triple helix may have different properties (Burganadze and Veis 1997).

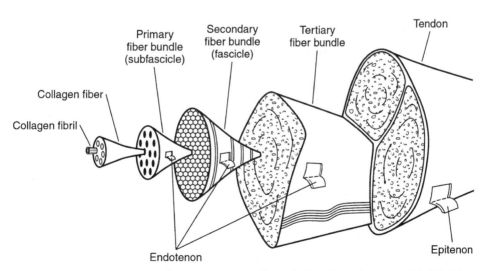

Figure 2-3. The organization of tendon structure from collagen fibrils to the entire tendon. (Modified from Kannus P. Structure of the Tendon Connective Tissue. Scandinav J Med Sci Sports 2000;10:312-320.)

Type II Collagen

Type II collagen is found in hyaline cartilage, cornea, and vitreous humor and is composed of three identical α chains. The differences in primary structure between the two most abundant fibril-forming collagens (types I and II) underlie the characteristic differences in morphology between these two kinds of fibrils. Type II collagen fibrils are smaller than type I and are oriented randomly within the surrounding viscous PG matrix. The property of strength and compressibility imparted by rigid macromolecules (both PGs and fibers) act to minimize large deformation in shape and absorb joint shock in the case of articular cartilage. Type II collagen commonly occurs in connective tissues subject to compressive forces, notably articular cartilage, and also in the intervertebral discs, and menisci (Eyre and Muir 1977). Fibrocartilage has properties intermediate between those of dense fibrous connective tissues containing both type I collagen and hyaline cartilage (type II collagen).

Type III Collagen

Type III collagen accounts for 10% to 50% of the total collagen in adult tissue. Type III collagen consists of three identical α chains (homotrimer of α1(III) collagen chains) and although expressed in many tissues, still is primarily a component of extensible connective tissues including skin, gut, lungs, vascular system (large arteries), muscle, liver, and uterus. Type III collagen is often co-expressed with type I collagen but is not found in mature bone and tendon fibrils (Kielty et al. 1993). Characteristic of this collagen is its relatively high proportion of Hyp, its high glycine content (greater than 33% of the residues), and the presence of intramolecular disulfide bonds involving two cysteine residues close to the C-terminal region of the triple helix. Hyp is crucial to the structural stabilization of the collagen triple helix, and intramolecular-interchain water bridges contribute importantly to stabilization of the collagen triple helix. The ability of this collagen to cross-link rapidly through intermolecular, disulfide bridge formation is remarkable in early development and wound healing where collagen is deposited at a rapid rate in an area previously deplete of connective tissue. Type III collagen is essential for the normal tensile strength of skin, aorta, and intestinal tissues.

Overview of Types I to III (Fibrillar/Interstitial) Collagen Organization

The most abundant collagen is type I, which assumes a long, thin rod shape. Type I collagen is the major structural element of skin, bone, tendon and other fibrous tissues where it forms large, banded fibers. Type II collagen is the major structural protein in cartilage. Type III collagen is present in a wide variety of tissues, usually in association with type I collagen with the exception of mature tendon and bone. All molecules of the interstitial collagens have a rodlike shape with a length of about 300 nm, diameter of 1.5 nm, and a molecular weight of about 280,000 Da.

Types I to III collagen, although biochemically distinct, demonstrate several common features. Each is derived from a precursor (procollagens I-III) that is converted to collagen by the proteolytic removal of amino and carboxyl peptides. Removal of the peptides permit the self-assembly of the collagen molecules into fibers. The length of the major triple helix of these collagens is 300 nm, and each molecule contains rather short nonhelical peptides at each end. These regions are known as the *telopeptides,* which are the sites where cross-linking of the collagen molecules occurs.

The interstitial collagens are composed of three α chains, each more than 1000 residues in length. These collagens, as noted before, contain two distinct types of structural domains: a triple-helical domain and globular domain. The size and distribution of these domains is variable between the individual collagen types. The α chains contain two structurally and functionally different sequence regions, the central triple helical part of 1014 residues and the nontriple-helical regions at both ends of the chain, whose length can vary in the range of nine to 50 residues. The nonhelical regions can be compared as flexible arms, bearing the functional groups for the intermolecular bonds lysine or hydroxylysine residues, which may be oxidized to lysylaldehydes. The triple helical region controls for the formation and stabilization of the triple helix and is responsible for the self-assembly of the molecules to form fibrillar structures.

The genetically defined sequence of amino acids in a polypeptide chain determines the folding of the chain into the three-dimensional conformation that is essential for the biologic activity of a protein. In the case of the interstitial collagens, the amino acid sequence determines the structure in two ways:

1. Three polypeptide (α) chains are folded into a rodlike triple-helical molecule about 300 nm long and 1.5 nm in diameter.
2. Lateral and longitudinal association of these triple-helical molecules into fibrils occurs.

Two controlling factors, ambient PG and fibril polarity, can work against the tendency of fibrils to fuse. This may account for the different distributions of collagen fibril diameters observed in diverse tissues and at different ages (Scott and Parry 1992).

Stabilization of Fibrillar Collagens

The stabilization of fibrillar collagen structure involves several closely related intra- and intermolecular interactions (Burganadze and Veis 1997). The fibrillar collagens, types I, II, III, V and XI, all have a single uninterrupted triple helical domain built from three α-chains, each with a mass of about 95,000 Da (Burganadze and Veis 1997). As mentioned earlier, an essential feature for the formation of the triple helical structure is that in the central part, every third position along the chains is occupied by the amino acid glycine (Gly). The occurrence of glycine (the smallest amino acid) in this position is essential, as it occupies "restricted" space in which the three helical alpha chains come together in the center of the triple helix. Any substitution of any of the glycines by any other amino acid will produce an interruption in the triple helix pattern. In addition, the positioning of glycine in the helix contributes to the stability of the collagen molecule by allowing hydrogen bonds to form between the three chains of the helix. The other important amino acid components for assumption of triple-helical conformation are proline, 4-Hyp and lysine or hydroxylysine in the polypeptide chains. Of the approximately 1000 residues in the alpha chain, about 100 of the X position amino acids are proline and about 100 of the Y position amino acids are 4-Hyp. These two amino acids limit rotation of the polypeptide chains, further stabilizing the triple helix. The triple helix is most stabilized by the Pro-rich tripeptide units such as Gly-Pro-Hyp and Gly-Pro-Y. Specifically, the

hydroxyl group of 4-Hyp plays a critical role in stabilizing the triple helix of collagen. Hyp and Pro form hydrogen bonds (intramolecular) within each chain. The triple helix is a relatively rigid structure, which explains the resistance of the molecule to extension or compression (Prockop and Kivirikko 1995). The other amino acids occupying the X-Y positions (other than Pro and Hyp) are essential for organization of collagen at the third organizational level, the assembly of three triple-helical molecules into collagen microfibrils (lateral and longitudinal arrangement) (Figure 2-4). The arrangement of these other amino acids cluster in groups of hydrophobic and charged residues, and because their side chains jut from the center of the triple helix, they can direct the association of individual collagen molecules.

Longitudinal Arrangement

A staggering of collagen molecules about 300 nm long by about one quarter of their length gives collagen fibrils a characteristic spacing and pattern of bands that is repeated about every 67 nm when observed by electron microscopy. Multiple three-stranded type I collagen molecules pack side-by-side in a module format, ultimately forming fibrils with a diameter of 50 to 200 nm. The collagen molecules are aligned end-to-end in overlapping rows; this longitudinal staggering of the molecules involves approximately one quarter of the length of the monomer and leaves a hole between the end of one triple helix and the commencement of the one following it (see Figure 2-4).

Cross-Sectional Arrangement

Microfibrils are discrete structures of five collagen molecules in cross-section, which create a basic unit for assembly of fibrils (see Figure 2-4). A crystal structure based on quasihexagonal packing has been developed from x-ray diffraction imaging of collagen fibrils (Wess et al. 1995). The structure of the collagen fibril presents a paradox in that most proteins are noncrystalline in vivo, but collagen fibrils seen in vivo are seemingly crystalline (Prockop and Fertala 1998). Aggregation of these microfibrils forms the fibril that displays a 640-degree Angstrom cross-banding pattern that may

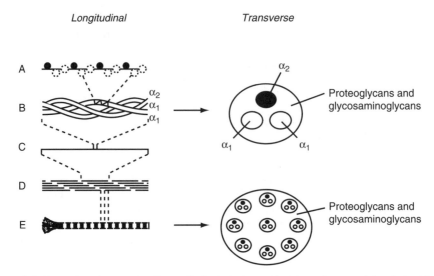

Figure 2-4. Formation of a type I collagen fibril. *A*, Amino acids join to form an alpha chain. Glycine occupies every third position (black circles). *B* and *C*, Three alpha chains coil to form the right-handed triple helix of a collagen molecule. The alpha chains are surrounded by a thin layer of proteoglycans and glycosaminoglycans. *D*, The collagen molecules link to form a tropocollagen molecule or microfibril. Within a microfibril and fibril, the collagen molecules pack in a quarter-staggered orientation (i.e., each collagen molecule overlaps its neighbour by a quarter of its length), producing the characteristic banding pattern of the final collagen fibril. *E*, The striated collagen fibril. The microfibrils are surrounded by proteoglycans and glycosaminoglycans. (Modified from Kannus P. Structure of the Tendon Connective Tissue. Scandinav J Med Sci Sports; 2000;10:312-320.)

be visualized ultrastructurally (Figures 2-4 and 2-5). Collagen fibrils assume a "crimped" posture that manifests itself functionally at the level of the fascicle (see Figure 2-3). An angle of 15 to 20 degrees exists between the fibril and the long axis of tendon (Betsch and Baer 1980). The combination of collagen-ground substance interaction, the molecular structure of the collagen molecule (microfibrils), and cross-linking properties resulting from microfibril aggregation all seem likely to contribute to this phenomenon (Gathercole and Keller 1968). The application of a tensile load placed on a ligament or tendon affects crimp at the level of the fascicle, which recovers once the load is relieved.

Radial growth of collagen fibrils takes place in all connective tissues according to the tensile stresses exerted on them and may proceed by aggregation of "protofibrils" (approximately 10 nm) and existing fibrils (Scott and Parry 1992). In young tissues, fibrils are prevented from making frequent intimate contacts that lead to aggregation by abundant interfibrillar PG that keeps the fibrils apart. The two controlling factors, ambient PG and

fibril polarity, working against the tendency of fibrils to fuse, account for many features of the observed distributions of collagen fibril diameters in diverse tissues and at different ages (Scott and Parry 1992). The assembly of the collagen fibrils continues to be of some dispute (Prockop and Fertula 1998). One favored theory about how collagen fibrils assemble is by an entropy-driven process involving specific binding sites on the monomers, which closely resembles crystallization (Prockop and Fertala 1998). The spontaneous self-assembly of collagen appears to be most similar to that seen in the formation of crystals that incorporates two steps, including the zipperlike folding of the monomer and the self-assembly of monomers into fibrils (Prockop 1998). The process of self-assembly is entirely spontaneous and appears to be driven by large entropy changes caused by loss of water from the surface of the monomer (Prockop 1998). Ultimately, collagen fibril diameters may increase during development to greater than 400 nm postmaturity, and those tissues subjected to the highest tensile loads contain the largest fibrils (Scott and Parry 1992).

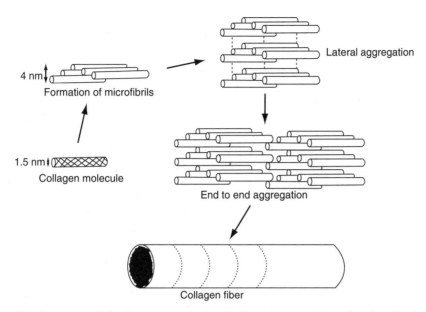

Figure 2-5. Formation of the five-membered microfibril and its potential for lateral and end-to-end aggregation to form fibers. (Modified from Burgeson R, Nimni M. Collagen types: Molecular Structure and Tissue Distribution. Clin Orthopaed Rel Res 1992; 282: 250-272.)

Box 2-3. Sequence of Intracellular → Extracellular Events in the Biosynthesis of Fibrillar Collagen

---

Transcription and Translation
 1. Synthesis of specific mRNAs for the different procollagen chains
 2. Translation of the message in the endoplasmic reticulum

Posttranslational Events
 3. Hydroxylation
    a. Hydroxylation of specific proline residues
    b. Hydroxylation of lysine by lysyl hydroxylase
 4. Glycosylation of hydroxylysine by galactosyltransferase and addition of glucose by a glucosyltransferase
 5. Removal of N-terminal signal peptide
 6. Release of completed alpha chains from ribosomes
 7. Recognition of three alpha chains through the C-terminal propeptide and formation of disulfide crosslinks
 8. Folding of the molecule and formation of a triple-helix
 9. Intracellular translocation of the procollagen molecules and packaging into vesicles
10. Fusion of vesicles with the cell membrane and extrusion of the molecule with the concurrent cleavage of the C-terminal nonhelical extension and selected portions of the N-terminal nonhelical extensions by peptidases

---

Collagen Biosynthesis

The intracellular and extracellular events leading to the assembly of collagen fibers that will be discussed pertains to the banded, fiber-forming collagens that display several unique features (Box 2-3). The corresponding events occurring in biosynthesis of the other collagens are less well known. The main intracellular steps in the assembly of a pro-

collagen molecule from pro-α chains are cleavage of the signal peptides, hydroxylation of certain proline and lysine residues to 4-Hyp, 3-Hyp, and hydroxylysine, glycosylation of some of the hydroxylysine residues to galactosylhydroxylysine and glucosogalactosyl-hydroxylysine, glycosylation of certain asparagine residues in one or both of the propeptides, and association of the C propeptides through a process directed by their structures, and formation of intrachain and interchain disulphide bonds (Myllyharju and Kivirikko 2001). Extracellular steps in biosynthesis include cleavage of the N and C propeptides (Prockop et al. 1998); self-assembly of the collagen molecules into fibrils by nucleation and propagation (Kadler et al. 1996; Graham et al. 2000); and the formation of covalent cross-links (Smith-Mungo and Kagan 1998).

At least eight enzymes modify the collagen protein during or after its synthesis (Prockop and Kivirikko 1995). A general overview of the sequence of events in the biosynthesis of collagen can be captured in Figure 2-6.

The Procollagen Molecule

The fibril-forming collagens first are synthesized as large precursor molecules referred to as *procollagens*. Procollagen later is trimmed enzymatically of its nonhelical ends, which allows for the spontaneous assembly of fibers in the extracellular space. The functional importance of the carbohydrate in the carboxy-end of procollagen is unknown but could be part of a recognition mechanism for alignment or assembly into microfibrils (Burgeson and Nimni 1992). The extensions play a role in the assembly of the trihelical collagen molecule. Once the molecule is completed and translocated to the cell surface, the extensions are cleaved enzymatically from some collagens and fibrillogenesis occurs.

Posttranslational Modifications

Collagen synthesis involves numerous posttranslational modifications. Posttranslational modification of procollagen is essential for the formation of mature collagen molecules and their assembly into fibrils. Collagen biosynthesis involves an unusually large number of posttranslational modifications that require at least eight specific enzymes (Kivirikko 1993), many of which are unique to collagens and a few other proteins with collagen-like amino acid sequences. This posttranslational processing occurs in two stages. *Intracellular* processing involves the synthesis of the alpha chains and results in the formation of triplehelical *procollagen* molecules. *Extracellular* processing converts these molecules into collagens and incorporates the col-

lagen molecules into stable crosslinked fibrils or other supramolecular aggregates (Figure 2-7).

Intracellular events

Intracellular modifications require at least five specific enzymes (e.g., three specific hydroxylases responsible for hydroxylation of certain proline and lysine residues to 4-Hyp, 3-Hyp, and hydroxylysine) and two specific glycosyltransferases (e.g., galactosyltransferase and glucosyltransferase for the glycosylation of some of the hydroxylysine residues to galactosylhydroxylysine and glucosylgalactosylhydroxylysine).

Cysteine residues need to be juxtaposed to enable formation of the disulfide bridges that link the individual pro-α chains at the C-terminal ends. Both inter- and intrachain disulfide bonds are formed. Intracellular translocation of procollagen occurs in the ribosome, endoplasmic reticulum, and the Golgi apparatus before its extrusion into the extracellular space.

Extracellular events

Extracellular events in collagen biosynthesis are described as follows:

1. Extracellular modifications require at least one specific oxidase and two proteinases to cleave the N-terminal (non-helical amino) and C-terminal (non-helical carboxyl) polypeptide extensions. Extracellular collagen fibrils are formed by secretion of a soluble procollagen that is then enzymatically processed into an insoluble collagen. Both the N- and C-propeptides of procollagens must be cleaved by specific proteinases for the proteins to self-assemble into fibrils under physiologic conditions (Prockop and Kivirikko 1995).

2. In fibrillogenesis, the extracellular events in the biosynthesis of a fibril-forming collagen include cleavage of the N and C propeptides, self-assembly into fibrils, and cross-link formation. The tendency of collagen molecules to form macromolecular aggregates is common to most fibrous proteins that form filaments with helical symmetry. Electron micrographic and x-ray diffraction data support the view that within

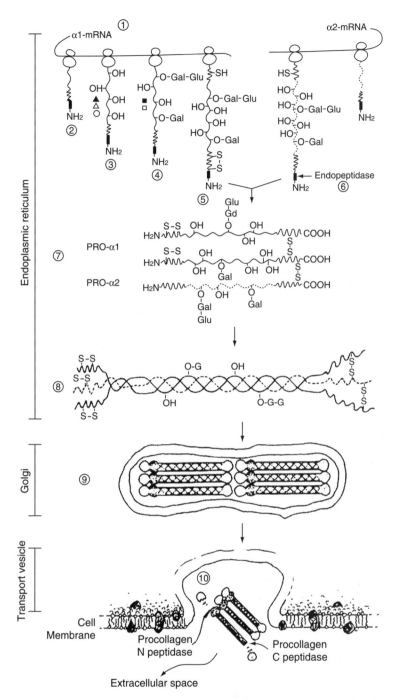

Figure 2-6. Sequence of events in the biosynthesis of collagen: *(1)* Synthesis of specific mRNAs for the different procollagen chains. *(2)* Translation of the message on polysomes of the rough ER. *(3)* Hydroxylation of specific proline residues by 3-proline hydroxylase and 4-proline hydroxylase and of lysine by lysyl hydroxylase. *(4)* Glycosylation of hydroxylysine by galactosyltransferase and addition of glucose by a glucosyltransferase. *(5)* Removal of the N-terminal signal peptide. *(6)* Release of completed alpha chains from ribosomes. *(7)* Recognition of three alpha chains through the C-terminal prepeptide and formation of disulfide cross-links. *(8)* Folding of the molecule and formation of a triple-helix. *(9)* Intracellular translocation of the procollagen molecules and packaging into vesicles. *(10)* Fusion of vesicles with the cell membrane and extrusion of the molecule accompanied by the removal of the C-terminal nonhelical extensions and part of the N-terminal nonhelical extensions by specific peptidases. (Modified from Burgeson R, Nimni M. Collagen types: Molecular Structure and Tissue Distribution. Clin Orthopaed Rel Res 1992;282:250-272.)

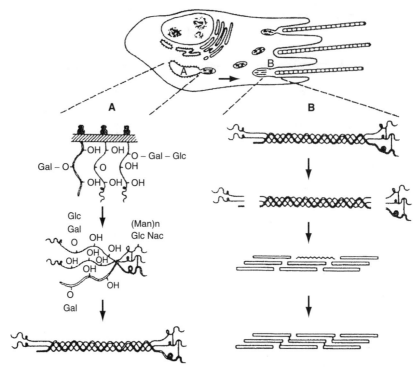

Figure 2-7. Fibroblast assembly of collagen fibers. **A**, Intracellular posttranslational modifications of pro-α chains, association of C-propeptide domains, and folding into triple-helical conformation. Gal denotes galactose, Glc glucose, GlcNac N-acetylglucosamine, and (Mann) mannose residues. **B**, Enzymic cleavage of procollagen to collagen, self-assembly of collagen monomers into fibrils, and cross-linking of fibrils. (Modified from Prockop DJ, Kivirikko KI. Heritable Diseases of Collagen. N Engl J Med 1984;311(6):376-386.)

collagen fibers, a regular arrangement of molecules results from such an assembly. After the removal of the nonhelical extensions the newly formed collagen molecules appear to organize into native fibers. Microfibrils in a quarter-staggered configuration have lost their C-terminal nonhelical extensions and part of their N-terminal extensions enabling a ready organization into small-diameter fibers that retain part of N-terminal nonhelical extensions. After being relieved of these peptides by a procollagen peptidase, fibers are able to grow in diameter by apposition of microfibrils, merging with other small-diameter fibers.

3. Formation of covalent cross-links is also a major extracellular event. During the process of extrusion, recently formed microfibrils must be recognized by the enzyme lysyl oxidase, which converts certain peptide-bound lysines and hydroxylysines to aldehydes. Lysyl oxidase

catalyzes the oxidative deamination of lysine and hydroxylysine. In this way, this enzyme initiates the biosynthesis of cross-links in collagen that give strength to the tissue and allows the fiber to function under mechanical stress. In newly formed collagen the cross-links are easily reducible because few exist. A decrease in the total number of reducible cross-links occurs when stable cross-links form as collagen matures. The evidence for the increase in stability is that mature collagen survives a higher denaturation temperature and is not soluble in neutral salt or acid solutions as it matures. The protein-lysine 6-oxidase (lysyl oxidase) is a cuproenzyme that is essential for stabilization of extracellular matrices, specifically the enzymatic cross-linking of collagen and elastin. The direct influence of dietary copper on the functional activity of lysyl oxidase is clear: copper is an essential cofactor for amine oxidases such as lysyl oxidase (Rucker et al. 1998). The side chain of glycine, a hydrogen, fits into the tightly packed center of the triple-stranded helix; hydrogen bonds linking the peptide bond (NH) of a glycine residue with a peptide carbonyl (C=O) group in an adjacent polypeptide contribute to holding the three chains together.

Summary of Collagen Biosynthesis

Collagen biosynthesis involves a large number of co-translational and posttranslational events of which many are particular to collagens. Interstitial collagen formation occurs initially in the rough endoplasmic reticulum (ER) of the connective tissue fibroblasts. A display of repeating (Gly-X-Y) sequences forms long non-helical polypeptide chains of the same length in which every third residue is glycine. In the endoplasmic reticulum, three polypeptide chains become attached together and eventually, through interchain disulphide bonds (between N- and C-terminal propeptides), form a triple helical procollagen molecule. These chains stay in proximity to one another because of the three-dimensional shape of each chain and the relative placement of radicals that chemically react with one another, allowing procollagen molecules to be synthesized into uniform molecules with fixed dimensions of length and width. Therefore collagen is first synthesized as procollagen, a longer molecule which contains additional propeptides. Propeptides are removed after secretion from the ER and collagen fibrils then self-assemble into a rodlike monomer through an entropy-driven process in the extracellular space. The propeptides, as only one of their functions, prevent premature formation of fibrils.

Therefore the usual sequence of intracellular events is hydroxylation of the pro-α chains, followed by synthesis of interchain disulfide bonds and the formation of the triple helix. Intracellular events during collagen formation are catalyzed by several specific enzymes. One enzyme, prolyl 4-hydroxylase is critical in the formation of 4-hydroxyproline residues that are essential constituents for the folding of the newly synthesized collagen polypeptide chains into triple-helical molecules. (*Intramolecular bonds* are formed in

the conversion of unstable hydrogen bonding to stable covalent bonding in the assembly of the procollagen molecule.) The procollagen molecule is transported to the cell membrane and extruded into the interstitial space. The extracellular processing involves the conversion of procollagen to collagen. A spontaneous assembly occurs of collagen molecules into fibrils that are considered immature only because they do not have the tensile strength until they are cross-linked by a series of covalent bonds. Briefly, this involves oxidative deamination of amino groups (lysyl and hydroxylysyl groups), which allows for *intermolecular* cross-linking. Cross-linking occurs approximately at the terminal 25% of the collagen molecule forming the collagen fibril. Hydroxylysine is necessary for the synthesis of a cross-link of maximal stability. Cross-links between adjacent molecules are a prerequisite for the collagen fibers to withstand the physical stresses to which they are exposed. *Intermolecular bonds* therefore are attachments made by the molecules of the ground substance that interact with the collagen and between collagen microfibrils in fibril/fiber formation.

Pathophysiology of the Fibrillar Collagens

Overview

Disorders of connective tissues provide insight into the biological functions of the collagens. Many diseases involve collagen either directly or indirectly. The critical role of collagens is evident in the spectrum of clinical manifestations found in the multiple gene mutations determined in the more than 25 types of collagen (Myllyharju and Kivirikko 2001). Many collagenopathies are known and are the result of mutations that alter the expression or primary structure of collagen that are the predominant causes of severe skeletal defects (Prockop 1998). The consequence of mutations in collagen is diverse, ranging from early lethal phenotypes to predisposition for certain disease states, including OI, many chondrodysplasias, subtypes of Ehlers-Danlos syndrome (EDS), some cases of osteoporosis, arterial aneurysms, osteoarthritis, and some conditions affecting the intervertebral disc (Myllyharju and Kivirikko 2001).

The special properties that enable collagen to act as the major supporting framework of the body are largely dependent on the high structural stability of the collagen fibers. Recall that in health, fibrillar collagen is structurally stable because of the inherent:

- unique molecular configuration
- highly specific alignment of the molecules during extracellular aggregation
- formation of cross-links

The formation of cross-links is particularly important in conferring on the collagen fibers the high tensile strength and resistance to chemical attack necessary for their function. A malfunction, genetic or otherwise, in any one of the complex sequence of events leading to the formation of the final cross-linked fiber could result in an impairment of the fiber strength.

A number of connective tissue diseases are evident in which the clinical symptoms suggest a cross-linking defect. The extent of cross-linking may be important in affecting the catabolic rate in the more common conditions involving fibrosis and degeneration of connective tissue.

Various conditions, both normal and pathologic, embrace the concepts of tissue repair and regeneration of their collagenous framework, and collagen is critical in its role in the healing of wounds and fractures. After trauma or surgery, abnormal deposition of collagen may cause impaired function, and a multitude of conditions causing considerable disability originate from changes in the nature and organization of collagen. For example after trauma or surgery, abnormal deposition of collagen may impair function (adhesions after repair of long tendons, excessive scar formation during healing). Excessive collagen formation also may lead to fibrosis in various organs and tissues. In contrast, all conditions that inhibit collagen formation result in delayed healing of tissues. Therefore on one hand cells may produce collagen in either reduced or increased amounts (altered quantity), while on the other they may produce structurally defective collagen (altered quality).

Altered Quantity

In some circumstances cells produce collagens in altered quantity, either a reduced or increased amount. In circumstances such as wound healing and fracture repair, which are dependent on excessive collagen synthesis, any condition that inhibits collagen formation will act to impede the healing process. Normal wound healing involves the formation of scar and fibrous tissue that largely consists of collagen fibrils. Wound repair benefits from a moderate degree of fibrous tissue; however, if developed in excess it may impair the normal function of tissue. Extreme collagen pathology is demonstrated in the case of excessive collagen accumulation, which is referred to as *fibrosis*. Excessive collagen accumulation is associated with scarring of the skin after burns or traumatic injury as well as fibrosis affecting the liver, lungs, and kidneys resulting from injury to these organs. These conditions are characterized by excessive deposition of collagen seen in liver cirrhosis, scleroderma, skin keloid, pulmonary fibrosis, and diabetes. Efforts to inhibit collagen synthesis under these conditions include targeting the processes involved in transcription of the genes, translation of the messenger ribonucleic acid (mRNA), and the unique posttranslational enzymes involved in the biosynthesis of the protein (Prockop and Kivirikko 1995). With respect to the latter approach, the most suitable targets appear to be prolyl 4-Hyp, procollagen N-proteinase, procollagen C proteinase, and lysyl oxidase (Myllyharju and Kivirikko 2001).

Altered Quality

Collagen mutations lead to heritable defects of connective tissues. Cells may produce structurally defective collagen. Mutations in collagen genes may predispose individuals to a wide spectrum of diseases. Mutations in collagen genes or deficiencies in the activities of specific posttranslational enzymes of collagen synthesis have been characterized in many heritable disorders affecting the musculoskeletal system such as OI, chondrodysplasias, and some subtypes of the EDS, to name a few. Mutations in the genes encoding the individual collagen α-chains often lead to defects of the extracellular matrix. These mutations are generally dominant with the more abundant collagen types such as may be seen with type I OI and EDS type IV collagen mutations. In addition, collagen mutations have been implicated in more prevalent diseases such as osteoporosis and osteoarthritis.

Where can things go wrong?

Mutations in collagen genes involve amino acid substitutions or amino acid deletions because of defects during the transcription and translation processes. More than 1000 mutations have been characterized in 22 genes encoding polypeptide chains for 12 out of the more than 25 collagen types (Myllyharju and Kivirikko 2001).

Mutations in Type I collagen. OI and EDS subtypes are examples of conditions resulting from the following mutations in type I collagen:

- Osteogenesis imperfecta: Defects in the chains of type I collagen that act to reduce their stability or amount are associated with fragile bones, a condition known as OI. OI and its clinical subtypes (Wenstrup 1997) is one of the most common heritable connective tissue disorders. The disease is characterized by brittle bones but also involves other tissues rich in type I collagen and weakens such tissues as the skin, ligaments, tendons, fasciae, sclerae, and teeth, and induces hearing loss by affecting the middle and inner ear. More than 90% of patients with OI have a mutation in one of the two genes for type I procollagen. To date, most of the mutations characterized in patients with the disease are single-base *substitutions* that convert a codon for glycine that occurs as every third amino acid in the collagen triple helix to a codon for a bulkier amino acid. Recall that glycine normally occupies every third amino acid position in each of the three alpha chains that is an essential requirement for triple helix formation of the collagen molecule. The ultimate effect is that conformational changes in the triple helix alter the self-assembly of the protein into fibers resulting in abnormal kinetics, thermodynamics, and structure (Prockop 1998).
- Ehlers-Danlos syndrome: A heterogeneous group of heritable connective tissue disorders characterized by articular hypermobility (some cases of joint laxity lead to congenital dislocation of the hips and other large joints), skin extensibility, and tissue fragility is known as the *Ehlers-Danlos syndrome* (EDS). The cardinal manifestations of EDS have been described

as hyperextensible skin with a soft, velvety, doughy texture; dystrophic scarring; easy bruising; joint hypermobility; and connective tissue fragility (McKusick 1993). This group is the most prevalent heritable disorder of connective tissue and is characterized by abnormal collagen synthesis and cross-linking (Stanitski et al. 2000). Although at least 10 types of EDS have been defined (Hamel et al. 1998), a simplified classification of EDS into six major types has been proposed, with the molecular basis of each of the types either being clearly defined or seen as emerging (Beighton et al. 1998). Lethal complications of EDS subtypes often are seen, such as the arterial rupture caused by an abnormality of collagen type III as a result of mutations in corresponding gene COL3A1 in the case of EDS subtype IV (Hamel et al. 1998). Secondary manifestations including vascular and colonic ruptures, ocular or dental problems, and platelet abnormalities distinguish the subtypes of EDS.
- Marfan syndrome is a condition in which the vast majority of cases are not a result of collagen mutations but rather result from mutations in the gene for fibrillin (attachment protein that interacts with collagen type I) on chromosome 15 (Dietz et al. 1991).

Mutations in Collagen Type II. Type II is the main collagenous constituent of cartilage. Abnormalities in type II collagen have been identified in several chondrodysplasias. Mutations in type II collagen have been characterized in achondrogenesis, hypochondrogenesis, and spondyloepiphyseal dysplasia. Mutations in type II collagen are not limited to chondrodysplasias but may also be found in association with osteoarthritis and intervertebral disc disease.

Mutations in Collagen Type III. Type III collagen is usually present in tissues that also contain type I collagen but is absent in mature bone and tendon fibrils. Tissues particularly rich in type III collagen include the vessel walls, skin, and gut. Mutations in type III collagen have now been identified in individuals with a variant of EDS, in some individuals who have sustained aneurysms, or who present with extremely fragile blood vessels.

Clinical Note

Physical Rehabilitation and Ehlers-Danlos Syndrome

Musculoskeletal problems associated with several of the Ehlers-Danlos syndrome (EDS) subtypes include joint pain, swelling, instability and spinal deformity (scoliosis). Ehlers-Danlos syndrome types I, III, VI (rare), and VII (rare) have been associated with major orthopaedic problems, including joint instability and secondary inflammation, diminished function and symptoms related to spinal malalignment. Functional orthopaedic problems of patients with EDS include joint pain, impaired ambulation, functional hand strength, upper extremity function, and back or neck pain, which may not correlate with the presence or absence of spinal deformity. Type III EDS may be considered the most debilitating form of EDS with respect to musculoskeletal function, particularly in terms of impaired upper extremity function and grip strength and abnormal ambulation (walking ability, stair climbing) (Stanitski et al. 2000). Use of assistive devices may be common among patients presenting with all types of EDS. An individual afflicted with Type III EDS is more likely to need surgery, and patients with Type III disorder report a higher incidence of pain and lower level of function with reasons attributed to a combination triad of joint pain, instability, and muscle weakness (Stanitski et al. 2000).

Posttranslational events. Collagen biosynthesis can be altered by defects in any of the enzymes or enzyme activity involved in the posttranslational process. Many genetic diseases involving collagen are attributed to defects in posttranslational reactions (recall that collagen synthesis involves a series of posttranslational modifications that require a minimum of eight specific enzymes). Deficiencies are particularly remarkable in the activities of the following enzymes:

- *Prolyl hydroxylase:* The enzyme prolyl 4-hydroxylase must convert about 100 prolyl residues in each polypeptide chain to 4-hydroxyproline so that the protein may fold into the triple-helical conformation at 37° C (98.6° F). Ascorbic acid is a required co-factor for prolyl hydroxylase, which is essential for the synthesis of hydroxyproline. *Scurvy* is the classic example of how collagen biosynthesis can be altered at the posttranslational level. A nutritional disorder of collagen metabolism, scurvy is caused by lack of vitamin C (ascorbic acid/ascorbate) where collagen fibers are produced in abnormally low amounts and associated with impaired wound healing processes. Ascorbate deficiency leads to synthesis of pro-α chains that have a low hydroxyproline content and therefore cannot form a stable triple helix at body temperature or normal fibrils. The non-hydroxylated procollagen chains are degraded

within the cell; tissues such as blood vessels, tendon, and skin become fragile without the structural support of collagen. Prolyl 4-hydroxylase acts on proline residues in the Y positions of the (Gly-X-Y) sequences in the procollagen alpha chains in a reaction that also requires ferrous iron, 2-oxoglutarate, molecular oxygen in addition to ascorbate.

- *Lysyl hydroxylase:* The *hydroxylysine* residues formed in the lysyl hydroxylase reaction have two important functions: (1) they act as attachment sites for carbohydrate units and (2) they are essential for the stability of *intermolecular collagen cross-links* (Kivirikko et al. 1992). A deficiency in lysyl hydroxylase activity therefore manifests in a number of connective tissue diseases.
- *Procollagen C-proteinase:* Procollagen C-proteinase is an enzyme required for cleavage of C-terminal propeptides in procollagen, an event essential for collagen fibril assembly.
- *Procollagen N-proteinase:* Altered levels of procollagen N-proteinase will manifest in impaired cleavage of the N-terminal propeptides from procollagen.
- *Lysyl oxidase:* Lysyl oxidase is a copper-dependent enzyme that initiates the cross-linking of collagens and elastin (Kivirikko and Kulvaniemi 1987). Therefore altered copper metabolism can affect lysyl oxidase activity and hence collagen cross-linking (Prockop and Kivirikko, 1984).

Excessive collagen formation: fibrotic diseases. The formation of scar and fibrous tissue is part of the normal healing process after injury. In some situations, however, excessive collagen accumulation leads to fibrosis and consequently impairs the normal functioning of the affected tissue. The goal of antifibrotic therapy is to arrest hydroxylation of proline residues to inhibit this co-translational and posttranslational modification, which ultimately prevents collagen triple helix formation so that a nonfunctional protein is formed and rapidly degraded (Kivirikko et al. 1993).

Other Fibrous, Noncollagenous Components of the Extracellular Matrix

Elastin

Elastin is made of fibers of rubberlike protein that impart resilience to the matrix. Elastic fibers are typically thinner than collagenous fibers, and they are arranged in a somewhat random manner with branches to form networks. Elastin is a cross-linked, random-coil protein that gives tissues their elasticity. Elastin fibers typically range in size from 0.2 to 1.0 μm in diameter but can increase in size to present from 5 to 15 μm in diameter in elastic ligaments. Tissues such as skin and blood vessels require elasticity in addition to tensile strength to function. Elastin is a 70,000 dalton protein, which like collagen, is unusually rich in proline and glycine but contains little hydroxyproline and no hydroxylysine.

Elastin molecules are secreted into the extracellular space, where they form filaments and sheets in which the elastin molecules are highly cross-linked to each other to generate an extensive network. (The cross-links between the two peptides known as *desmosine* and *isodesmosine* are unique to elastin.) Elastin can be degraded by the pancreatic enzyme elastase but is otherwise difficult to break down. Elastic material is the major extracellular substance in the elastic ligaments (in the form of elastic fibers) associated with the spinal column and in elastic arteries (assuming the form of fenestrated lamellae arranged as concentric layers within the vessel wall). In elastic ligaments, such as the *ligamentum flava* in the vertebral column, many thick elastic fibers lie in a parallel arrangement.

Reticulin

Reticular fibers form delicate networks unlike the bundlelike presentation of collagenous fibers. Reticulin is observed to be a variation of collagen as its ultrastructural presentation shares similar periodic structure with collagen, even though its fibrils are always of narrow diameter (about 20 nm) and they do not form large bundles. Reticular networks are found in close proximity to cells and can be observed surrounding adipocytes and smooth muscle cells and assuming a supportive position under the capillary endothelium. Reticular fibers also contribute to the formation of the reticular lamina component of the basement membranes in epithelium.

Changes in the Nonmineralized Connective Tissues across the Lifespan: Growth, Development, and Age-Related Processes

With age are changes that occur at the cellular, matrix, tissue, organs, and systemic levels that all play a role in the deterioration of musculoskeletal function. The multifactorial nature of the causes of decline act to alter the integrity of the dense fibrous tissues and lend them to injury, as well as have the potential to impede healing processes. The following discussion focuses on the changes in structure and function of ligaments, tendons and capsules, intervertebral discs, and articular cartilage after skeletal maturity.

Some general principles apply to connective tissues in terms of maturation and age-related processes. Generally, a decrease in musculoskeletal function results from development of age-related degenerative disorders in addition to a general loss of tissue strength observed with age (Yamada 1970). This age-related decline in musculoskeletal function may be attributed to changes in behavior (mechanical and pathobiologic) of the supporting tissues such as articular cartilage, intervertebral disc, tendons, ligaments and joint capsules. The combination of such effects is such that an increased likelihood and severity of damage is incurred in many structures of the musculoskeletal system as the individual ages. With advancing age, clinical evidence supports that a longer time is assumed to recover from acute and repetitive musculoskeletal injuries, often necessitating extended rehabilitation after operative repair or reconstructive surgery of joints, tendons, and ligaments (Buckwalter and Cruess 1991). Therefore as a cell, tissue, or organ system ages, function gradually declines, susceptibility to disease and injury increases, and the ability to recover from disease of injury decreases (Buckwalter et al. 1993) (Figure 2-8). Well recognized is that the physiologic and biomechanical properties of the dense nonmineralized tissues change in a similar manner with age, even though the internal composition and proportion of constituents of each structure (e.g., ligaments and tendon, intervertebral discs, articular cartilage, joint capsule) differs. The age-related changes in these specific tissues in terms of composition, structure, and function are discussed in Chapters 3 to 5.

General Principles

Growth, development, and aging involve major changes in collagen biosynthesis and metabolism. The mechanisms underlying age-related changes in the nonmineralized connective tissues involve decreased numbers and function of cells and corresponding production of ECM (proliferation and synthetic capacity), which ultimately increase tissue susceptibility to injury as well as deterred and/or ineffective healing processes.

Cells

A decrease in mesenchymal stem cell population potentially leads to diminished ability and resource to heal, repair, and replace injured tissue. Normal differentiated cells have a limited division capacity, and these senescent cells, although viable, have lost the capacity to replicate (McCormick and Campisi 1991). Altered ability

of the cell to participate in synthetic events or other functions may be part of this senescent process (Seshadri and Campisi 1990; Buckwalter and Cruess 1991).

ECM Components

Many changes in the macromolecular framework of connective tissues may limit the ability of cells to replace degraded molecules or less functional PGs, which ultimately compromises the ability of cells to repair the matrix after injury to the joint complex or with repetitive impact loading (Buckwalter et al. 1994). Any decrease in the organization of the PG component of the matrix macromolecular framework alters the stability of the tissue and may contribute to the decline in the mechanical strength of connective tissues seen with aging, as may be witnessed in articular cartilage (Yamada 1970).

Altered posttranslational events of matrix proteins (e.g., collagen) may lead to altered turnover of matrix macromolecules, including formation and removal of byproducts. This alters composition that ultimately changes structural and functional properties of the ECM. Evidence exists that partially degraded molecules may accumulate with age in the matrix with an example being the accumulation of hyaluronic acid–binding fragments of the aggrecan PG in articular cartilage (Buckwalter et al. 1994). This may ultimately alter the mechanical properties and physiological role of the tissue. Intracellular degradation of collagen by phagocytosis in fibroblasts occurs in physiological remodeling of the ECM in many connective tissues with imbalances between degradation and synthesis leading to loss of tissue collagen. Aging is associated with an overall loss of collagen in dense connective tissues and with

Clinical Note

An appropriate exercise prescription for regular physical activity is believed to help maintain or restore musculoskeletal system function. Practitioners of orthopaedic physical therapy must assess the level of musculoskeletal function, particularly in the older person, for risk of injury and to design the appropriate prescription for type and intensity of physical activity. An emphasis on mobilizing soft tissues through stretching and range of motion regimens in addition to muscle strengthening programs (graduated resistance exercises) is important to maintaining integrity of the dense fibrous tissues and to promote optimal healing of injured soft tissues at any age.

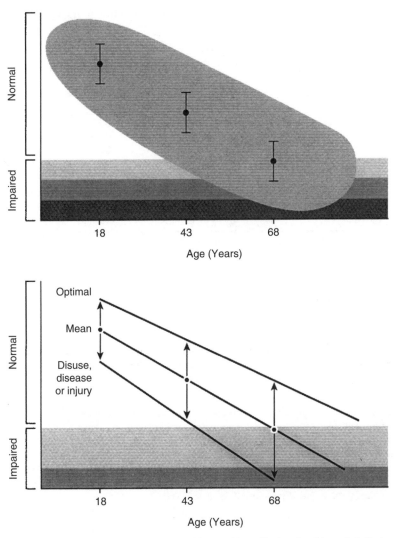

Figure 2-8. Decline in musculoskeletal function with age. (From Buckwalter JA et al. Soft-tissue Aging and Musculoskeletal Function. J Bone Joint Surg 1993;75A(10):1533-1548.)

Clinical Note

A direct correlation exists between increasing age and an increased prevalence of musculoskeletal impairment (Jette 1993). However, age-related changes in musculoskeletal function do not necessarily either progress uniformly in all individuals or cause impairment (Buckwalter et al. 1993). While altered or declining levels of circulating hormones (e.g., growth hormone and insulin growth factor I) target the musculoskeletal tissues, exercise and hormonal replacement have a role in attenuating disuse or disease and may maintain or improve elements of musculoskeletal function. A number of other age-related processes affect the central nervous system including proprioception and balance, vision and hearing, and cardiovascular functioning, all of which contribute to declining mobility. Furthermore, healing after soft-tissue injuries or surgical repair or reconstruction of joints, tendons, and ligaments often requires an increased period of time with advanced age (Buckwalter et al. 1996).

Table 2-1. Changes in the Interstitial Collagens (Types I-III) with Growth, Development, and Aging

Property	Change
Ratio of Type III to Type I collagen	Decreases in skin after birth
Rates of Synthesis and Degradation	
Rate of translation of pro-alpha chains	Decreases with age
Activities of prolyl and lysyl oxidases	Decreases with age
Activities of hydroxylysyl glycosyltransferases	Decreases with age
Rate of collagen degradation	Decreases after puberty
HyPro and HyLys excretion	Decreases after puberty
Quality of Collagen:	
Hydroxylysine and glycosylated hydroxylysine content	Decreases with age
Hydroxylysine-derived cross-links	Decreases with age
Immature reducible cross-links	Decreases with age

Modified from Prockup, DK, Kiririkko, KI, Tuderman, L, Guzman, N. 1979. The Biosynthesis of Collagen and Its Disorders. New England Journal of Medicine 301:13-23.

Clinical Note

The clinical reality is that aging and disease processes often co-present and are difficult, at best, to differentiate. Aside from the difficulty in distinguishing age and age-associated connective tissue pathologies from one another, the physical therapist is further faced with the clinical implications of physical management of these conditions in two ways:

• Can the course of events destined to occur in connective tissue because of the aging process be modified? This is important in determining best practice measures and identifying where the weight of physical medicine practice ideally should lie: e.g., in management versus the role of education and prevention of disease.

• How can the optimal repair of injured musculoskeletal tissues be facilitated and how is the course of events affected by the aging process with or without superimposed pathology? Inherent to this is determining the efficacy of and how the response to physical (mechanical/electrochemical) measures may be affected by age and age-associated pathologies of the musculoskeletal system.

---

increased lysosomal enzyme content in fibroblasts (McCulloch 1997). Age-related loss of collagen in connective tissues undergoing turnover may therefore be a manifestation of a deregulated increase of collagen phagocytosis in which the net loss of degraded collagen exceeds new synthesis (McCulloch 1997).

Decreased collagen degradation parallels the decrease in collagen synthesis seen with age, indicating an overall diminished turnover of collagen (Tuderman and Kivirikko 1977). The chemical characteristics and even the function of collagen changes with age (Table 2-1). The extent to which these changes are integral to the aging process remains unknown. Although the bulk of body collagen in adults is relatively stable, a portion of the collagen in all tissues is continually degraded and replaced even into old age. With increasing age, a loss in elasticity and strength of the nonmineralized soft tissues occurs (Yamada, 1970). Changes in posttranslational processes for the production of elastin, collagen, and the synthesis of PGs have been observed. With age, collagens are known to become less soluble (Schnider and Kohn 1981), more resistant to digestion by collagenase (Hamlin and Kohn 1971), and increasingly resistant to denaturation by heat (Everitt 1971) (because of the relative increase of cross-linked fibers). An increase in collagen cross-links occurs, particularly in periarticular fibrous tissue in the intervertebral disc (Hormel and Eyre 1991) and articular cartilage (Sell and Monnier 1989), which may contribute to altered mechanical properties and tissue degeneration with age (Buckwalter et al. 1993).

The greatest number of disorders of the noncalcified articular tissues are degenerative, metabolic or idiopathic and are often chronic. In an effort to delineate age-related versus pathologic processes, risk factors for the development of a disease are sought. To make the story fully circular, age is the greatest risk factor for many of the diseases that affect the tissues of the musculoskeletal system. For example, osteoarthritis is an example of pathology of the joint complex that manifests with advancing age (Chapter 4).

Summary

Connective tissues have important functions that include the following:

- Mechanical support and transmission of mechanical forces
- Being a medium within which substances are exchanged between blood and tissue (perfusion)
- Storage
- Vital immunologic protection against foreign microorganisms
- Provision of integral repair responses after insult to body tissues

To date, more than 25 collagen types have been identified, with 38 genetically distinct alpha chains differing in their length and in the precise amino acids involved. The ability of the helical and non-helical regions of various collagens to associate into fibrils or sheets or form cross-linking arrangements distinguish the different collagen types. The interstitial or fibrillar (types I-III) collagens that are the basis of the nonmineralized connective tissues encountered in orthopaedic physical therapy practice contain a repeating (Gly-X-Y) sequence that ultimately permits the folding of chains into a characteristic triple helix. The majority of the body's collagen is fibrillar in nature with these fibrous collagens comprising fibrils stabilized by covalent cross links.

Types I, II and III are the most common fibrillar collagens. Type I collagen is the most abundant collagen. Type I collagen is made of three subunits that form from a precursor procollagen molecule. After polypeptide synthesis, many posttranslational modifications occur where many proline and lysine residues are hydroxylated and selected hydroxyslysines are glycosylated. Type I collagen is the main fiber-forming collagen in tendon, ligament, and bone with two pro-alpha 1 (I) chains and one pro-alpha 2 (I) chain that form a triple helix from carboxy terminus to amino terminus. Procollagen peptidases act to remove peptides at the N-terminal and C-terminal ends to yield a type I collagen molecule that subsequently assembles into collagen fibrils. Type II is found primarily in hyaline cartilage. Type III is usually associated with type I collagen except in mature tendon and bone. Type IV is the most common non-fibrillar collagen and is a major constituent of all basement membranes. The insoluble fibrils (mainly collagen) of connective tissue act to transmit tensile forces as opposed to the interfibrillar soluble polymers of the ECM (PGs, HA) that elastically absorb compressive stresses.

Many diseases directly or indirectly involve collagen, the most abundant protein in the human body and the main constituent of skin, tendons, ligaments, demineralized bone and most blood vessels. Genetic "collagen disease" now includes the multiple variants of OI, Marfan syndrome and Ehlers-Danlos syndrome, all of which display considerable variability but are related to specific defects in collagen that result in disabling conditions based on changes in the nature and organization of collagen. Many diseases involve collagens in either a direct or indirect manner. Age-related changes affect the proliferative capacity of cells and a decrease in numbers of mesenchymal stem cells may affect the ability of dense fibrous connective tissues to maintain or repair themselves efficiently after injury.

References

Armstrong CG, Mow VC. Variations in the intrinsic mechanical properties of human articular cartilage with age, degeneration, and water content. J Bone and Joint Surg 1982;64-A:88-94.

Ayad S et al. The Extracellular Matrix. New York: Academic Press, 1994.

Beighton P et al. Ehlers-Danlos syndromes: revised nosology, Villefranche, 1997. Am J Med Genet 1998;77: 31-37.

Betsch D, Baer E: Structure and mechanical properties of rat tail tendon. Biorheology 1980;7:83-94.

Binkley J. Overview of ligament and tendon structure and mechanics: Implications for clinical practice. Physiother Can 1989;41(1):24-30.

Binkley J, Peat M. The effect of immobilisation on the ultrastructure and mechanical properties of the rat medial collateral ligament. Clin Orthopaed 1986;203:301-308.

Buckwalter JA. Fine Structural Studies of Human Intervertebral Disc. In AA White, Sl Gordon (eds), Proceedings of the Workshop on Idiopathic Low Back Pain. St. Louis: Mosby, 1982;108-143.

Buckwalter JA et al. Proteoglycans of human infant intervertebral disc. Electron microscopic and biochemical studies. J Bone Joint Surg [Am] 1985;67:284-294.

Buckwalter JA, Cruess R. Healing of Musculoskeletal Tissues. In CA Rockwood, Jr et al. (eds), Fractures. Philadelphia: JB Lippincott, 1991;181-222.

Buckwalter JA et al. Soft-tissue aging and musculoskeletal function. J Bone Joint Surg 1993;75A(10):1533-1548.

Buckwalter JA et al. Age-related changes in cartilage proteoglycans: quantitative electron microscopic studies. Microscopy Res Technique 1994;28:398-408.

Buckwalter JA et al. Healing of the Musculoskeletal Tissues. In CA Rockwood, Jr et al. (eds), Fractures (4th ed). Philadelphia: Lippincott-Raven, 1996;261-304.

Bullough P, Brauer F. Age-Related Changes in Articular Cartilage. In JA Buckwalter, VM Goldberg, SLY Woo (eds), Musculoskeletal Soft Tissue Aging: Impact on Mobility. Rosemont, Ill.: American Academy of Orthopaedic Surgeons, 1993;117-135.

Burganadze TV, Veis A. A thermodynamic analysis of the contribution of hydroxyproline to the structural stability of the collagen triple helix. Connect Tissue Res 1997;36(4):347-365.

Burgeson R, Nimni M. Collagen types: molecular structure and tissue distribution. Clin Orthopaed Rel Res 1992;282:250-272.

Butler D et al. Biomechanics of ligaments and tendons. Exer Sport Sci Rev 1978;6:125-181.

Cancedda R et al. Chondrocyte differentiation. Int Rev Cytol 1995;159:265-357.

Chazal J et al. Biomechanical properties of spinal ligaments and a histological study of the supraspinal ligament in traction. J Biomechanics 1985;18:167-176.

Cohen MM. Merging the old skeletal biology with the new. II. Molecular aspects of bone formation and bone growth. J Craniofac Dev Biol 2000;20:94-106.

Currier D, Nelson R. Dynamics of Human Biologic Tissues. Contemporary Perspectives in Rehabilitation. Philadelphia: F.A. Davis, 1992.

Dahners LE et al. The relationship of actin to ligament contraction. Clin Orthopaed 1986;210:246-251.

Dalgleish R. The human collagen mutation database. Nucleic Acids Res 1998;26(1):253-255.

Diament J et al. Collagen: ultrastructure and its relation to mechanical properties as a function of aging. Proceed Royal Society London 1972;180:293-315.

Dickson IR et al. Variations in the protein components of human intervertebral disk with age. Nature 1967;215:52-53.

Dietz HC et al. Marfan syndrome caused by a recurrent de novo missense mutation in the fibrillin gene. Nature 1991;352:337-339.

Donahue PJ et al. Characterization of link protein(s) from human intervertebral-disc tissues. Biochem J 1988;251:739-747.

Engel J. Does bound water contribute to the stability of collagen? Matrix Biol 1998;17:679-680.

Engvall E. Laminin variants: Why, where and when? Kidney Int 1993;43:2D6.

Enwemeka CS. Ultrastructural changes induced by cast immobilization in the isolated soleus tendon. APTA Annual Conference Abstr R-123. Anaheim, CA, June 24-28, 1990;65.

Erlebacher A et al. Toward a molecular understanding of skeletal development. Cell 1995;80:371-378.

Everitt AV. Food intake, growth and the aging of collagen in rat tail tendon. Gerontologia 1971;17:98-104.

Eyre DR, Muir H. Quantitative analysis of types I and II collagen in human intervertebral discs at various ages. Biochim Biophys Acta 1977;492(1):29-42.

Eyre DR et al. The cartilage collagens and joint degeneration. Brit J Rheumatol 1991;30(Suppl 1):10-15.

Frank C et al. Normal Ligament: Structure, Function and Composition. In SLY Woo and JA Buckwalter (eds), Injury and Repair of the Musculoskeletal Soft Tissues. Park Ridge, Illinois: American Academy of Orthopaedic Surgeons, 1988;45-101.

Galou et al. The importance of intermediate filaments in the adaptation of tissues to mechanical stress: evidence from gene knockout studies. Biology Cell, 1997;89(2):85-97.

Gathercole LJ, Keller A; Early development of crimping in rat tail tendon. Micron, 1968;9:83-89.

Geneser F. Textbook of Histology. Philadelphia: Lea & Febiger, 1986;157-184, 219-257.

Gower WE, Pedrini V. Age-related variations in protein-polysaccharides from human nucleus pulposus, annulus fibrosus, and costal cartilage. J Bone Joint Surg 1969;51-A:1154-1162.

Graham HK et al. Identification of collagen fibril fusion during vertebrate tendon morphogenesis. The process relies on unipolar fibrils and is regulated by collagen-proteoglycan interaction. J Mol Biol 2000;295:891-902.

Hamerman D. Aging and osteoarthritis: basic mechanisms. JAGS 1993;41(7):760-770.

Hamel BCJ et al. Ehlers-Danlos syndrome and type III collagen abnormalities: a variable clinical spectrum. Clin Genet 1998;53(6):440-446.

Hamlin CR, Kohn RR. Evidence for progressive, age-related structural changes in post-mature human collagen. Biochim Biophys Acta 1971;236:458-467.

Hassler O. The human intervertebral disc. A micro-angiographical study on its vascular supply at various ages. Acta Orthop. Scandinavica 1969;40:765-772.

Heikkinen J et al. Duplication of seven exons in the lysyl hydroxylase gene is associated with longer forms of a repetitive sequence within the gene and is a common cause for the type VI variant of Ehlers-Danlos syndrome. Am J Hum Genet 1997;60:48-56.

Holm S, Nachemson A. Nutrition of the intervertebral disc: acute effects of cigarette smoking. An experimental animal study. Uppsala J Med Sci 1988;93:91-99.

Hocking AM et al. Leucine-rich repeat glycoproteins of the extracellular matrix. Matrix Biol 1998;17(1):1-19.

Hormel SE, Eyre DR. Collagen in the aging human intervertebral disc: an increase in covalently bound flurophores and chromophores. Biochim. Biophys Acta 1991;1078(2):243-250.

Jackson D, Bentley J Collagen-glycosaminoglycan interactions. In Ramachandran GN (ed), Treatise on Collagen V2A. London: Academic Press, 1968;300-321.

Jette AM Using health-related quality of life measures in physical therapy outcomes research. Phys Ther 1993;73(8):528-537.

Kadler KE et al. Collagen fibril formation. Biochem J 1996;316:1-11.

Karpakka J. Effects of physical activity and inactivity on collagen synthesis in rat skeletal muscle and tendon (Dissertation). Oulu: University of Oulu, Finland. Acta Univ Oul D 1991;231:1-52.

Kennedy J et al. Tension studies of human knee ligaments. J Bone Joint Surgery 1976;58-A:350-355.

Kielty CM et al. In PM Royce and B Steinmann (eds), Connective Tissue and Its Heritable Disorders: Molecular, Genetic and Medical Aspects. New York: Wiley-Liss, 1993;103-147.

Kivirikko KI. Collagen biosynthesis: a mini-review cluster. Matrix Biol 1998;16:355-356.

Kivirikko KI. Collagens and their abnormalities in a wide spectrum of diseases. Annals Med 1993;25:113-126.

Kivirikko K, Kulvaniemi H. Posttranslational Modifications of Collagen and Their Alterations in Heritable Diseases. In J Uitto and A Perejda (eds), Connective Tissue Disease. Molecular Pathology of the Extracellular Matrix. New York: Marcel Dekker, 1987;263-292.

Kivirikko K et al. Hydroxylation of Proline and Lysine Residues in Collagens and Other Animal and Plant Proteins. In JJ Harding and M Crabbe (eds), Post-translational Modifications of Proteins. Boca Raton, FL: CRC Press, 1992;1-51.

Kuc IM, Scott PG. Increased diameters of collagen fibrils precipitated in-vitro in the presence of decorin from various connective tissues. Connect Tissue Res 1998;36(4):287-296.

Larson N, Parker WW. Physical Activity and its influence on the strength and elastic stiffness of knee ligaments. In ML Howell and AW Parker (eds), Sports Medicine: Medical and Scientific Aspects of Elitism in Sport, Vol.

8. Brisbane, Australia: Australian Sports Medicine Federation, 1982;63-73.

Little B et al. The effect of strenuous versus moderate exercise on the metabolism of proteoglycans in articular cartilage from different weight-bearing regions of the equine 3rd carpal bone. Osteoarth Cartilage 1997;5(3):161-172.

Madden JW, Peacock EE. Dynamic metabolism of scar collagen and remodeling of dermal wounds. Annals Surg 1971;174:511-520.

Martin G et al. The genetically distinct collagens. TIBS, July 1985:285-288.

McCormick A, Campisi J. Cellular aging and senescence. Curr Opin Cell Biol 1991;3:230-234.

McCulloch, CAG. Deregulation of collagen phagocytosis in aging human fibroblasts: effects of integrin expression and cell-cycle. Experimental Cell Res 1997;237(2):383-393.

McKusick VA. The Ehlers-Danlos Syndromes. In P Beighton (ed), Heritable Disorders of Connective Tissue. St. Louis, Mosby, 1993;189-251.

Mohamedali V et al. Adipose-tissue as an endocrine and paracrine organ. Internat J Obesity 1998;22(12):1145-1158.

Mow VC et al. Biomechanics of Articular Cartilage. In M Nordin and VH Frankel (eds), Basic Biomechanics of the Musculoskeletal System. Philadelphia: Lea & Febiger, 1989;31-57.

Myllyharju J, Kivirikko KI. Collagens and collagen-related diseases. Ann Med 2001;33:7-21.

Nimni M. Collagen: Structure, function, and metabolism in normal and fibrotic tissues. Semin Arthr Rheumat 1983;11(1):1-66.

Ottani V et al. Collagen structure and functional implications. Micron 2001;32(3):251-260.

Poole AR. Proteoglycans in health and disease: Structures and functions. *Biochem J* 1986;236:1-14.

Pope MH et al. Structure and Function of the Lower Spine. Occupational Low Back Pain: Assessment, Treatment, and Prevention. St. Louis: Mosby, 1991;562.

Prockop DJ et al. The biosynthesis of collagen and its disorders. N Engl J Med 1979;301:13-23.

Prockop DJ, Kivirikko KI. Heritable diseases of collagen. N Engl J Med 1984;311(6):376-386.

Prockop DJ, Kivirikko KI. Collagens: molecular biology, diseases, and potentials for therapy. Ann Rev Biochem 1995;64:403-434.

Prockop DJ. What holds us together? Why do some of us fall apart? What can we do about it? Matrix Biol 1998;16:519-528.

Prockop DJ, Fertala A. The collagen fibril: the almost crystalline structure. J Struct Biol 1998;122:111-118.

Prockop et al. Procollagen N-proteinase and procollagen C-proteinase. Two unusual metalloproteinases that are essential for procollagen processing probably have important roles in development and cell signaling. Matrix Biol 1998;16:399-408.

Quarto R et al. Modulation of commitment, proliferation, and differentiation of chondrogenic cells in defined culture medium. Endocrinology 1997;138(11):4966-4976.

Rigby BJ et al. The mechanical behaviour of rat tail tendon. J Gen Physiol 1959;43:265-283.

Rousselle P, Garrone R. Collagens and laminins: which messages for which cells. Pathologie Biologie 1998;46(7):543-554.

Rucker RB et al. Copper, lysyl oxidase, and extracellular-matrix protein cross-linking. Am J Clin Nutrit 1998;67(5):996-1002.

Ryan MC, Christiano AM. The functions of laminins: lessons from in vivo studies. Matrix Biol 1996;15: 369-381.

Sakai LY et al. Current knowledge and research directions in heritable disorders of connective tissue. Matrix Biol 1996;15:211-229.

Schnider S, Kohn RR. Effects of age and diabetes mellitus on the solubility and nonenzymatic glucosylation of human skin collagen. J Clin Invest 1981;67:1630-1635.

Scott JE, Parry DA. Control of collagen fibril diameters in tissues. Internat J Biol Macromol 1992;14:292-293.

Sell DR, Monnier VM. Structure elucidation of a senescence cross-link from human extracellular matrix. Implication of pentoses in the aging process. J Biol Chem 1989;264:21597-21602.

Seshadri T, Campisi J. Repression of c-fos transcription and an altered genetic program in senescent human fibroblasts. Science 1990;247:205-209.

Shyy JYJ, Chien S. Role of integrins in cellular-responses to mechanical stress and adhesion. Curr Opin Cell Biol 1997;9(5):707-713.

Smith-Mungo LI, Kagan HM. Lysyl oxidase: properties, regulation and multiple functions in biology. Matrix Biol 1998;16:387-398.

Stanitski et al. Orthopaedic manifestations of Ehlers-Danlos syndrome. Clin Orthop 2000;376:213-221.

Trout JJ et al. Ultrastructure of the human intervertebral disc. II. Cells of the nucleus pulposus. Anat Rec 1982;204:307-314.

Tuderman L, Kivirikko K. Immunoreactive prolyl hydroxylase in human skin, serum and synovial fluid: changes in the content and components with age. Europ J Clin Invest 1977;7:295-299.

Vaatainen U et al. Collagen cross-links in chondromalacia of the patella. Internat J Sports Med 1998;19(2): 144-148.

Vernon-Roberts B, Pirie CJ. Degenerative changes in the intervertebral discs of the lumbar spine and their sequelae. Rheumat Rehab 1977;16:13-21.

Warren CG et al. Elongation of rat tail tendon: effect of load and temperature. Arch Phys Med Rehabil 1972;50: 481-487.

Watanabe H et al. Roles of aggrecan, a large chondroitin sulfate proteoglycan, in cartilage structure and function. J Biochem, 1998;124:687-693.

Wenstrup R. From Genes to Tissue in Osteogenesis Imperfecta: A Long and Winding Road. In MM Cohen, Jr and BJ Baum (eds). Studies in Stomatology and Craniofacial Biology. Amsterdam: IOS Press, 1997; 191-207.

Wess TJ et al. Type I collagen packing, conformation of the triclinic unit cell. J Molec Biol 1995;248:487-493.

Woo SL-Y et al. Connective tissue response to immobility. Arthr Rheumatol 1975;18:257-264.

Woo SL-Y et al. The biomechanical and morphological changes in the medial collateral ligament of the rabbit after immobilization and remobilization. J Bone Joint Surg 1987;69-A:1200-1211.

Yamada H. Strength of Biological Materials. In FG Evans (ed), Baltimore: Williams and Wilkins, 1970.

Yamauchi M et al. Cross-linking and the molecular packing of corneal collagen. Biochem Biophys Res Commun 1996;219:311-315.

Chapter 3

The Nature of the Dense Connective Tissues of the Musculoskeletal System: Structure, Function, and Biomechanics of Tendon, Ligament, and the Joint Capsule

Ligament, tendon, and capsule are similar tissues in that they are composed of densely packed collagen fibers associated with connective tissue cell types of which the majority are fibrocytes/fibroblasts. These tissues are poorly vascularized and hence are relatively metabolically stable tissues. A poor vascular supply in addition to the dense packing of collagen fibers bestows a limited ability of these stable tissues to undergo acute change in terms of their length, strength, and extensibility properties under normal physiologic conditions. However, some basic differences exist in the arrangement of collagen fibers and other ultrastructural components between ligaments, tendons and capsules that is ultimately reflected in their biomechanical properties.

Tendon and Ligament: General Characteristics

Tendon is composed of dense connective tissue in which cells are surrounded by an extensive, predominantly collagen-based extracellular matrix (ECM). Tendons are structures that act to join skeletal muscle to bones. Each muscle usually has two tendons, proximal and distal, each of which is generally cordlike in nature. The site of muscle and tendon union is referred to as the *myotendinous* junction (Figure 3-1), whereas the bone-tendon union is referred to as the *osseotendinous* junction. Tendons are designed to transmit longitudinal as well as transverse and rotational forces created in the muscle to bone. They are tough structures capable of withstanding direct pressure and high

mechanical loads yet can maintain internal fiber connections. A tendon consists of parallel bundles of collagen fibers between which are rows of fibroblasts (Figure 3-2).

The function of ligaments is to join bone to bone. Ligaments also consist of roughly parallel bundles of fibers and fibroblasts (fibrocytes); however, the fibers are arranged in a less regular manner than tendon.

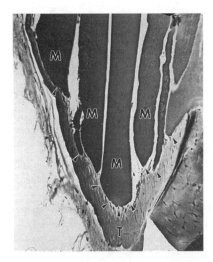

Figure 3-1. Light micrograph of longitudinal section through several frog semitendinosus muscle cells (M) attached to their tendon of insertion (T) at myotendinous junctions (arrowheads, magnification X250). (From Garrett W, Tidball J. Myotendinous Junction: Structure, Function and Failure. In SL-Y Woo, JA Buckwalter. Injury and Repair of the Musculoskeletal Soft Tissues. Rosemont, Ill: American Academy of Orthopaedic Surgeons, 1988;174.)

Tendon: Specific Characteristics

Gross Structure

Tendons appear white in color and are elastic in texture. Great variation exists in their presentation in terms of shape and the means by which they make their attachment to bone. Some tendons present as wide and flat (quadriceps or triceps surae muscle tendons). Others may be cylindrical (biceps muscle tendons) or ribbon shaped (plantaris, finger flexor muscle tendons). The gross morphology of each tendon reflects the function of its muscle. For

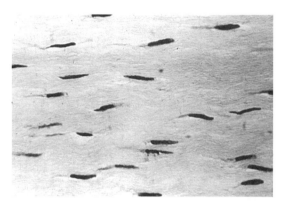

Figure 3-2. Photomicrograph of a longitudinal section of a human flexor tendon showing the spindle-shaped fibroblasts (**H** and **E**, magnification X250). (From Woo SL-Y et al. Anatomy, Biology and Biomechanics of Tendon, Ligament, and Meniscus. In SR Simon. Orthopaedic Basic Science. Rosemont, Ill: American Academy of Orthopaedic Surgeons, 1994;47.)

example, the quadriceps tendon is attached to a powerful muscle that acts to resist forces as opposed to fine motor movement required of the tendons in the hand and fingers.

Ultrastructure

Tendons consist of collagen (65% to 80%) and elastin (2%) fibers by dry weight that are embedded in a proteoglycan water-based matrix (Curwin 1997). While elastic fibers do occupy a portion of the ECM of tendon, the mechanical stability of the collagen plays the most important role in imparting mechanical strength to a tendon. Of the collagenous component, normal adult tendons are composed largely of type I collagen (95%) and the remaining 5% consist of types III, V, VI and IX collagen (Gelberman et al. 1988; Vogel and Koob 1989). Types III and V collagens form heterotypic fibers with type I collagen fibers (Fleischmajer et al. 1990) and may serve to regulate type I collagen fiber diameter (Birk et al. 1990). The three-dimensional ultrastructure of a collagen fiber from tendon (Figure 3-3) is complex in that the fibrils within one collagen fiber are oriented not only longitudinally but also transversely and horizontally (Kannus 2000). In fact, along the whole length of tendons the ratio of longitudinally to transversely or horizontally running fibers ranges between 10:1 and 26:1 (Jozsa et al. 1991). X-ray diffraction of rat tail tendon supports that type I collagen fibrils contain regions of three-dimensional crystalline arrays

---

Clinical Note

Response of Tendon and Ligament to Physical Stress and Immobilization

Altered mechanical stress levels experienced in extreme levels of physical activity such as immobilization and exercise are known to result in changes in the mechanical properties of ligament and tendon. Changes in the connective tissues associated with immobilization that occur with casting, weakness, and pain are of direct importance to the physical therapist. The effects of immobilization on tendons include significant loss of water content, glycosaminoglycan concentration and strength. The clinical implication of immobilized tendon or ligament is that it becomes unable to withstand high loads and reaches yield points significantly earlier than tendon/ligament that is mobilized or is from a younger but mature specimen. Mechanical stress is therefore important in enhancing fibril alignment in both tendon and ligament, which ultimately imparts tissue strength. Physical management strategies should be driven by the application of appropriate levels of mechanical stimulation in the form of therapeutic exercise or joint mobilization as movement is reintroduced.

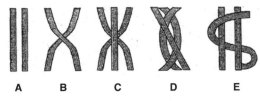

A   B   C   D   E

Figure 3-3. Collagen fiber crossing. The types of collagen fiber crossing in tendons: **A**, Parallel running fibers; **B**, simply crossing fibers; **C**, crossing of two fibers with one straight-running fiber; **D**, a plait formation with three fibers; **E**, up-tying of parallel running fibers. (From Kannus P. Structure of the Tendon Connective Tissue. 2000. Scand J Med Sci Sports 2000;10:312-320.)

where molecular packing is speculated to be by a staggered sheet or microfibril arrangement (Wess et al. 1998).

Proteoglycans (PGs) in tendon play an important role in regulating the nature of the ECM in both the tendon and its associated fibrocartilage (Waggett et al. 1998). Small quantities of PGs are present in tendon, with decorin being the major small PG in the purely tensional regions of a tendon (Vogel and Heinegard 1985). Decorin, lumican, and fibromodulin are thought to play a role in collagen fibrillogenesis and their expression is probably important in regulating this in the midtendon and the fibrocartilages (Vogel et al. 1984). In other connective tissue-based structures such as articular cartilage, aggrecan is well represented with its function being to resist compressive forces because of the large amount of water associated with its charged glycosaminoglycan (GAG) chains (Wight et al. 1991).

Diversity exists within a tendon in terms of collagen content and distribution of other associated ECM components because of the diverse forces imposed upon tendons at specific sites along its structure. Researchers have determined that the biochemistry of the ECM changes and tendons are frequently cartilaginous at certain regions (Vogel and Koob 1989). For instance, striking differences exist in the ECM between the midtendon region of the Achilles' tendon and its insertion. Types I, III, V and VI collagens, decorin, biglycan, fibromodulin and lumican have been found in both the midtendon and the fibrocartilaginous insertion regions. A consistent presence of messenger ribonucleic acid (mRNA) is found for type II collagen in the fibrocartilage region that is rarely found in the midtendon region. The transitional character of fibrocartilage can be observed in that representation exists of type II collagen, a prominent component of the fibrocartilage regions of the tendon, as well as types I and III collagen. Fibrocartilage is characterized by having properties intermediate between those of dense fibrous connective tissue (type I) and hyaline cartilage (type II) collagen. Aggrecan mRNA is present in the fibrocartilage region and is typically absent from the midtendon region. The localization of GAGs appears to be site specific in that high representation of dermatan sulphate may be present in a tensional zone of tendon while at a pressure zone such as an insertion site, there may be high representation of chondroitin sulphate (Merrilees and Flint 1980). The large aggregating PGs (e.g., aggrecan) present in tendons are similar to those PGs of cartilage. These aggregates may contribute to dissipating loads since they are more abundant in those parts of the tendon subjected to increased pressure (Poole 1986). The presence of type V collagen in both the midtendon and fibrocartilage is linked to the occurrence of type I collagen found in both regions (Waggett et al. 1998). Thus the range and distribution of ECM molecules detected in the Achilles tendon reflect the different forces acting on it. The mid-tendon largely acts to transmit tension and is characterized by molecules typical of fibrous tissues; the fibrocartilage also resists compression and thus contains, in addition, molecules typical of cartilage (type II collagen and aggrecan) that function to resist these forces (Waggett et al. 1998). Fibrocartilage is well described at tendon insertion sites known as *entheses,* where it may reduce stress concentration at the insertion site of a tendon into bone, or bone-tissue interface (Benjamin and Ralphs 1995). Here enthesial-fibrocartilage permits a transition in mechanical properties between tendon and bone (Benjamin and Ralphs 1995) via the following tissue types: pure tendon, uncalcified fibrocartilage, calcified fibrocartilage, and bone. Sesamoid fibrocartilage is believed to facilitate withstanding compression of the Achilles tendon as it presses against the heel during walking and running (Waggett et al. 1998). In the case of the Achilles tendon, periosteal fibrocartilage lies on the bony surface of the heel that is compressed by tendon, separated from the sesamoid fibrocartilage by a synovial bursa (Figure 3-4).

In summary, the properties of tendon depend mainly on the properties and architecture of the collagen and elastin fibers that interact with each other. Proteoglycans, as noncollagenous macromolecules interwoven with collagen fibers and elastin, also contribute to the viscoelastic properties of tendon. Because of their high fixed charge density and internal repulsion forces, PGs are rigidly extended and impart high capacity to the neighboring collagen fibers to resist high levels of compressive and tensile forces. The concentration of GAGs is, however, relatively smaller in tendinous tissue than is found in cartilage or other connective tissues. Aggrecan is most clearly represented in tendons that wrap around bony pulleys (Vogel and Heinegard 1985) and at tendon insertions (Waggett et al. 1998).

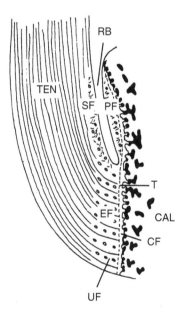

Figure 3-4. A diagrammatic representation of the attachment of the human Achilles tendon (TEN) to the calcaneus (CAL). Note the three fibrocartilages at the insertion site: enthesial fibrocartilage (EF) at the bone-tendon junction, sesamoid fibrocartilage (SF) on the adjacent, and deep surface of the tendon and periosteal fibrocartilage (PF) on the opposing surface of the calcaneus. SF and PF are separated by the retrocalcaneal bursa (RB), but they are pressed against each other during ankle movements. EF has a zone of uncalcified fibrocartilage (UF) which is separated from a zone of calcified fibrocartilage (CF) by a tidemark (T), indicated by the broken line. (From Waggett AD et al. Characterization of Collagens and Proteoglycans at the Insertion of the Human Achilles Tendon. Matrix Biol 1998;16: 457-470.)

The Cellular Component of Tendon

Tenoblasts and tenocytes, which are the elongated fibroblasts and fibrocytes that lie interspersed between collagen fibers (Figure 3-5), are responsible for producing the extracellular matrix characteristic of tendons. These cells assume a complex hierarchical organization within the tendon. The tenoblasts and tenocytes comprise approximately 90% to 95% of the cellular elements in tendon. In addition, the remaining 5% to 10% of cells include chondrocytes that are present at pressure and insertion sites, synovial cells on tendon sheaths, and vascular cells that may be found in the endotenon and epitenon (Figure 3-6).

In newborn tendon, a high cell-to-matrix ratio exists with the cells arranged in long parallel chains. As tendon matures in the adult human, the cell-to-matrix ratio decreases, and the tenocytes become elongated (Ippolito et al. 1980). Intercellular contacts assume desmosomal junctions, tight junctions or gap junction forms (Jozsa and Kannus 1997). Tenocytes continue to be metabolically active cells, although however, not at the same capacity as tenoblasts. Both are active in energy production and biosynthesis of collagen and other matrix components (Jozsa and Kannus 1997). In terms of matrix metabolism, which is highest during growth and diminishes with age, the tendon cells are capable of synthesizing all components of

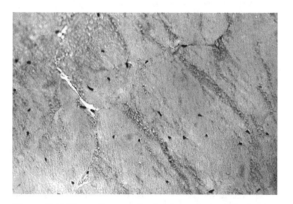

Figure 3-5. Photomicrograph of a cross section of a human flexor tendon showing the star-shaped fibroblasts with cytoplasmic processes between collagen bundles (**H** and **E**, magnification X250). (From Woo SL-Y et al. Anatomy, Biology and Biomechanics of Tendon, Ligament, and Meniscus. In SR Simon. Orthopaedic Basic Science. Rosemont, Ill: American Academy of Orthopaedic Surgeons, 1994;48.)

the tendon matrix including the collagen and elastic fibers, proteoglycans, and structural glycoproteins (Curwin 1997). However, the low metabolic rate of adult tendon tissue is important for the tendon to assume loads and remain in periodic tension without becoming ischaemic and undergoing necrosis (Kannus 2000). The tradeoff for this characteristic may be witnessed clinically in that once injured, tendon demonstrates a slow rate of recovery and healing (Williams 1986).

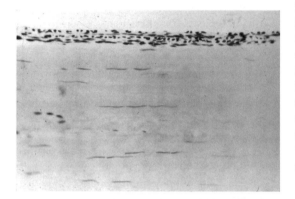

Figure 3-6. Longitudinal section of a human flexor tendon illustrating the epitenon on the surface of the tendon (**H** and **E**, magnification X125). (From Woo SL-Y et al. Anatomy, Biology and Biomechanics of Tendon, Ligament, and Meniscus. In SR Simon. Orthopaedic Basic Science. Rosemont, Ill: American Academy of Orthopaedic Surgeons, 1994;50.)

As discussed in Chapter 2, collagen fibrils consist of aggregated microfibrils whose base is the insoluble, cross-linked collagen molecule. A collection of collagen fibrils forms a collagen fiber that is the fundamental unit of tendon (Figures 3-7 and 3-8). The proportions of these ultrastructural components vary slightly from tendon to tendon and with age. The diameter of the tertiary fiber bundles of human tendons varies from 1000 to 3000 μm, whereas the diameter of the secondary bundles ranges from 150 to 1000 μm. The collagen fiber diameter also varies ranging from 5 to 300 μm. Collagen concentration in each fiber is directly related to the fiber diameter, which depends more on the number as opposed to the size of constituent microfibrils (Elliott 1965). The diameter of both the secondary and tertiary bundles of human tendons is related to the macroscopic size of the tendon so that the lowest values may be observed in small tendons (e.g., the finger flexors) and largest values seen in large tendons (e.g., Achilles tendon) (Jozsa and Kannus 1997).

Inorganic Composition of Tendon

Inorganic components comprise less than 0.2% of the dry weight of tendon and may include calcium, magnesium, manganese, cadmium, cobalt, copper, zinc, nickel, lithium, lead, fluoride, and silicon

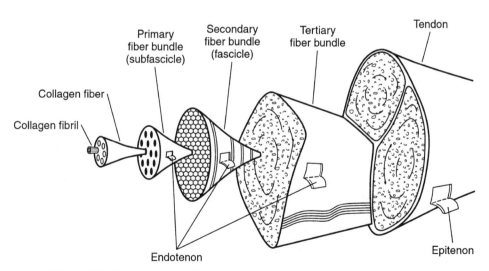

Figure 3-7. The organization of tendon structure from collagen fibrils to the entire tendon. (From Kannus P. Structure of the Tendon Connective Tissue. Scand J Med Sci Sports 2000;10:312-320.)

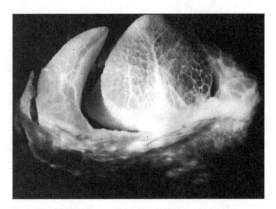

Figure 3-8. Cross section of human flexor tendon (flexor digitorum superficialis, flexor digitorum profundus) at the midportion of the proximal phalanx of the third digit. The endotenon tissue of the profundus is clearly visible. (From Woo SL-Y et al. Anatomy, Biology and Biomechanics of Tendon, Ligament, and Meniscus. In SR Simon. Orthopaedic Basic Science. Rosemont, Ill: American Academy of Orthopaedic Surgeons, 1994;50.)

(Spadaro et al. 1970). Calcium, as the most highly represented inorganic component in tendon is found in concentrations ranging from 0.001% to 0.01% in the tensional area of normal tendon, and 0.05% to 0.1% at insertion sites (Kannus 2000). In pathologic conditions where the tendon calcifies (calcifying tendinopathy) a tenfold to twentyfold increase in calcium levels may be determined (Jozsa et al. 1989).

Tendon Structure and Structures that Surround Tendon

Although tendon is described often in terms of its composition as a single structure it is better observed as a composite unit consisting of the main tendon body that has a synovial tissue covering. The synovial tissue is in the form of a distinct fibro-osseous sheath in certain regions (where a true synovial space exists); in other regions the synovial cells may be found intermittently distributed along the outer surface of tendon (Henderson and Edwards 1987). Structures that surround tendons may assume different forms (Kannus 2000):

1. Long tendons glide through canals made of fibrous sheaths that may also be referred to as *retinacula*. They are essential to reduce friction as tendons glide through bony grooves and notches. This is typical of the flexor and extensor tendons in the hands and feet.
2. Where curves occur along the course of a tendon, "reflection pulleys" exist that are anatomic reinforcements of the fibrous sheaths in (1).
3. Synovial sheaths, consisting of an outer fibrous layer under which there are two thin and serous sheets (parietal and visceral), surround the tendons in a tunnel form at bony or other friction bearing surfaces. Once again this is typical around the tendons of the hands and feet.
4. In some tendons where no true synovial sheath exists, a paratenon, which is an elastic sheath made of loose fibrillar tissue, acts to reduce friction. The Achilles tendon is characterized by a paratenon with thin gliding membranes (Jozsa and Kannus 1997).
5. Bursae associated with tendons are critical in their role to reduce friction as the tendon courses along bony prominences. Many examples of these extratendonous structures in the body exist, including the subacromial, infrapatellar, and deep trochanteric bursae.

Organization of Tendon: Paratenon, Epitenon, Endotenon

Paratenon is loose areolar connective tissue that surrounds most tendons. Within the paratenon are type I and type III collagen as well as elastin fibrils, with its inner surface lined by synovial cells (Williams 1986). The *epitenon* is a fine connective tissue sheath found under and contiguous with the paratenon on its outer surface as well as the *endotenon* in its inner surface (see Figures 3-6 to 3-8). The endotenon (Figure 3-9) invests the tendon fibers and acts to bind individual fibers, and in larger units, fiber bundles together (Jozsa et al. 1991). High levels of hydroxylated PG components are found between the endotenon and the tendon fascicle surfaces that permit both the binding of individual fibers and the fiber groups to glide on each other (Rowe 1985). Blood vessels, nerves and lymphatics are carried within the endotenon network to invest in the deep tendon (Figures 3-10 to 3-12).

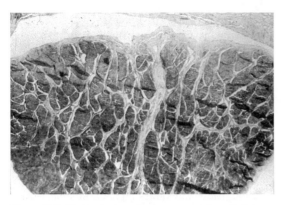

Figure 3-9. Photomicrograph of a cross section of a human flexor tendon showing the connective tissue (endotenon) that surrounds the fascicles of the tendon (*H* and *E*, magnification X25). (From Woo SL-Y et al. Anatomy, Biology and Biomechanics of Tendon, Ligament, and Meniscus. In SR Simon. Orthopaedic Basic Science. Rosemont, Ill: American Academy of Orthopaedic Surgeons, 1994;50.)

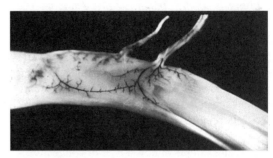

Figure 3-11. India ink injected specimen illustrating the vascular supply of the flexor digitorum profundus in a human through the vinculum longus. (From Woo SL-Y et al. Anatomy, Biology and Biomechanics of Tendon, Ligament, and Meniscus. In SR Simon. Orthopaedic Basic Science. Rosemont, Ill: American Academy of Orthopaedic Surgeons, 1994;51.)

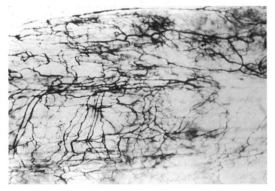

Figure 3-10. India ink injected (Spalteholz technique) calcaneal tendon of a rabbit, illustrating the vasculature of a paratenon-covered tendon. Vessels enter from many points on the periphery and anastomose with a longitudinal system of capillaries. (From Woo SL-Y et al. Anatomy, Biology and Biomechanics of Tendon, Ligament, and Meniscus. In SR Simon. Orthopaedic Basic Science. Rosemont, Ill: American Academy of Orthopaedic Surgeons, 1994;50.)

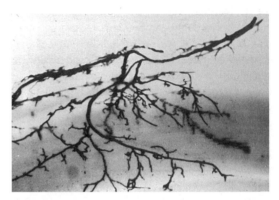

Figure 3-12. Close-up of specimen (Spalteholz technique) showing the extent of the blood supply from the vinculum longus. The vessels in the vinculum divide into the dorsal, proximal, and distal branches, giving off vertical vascular loops into the tendon substance. (From Woo SL-Y et al. Anatomy, Biology and Biomechanics of Tendon, Ligament, and Meniscus. In SR Simon. Orthopaedic Basic Science. Rosemont, Ill: American Academy of Orthopaedic Surgeons, 1994;51.)

Biomechanical Properties

Tendons are characterized by their ability to resist lengthwise pulling forces. Tendons are tough structures and are thus able to sustain significant stresses. They allow high tensile forces to be generated through muscle. Within tendon, collagen fibrils are closely packed, oriented roughly in parallel along their length to impart resistance to high, uniaxial tensile forces typically sustained by these structures. An understanding of the structure, function, and properties of normal tendon in biomechanical and biochemical terms is essential for a discussion of tendon injury and comprehension of both invasive and noninvasive repair processes.

Connective Tissue Adaptation to Mechanical Stress: The Association between Ultrastructure and Biomechanical Requirements of Tendon

A positive effect exists of physical strain on maintaining the integrity of tendon tissue; however, less is known about how mechanical strain specifically affects tendon cells (Zeichen et al. 2000). Tendon regions subjected almost exclusively to tension differ from regions subjected to high levels of compression in addition to tension (Mehr et al. 2000). This is an example of how a type of connective tissue adapts to specific mechanical stresses imposed on it when subjected to a variety of loading conditions. The majority of regions within tendon consist of spindle-shaped fibroblasts surrounded by densely packed, longitudinally oriented type I collagen fibrils and are represented in regions of the tendon exposed almost exclusively to tensile loading (Gelberman et al. 1988). In contrast, and as discussed before, fibrocartilaginous tissue of tendon that is typical of regions of tendon subjected to repeated compression presents with spherical cells surrounded by matrix containing hyaline cartilage proteoglycans (aggrecan) and both types I and II collagen (Giori et al. 1993). The presence of tenascin-C, an antiadhesive protein, is considered an important cellular adaptation to compressive forces imposed upon tendon that help to establish and maintain fibrocartilagenous regions by decreasing cell-matrix adhesion.

The primary function of tendons is to transmit muscle force to the skeletal system while allowing limited elongation. Where tendons wrap around bony pulleys, they must be able to withstand compression and shear in addition to tension. Tendons possess one of the highest tensile strengths of all the soft tissues in the body because collagen is the strongest fibrous protein and also because these fibers are arranged longitudinally as well as transversely and horizontally (see Figure 3-3) forming spirals and plaits (Jozsa et al. 1991). The arrangement of collagen fibers within tendon enables tensile forces as well as rotational forces to be accommodated during motion and general activity. Therefore the internal arrangement of collagen fibers is related to optimal transmission of forces of the muscle contractions via increasing the tensile strength of the tendon as well as is associated with specific anatomic points along the tendon (Kannus 2000).

Most biomechanical studies of tendon have focused on its ultimate tensile strength and strain properties. While the stress-strain relationship in the tendon is generally similar to that of other collagen-based soft tissues such as ligaments (see Figure 3-19) and skin, each structure maintains its own inherent material properties. For both tendons and ligaments, factors such as age, species, and type of structure contribute to differences in reported ultimate strain values (Woo et al. 1982). Such factors contribute, in addition to different test environments, to the divergent ultimate strain values reported in tendon ranging from 9% to more than 30%, while that reported for ligaments ranges from 12% to more than 50% (Abrahams 1967; Kennedy et al. 1976; Woo et al. 1979). The ultimate stress and strain values of digital flexor tendons demonstrated that they were much stiffer (3% to 4% strain) and stronger than their compensatory extensor tendon with the ultimate tensile strength for the flexor tendons measured at twice that of the extensors (Woo et al. 1982). The digital flexors notably have much higher collagen concentration (29%) per wet weight of tissue than that of the digital extensors (23%) (Woo et al. 1981).

Crimp

The phenomenon of *crimp*, which is a wavy formation of the collagen fibers, exists within or between fascicles (Figure 3-7). The crimp angle may vary from between 0° to 60° and is considered attributable to the varying contribution of the proteoglycans and collagen cross-linking (Jozsa and Kannus 1997; Rowe 1985). The crimped configuration disappears if the tendon is stretched slightly and is the result of straightening of the collagen fibers (Elliot 1965). If the tension is applied to result in less than 4% elongation and is subsequently released, the normal wavy appearance of the tendon is regained. The presence of elastic fibers also is believed to contribute to the recovery of the wavy configuration of the collagen fibers after tendinous stretch (Butler et al. 1978). During normal physiologic movements, the elongation of the tendon functions within this limit of 4% strain. However, once this limit of 4% elongation is exceeded the wavy crimped form is dissolved; if the stress results in an elongation of original tendon length greater than 8%, the tendon typically will rupture (Jozsa and Kannus 1997). The ultimate strain values for tendons is considered to range from 8% to 13% (Woo 1982).

Effects of Mechanical Loading on Tendon: Cellular Mechanisms

Fibroblasts respond to different stresses, such as tension and compression, by mechanisms not fully known. Cellular responses to loading include cytoskeletal remodeling and altered ion transport (Bershadsky et al. 1980) as well as diminished cell-matrix adhesion by creating conditions that influence the properties of cell-surface matrix receptors and integrins (Banes et al. 1995). For instance, tenascin-C, an anti-adhesive protein, was shown to play a physiologic role in the tendon by inhibiting cell-matrix binding in regions of tendon subjected to compression (Mehr et al. 2000).

Reduced strain stimulus leads to a rapid loss of cross-sectional area, modulus and strength of both tendon and ligament (Wren et al. 2000). When loading is restored through remobilization, the strain stimulus is elevated and the properties rapidly recover as the immobilization effects are reversed. Similar changes occur in immature animals; however, the difference between immature and mature animals can be attributed to baseline biologic growth that occurs independently from mechanical loading. Overall, the mechanical properties of tendons and ligaments are determined by microstructural parameters including collagen fiber content, fiber orientations, and cross-link density (Wren and Carter 1998). Fibroblasts change these parameters through altered biosynthetic activity stimulated by mechanical loading. Cyclic tensile strains stimulate an up regulation of type I collagen production (Sutker et al. 1990) and alignment of the collagen fibers in directions of principle tensile strain (Harris et al. 1981; Nakatsuji and Johnson 1984). Once loading is removed, degradation of the extracellular matrix (Aggeler et al. 1984) ensues and collagen fiber alignment becomes disrupted (Hayashi 1996) and inappropriate cross-linking may be effected (Harwood and Amiel 1992).

Overuse Injury

Tendons are vulnerable to mechanical overload or overuse from repetitive trauma. The most common site of injury is at the Achilles tendon (Orava et al. 1991). Injuries attributed to the overuse of tendons increase with age. Researchers have suggested that this may correlate with increased hypovascularity of the tendon. One study demonstrated, however, that the peritendinous blood flow to the zone of the tendon that sustains the highest incidence of injury from overuse is unaltered by age during exercise, indicating that factors other than blood flow are important for the increased incidence with age of injuries from overuse (Langberg et al. 2001).

Healing and Repair in Tendon Injury

An understanding of structure and function of components of tendon tissue is essential to the comprehension of mechanisms underlying the basis of healing and repair processes involved after injury. The tendon healing process can be divided into inflammatory, fibroblastic/proliferative, and remodeling/organizational stages. Injured and surgically repaired tendons heal via the formation of scar tissue, a process referred to as *fibrosis*. This event, while an essential part of the healthy healing process also can represent an unpredictable factor that when uncontrolled, contributes to morbidity, particularly after surgery or injury. Dense adhesions may be produced that act to limit, if not prevent, joint excursion. This presentation is most evident in the region of the synovial flexor sheaths (Potenza 1962; Strickland 1986). Potenza (1962) originally theorized that the tendon proper possesses no powers of regeneration and the ingrowth of granulation tissue from within the synovial sheath represents the healing process. However, authorities currently believe that the intrinsic tendon cells, in fact, have the capacity to proliferate and to heal via intra-tendinous processes (DeKlerk and Jonck 1991). A high proliferation of both synovial cells and an initial but much lower rate of activity of intrinsic tendon cells appear to have a direct bearing on the end result of the repair process after injury (DeKlerk and Jonck, 1991). In an attempt to achieve early and better functional outcome, protected mobilization after surgery is advocated as well as specific approaches to suture techniques (Messina 1992). Certain cases, such as the management of severed flexor tendons within the digital sheath, continue to present a challenge in that dense adhesions form

Clinical Note

Tendinopathy

The Achilles tendon is vulnerable to overuse injuries that are commonly associated with physical activities such as running and jumping (Kvist 1994). The clinical presentation is characterized by pain, edema that may be localized or diffuse in nature, and an impairment of physical performance. In the acute phase of Achilles tendinopathy, the tendon is diffusely swollen and edematous, and the middle third of the tendon is typically tender to palpation (Paavola et al. 2000). Pain and stiffness present upon mobilization in the morning with a progressive decrease in these symptoms as, for instance, a runner warms up (Leach et al. 1981). While no significant restriction may occur in normal activities of daily living, an athlete may report pain-induced limitation in sports and related activities that persist as the condition becomes chronic (Paavola et al. 2000). Chronic Achilles tendinosis is a condition with an unknown etiology and pathogenesis that is often, but not always, associated with pain during loading of the Achilles tendon (Alfredson and Lorentzon 2000). Chronic Achilles tendinopathy is characterized by decreased swelling, persistent exercise-induced pain that may become constant with walking, and the frequent presentation of tender nodules and thickening of the tissues surrounding the tendon (Kvist 1991). Histologically, no inflammatory cells are present, but increased amounts of interfibrillar glycosaminoglycans and changes in the collagen fiber structure and arrangement may be seen (Alfredson and Lorentzon 2000). Management of Achilles tendinopathy includes restriction of activity (Kvist and Kvist, 1980), cryotherapy (Clement et al. 1984), nonsteroidal anti-inflammatory drugs (Clement et al. 1984), intravenous injections of heparin (Larsen et al. 1987), local corticosteroid injection (Kvist and Kvist 1980), heel lifts and orthoses (Clement et al. 1984), and physical therapy/exercise to improve strength and flexibility (Kellett 1986). Judicious use of locally injected (peritendinous) corticosteroid (limited to 1-3 injections) is currently employed in the management of acute tendinopathy for rapid pain relief and anti-inflammatory effect enabling quick return to strenuous physical activity (Leadbetter 1995). Eccentric strengthening programs have been reported to help resolve chronic tendinitis affecting the Achilles tendon (Alfredson et al. 1998). Surgical intervention may be advised for individuals with chronic Achilles tendinopathy and in whom conservative management has been unsuccessful (Kvist 1994). In an 8-year follow-up of individuals with acute or subchronic (duration of symptoms before initiation of treatment less than 6 months) Achilles tendinopathy, the long-term prognosis of patients (in whom 29% had to be operated upon during the follow-up period), regardless of management strategy, was reported as favorable (94% subjects were asymptomatic) as determined by subjective and functional assessments (Paavola et al. 2000). Furthermore, 41% of these subjects experienced overuse symptoms (exertional pain with or without swelling and stiffness) in the initially uninvolved Achilles tendon (Paavola et al. 2000).

Traditional theory would hold that pain in tendinopathy arises through one of two mechanisms: inflammation in tendinitis or separation of collagen fibers in more severe forms of tendinopathy. The latter may resemble the pain incurred in association with collagen separation after an acute grade I or II ligament injury (Khan et al. 2000). Histopathologic examination of surgical specimens from patients with chronic tendon pain arising at the Achilles, patellar, lateral elbow, medial elbow, and rotator cuff tendons demonstrated the absence of inflammatory cells (Khan et al. 1999). Furthermore, prostaglandin E2, an indicator of inflammation, is not elevated in patients with Achilles tendon pain beyond that of normal controls (Alfredson 1999). However, nociceptors provide significant afferent pain pathways and in sites, such as the knee, are located in the retinaculum, fat pad, synovium, and periosteum (Witonski and Wagrowska-Danielewicz 1999). Secondly, biochemical irritants may include extravasation of glycosamines, including chondroitin sulphate, that may be released from damaged tendon (Witonski and Wagrowska-Danielewicz 1999). Therefore support exists for a biochemical cause of pain in tendinopathy. Treatment efforts at resolving the pain associated with this condition might be improved by addressing the biochemical milieu rather than focusing on the reduction of inflammation or augmenting collagen repair (Khan et al. 2000).

between the tendon and the sheath and ultimately impede restoration of normal range of movement (DeKlerk and Jonck, 1991).

Mechanism of Scar Tissue Formation

The clinician must appreciate how scar tissue is both initiated and perpetuated. An important fundamental characteristic of connective tissue is demonstrated during its repair after injury. Fibroplasia is one component of scar formation with other aspects involving a degree of matrix contraction and reorganization (Bell et al. 1979). Scar formation in tissues that do not inherently have significant regenerative capacity (e.g., cartilage) also occurs by stimulation of undifferentiated mesenchymal cells that ultimately replace tissue defects with fibrous connective tissue. Recent efforts have tried to improve tendon healing by extrinsic means, including specific growth factor (known to induce bone and cartilage) injection into sites of injured tendon (Forslund and Aspenberg, 2001). Simultaneous mechanical stimulation via loading was noted to be of great importance for tissue differentiation and tendon repair in the growth factor injected group inducing a strong tendon-like tissue instead of bone or cartilage (Forslund and Aspenberg 2001).

Basic Principles

A sequence of cellular and biochemical events occurs during the repair of dense connective tissues that is essential knowledge for the physical therapist. For instance, an understanding of the pathophysiology underlying scar tissue formation is necessary for optimal clinical management of fibrotic adhesions. The understanding of scar tissue composition and dynamics is vital to appreciate and predict its response to physical management as well as to guide its maturation and resolution.

Stage 1: Inflammation (1 to 4 days)

General. Inflammation is a local defense reaction made by an organism in response to a noxious (harmful) event. Insulting agents to the organism include chemically irritating compounds, micro-

organisms such as foreign bacteria, and physical trauma causing disruption to the tissue (Box 3-1).

A sequence of cellular and biologic events occurs after injury to and during the repair of dense connective tissue. In addition to the tenoblasts (fibroblasts), tenocytes, chondrocytes, synovial cells, and vascular cells that are native to tendon, inflammatory cells, macrophages, and myofibroblasts are hallmark cells present in pathologic conditions affecting tendon tissue (Jozsa and Kannus 1997). The development of fibrosis usually is preceded by an accumulation of inflammatory cells within a tissue. Cells mediating inflammation, such as the activated macrophage, stimulate the migration of fibroblasts into the area of insult, ultimately resulting in an increase in collagen synthesis.

The Fibroblast. The fibroblast is considered the culprit cell around which the cascade of events involved in scar tissue formation revolves. The fibroblast is a component of all connective tissues and while it may assume a different form across these diverse tissues it has the common quality of being able to form and re-organize structural proteins to varying extent and degrees depending on the site (Couchman et al. 1983). Once an insult has occurred to a tissue, the wound space fills with blood products, which form a clot almost immediately. The first line of defence is provided by leukocytes and macrophages. Only after a period of at least 48 hours do fibroblasts become active in collagen production. The fibroblast, as the cell central to scar tissue formation processes, not only is known to proliferate in response to a given stimulus but also degrades and disorganizes the extracellular matrix (Khan et al. 1998). In the uninjured state, fibroblasts are typically metabolically quiescent; however, once a stimulus is received, proliferation of local and recruited fibroblasts may occur that ultimately results in cell migration, division, and ECM synthesis and remodeling

Box 3-1. General Principles of Inflammation

Acute vs. Chronic Inflammation

- Trauma → acute inflammation
- Trauma → inflammation > 2 weeks = chronic inflammation

(Morgan and Pledger 1992). Enzymes released that act to degrade and ultimately re-organize the ECM are referred to as matrix metalloproteinases (Hembry et al. 1985). Growth regulatory factors (e.g., TGF-β1, EGF, IGF-1, b-FGF) are evident in the wounded-tissue environment, all having far-reaching effects on fibroblast cell behavior in terms of extent of stimulation of both cell proliferation and matrix reorganization (Roberts and Sporn 1993). Both TGF-β1 and EGF are known to induce fibroblast matrix production, and b-FGF is regarded as a potent neovascular agent (Folkman and Klagsburn 1987). The establishment of a significant population of fibroblasts requires two to three days, and the peak of collagen production and deposition occurs only after this period of cellular recruitment and activation. During the first few days of wound healing, the scar has no significant extracellular matrix with collagen fibers to provide strength and stability. At this stage, the fragile scar tissues are held together predominantly by intercellular attachments and the formation of fibroblast-reticulin networks (Tillman and Cummings 1992).

The source and extent of fibroblast involvement from synovial sheath or fibro-osseous sheath (extrinsic) compared to endotenonon tendon core (intrinsic) in scar tissue response after tendon injury was investigated in one study (Khan et al. 1998). Traditionally, the formation of dense adhesions and scar tissue has been reported to be more extensive when the injury is in the vicinity of fibro-osseous sheaths (Potenza 1962); however, excessive removal of the sheath in the management of tendon lacerations does not appear to lead to better functional results (Peterson et al. 1990). Researchers have determined that fibroblasts from both the epitenon

(Manske and Lesker 1984), and endotenon (Khan et al. 1998) play a role in the biology of healing tendon; however, the synovial (fibro-osseous) sheath appears to be the most potentially liable source of very reactive and aggressive fibroblasts and contributes to an even greater extent in terms of matrix production, contraction, and reorganization of scar (Khan et al. 1998). The delivery of mesenchymal stem-cell organized collagen implants to a large (Achilles) tendon gap defect in an animal model also has been shown to improve tendon biomechanics and structure when compared to controls at all points across a three-month period (Young et al. 2000).

Stage 2: Proliferation/Fibroplasia: The Growth Phase of Scar (Days 5-21)

Scar tissue rapidly increases in bulk within 21 days, which is a process known as *fibroplasia*. The fibroplastic phase typically spans a 3- to 4-week period. As the scar tissue enters the fibroplastic stage, its composition becomes altered. Collagen first appears around day 4 or 5. Until approximately day 21 of this stage, the quantity of collagen present increases (Figure 3-13). A parallel exists between the size of the scar and the quantity of collagen, implying that the percentage of collagen remains relatively constant through this period. Hence simultaneous collagen degradation occurs during this period, resulting in large amounts of collagen remodeling. Lysis of some fibers, aggregation of new fibers, and increases in the size of other fibers occur. The hallmark of the fibroplastic stage is intensive collagen synthesis and degradation during which significant architectural changes occur, and the fibers attach and align themselves. Initially the fibers are small and ran-

---

Clinical Note

The Inflammatory Phase:

Implications for Clinical Practice

This stage of healing is highly cellular and is characterized by the presence of extremely fragile scar tissue. Any efforts to stretch the repair tissue will cause elongation of the scar with the following results:
   Negative: potential exists for disruption in cell membranes leading to cell death of essential connective tissue forming cells if the structure is moved too abruptly (e.g., high or sudden loading)
   Positive: gentle inner range movement promotes cell migration in response to protected loading

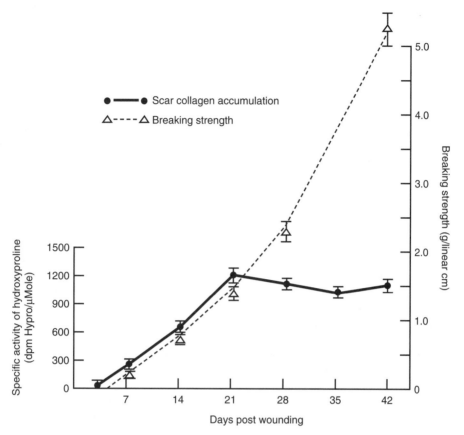

Figure 3-13. Comparison of scar collagen accumulation and breaking strength of wounds. (From Levenson SM et al. The healing of rat skin wounds. Ann Surg 1965;161:293.)

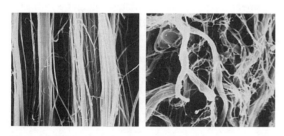

Figure 3-14. Normal ligament (left) and healing scar at 2 weeks (right) (magnification X7000). (From Andriacchi T et al. Ligament: Injury and Repair. In SLY Woo, JA Buckwalter (eds), Injury and Repair of the Musculoskeletal Soft Tissues. Rosemont, Ill: American Academy of Orthopaedic Surgeons, 1988;112.)

domly aligned (Figure 3-14). In time, larger bundles of fibers are formed, alignment becomes more parallel, and spaces appear between them.

Inflammatory cells gradually disappear, with fibroblasts becoming the predominant cell from approximately day 5 onward. *Myofibroblasts* constitute the bulk of the cells observed at the peak of fibroplasia, along with other fibroblasts. Fibroblasts are responsible for remodeling without shrinkage, whereas myofibroblasts can cause scar tissue shrinkage. Diminishing levels of myofibroblasts mark the termination of the contraction phase and beginning of the maturation phase.

Clinical Implications: Treatment to increase range of motion and function of a joint can be very effective at this stage because of the opportunity to modify the outcome of the intense collagen remodeling processes. The application of appropriate physical movement during this phase makes a difference in the ultimate tissue healing process outcome.

Scar Tissue Contraction and Shrinkage. Once scar tissue has formed, it begins to shrink within five days. This shrinking is an active process in which the scar develops significant centripetal forces, allowing the wound edges to be pulled together. It is the actual contraction of the myofibroblasts that arrive at the scar site during the 5-21 day period that causes the shrinkage. The myofibroblasts appear to cling on to one another and the fibrillar structures in the extracellular matrix, so that the individual contraction of each cell is transmitted to the tissue as a whole. In untreated, newly formed scar, normal contraction will occur for about 3 weeks. In some cases, this prolonged shrinkage results in the development of a very large, tense scar referred to as *keloid*.

Stage 3: Remodelling/Consolidation Phase (Days 21-60)

A scar will stop increasing in size at about 21 days, providing normal healing has ensued. Scar tissue shrinkage diminishes rapidly and myofibroblasts disappear, leaving behind a predominant population of fibroblasts. During the consolidation phase, the tissue changes from a predominantly cellular tissue to a less cellular fibrous tissue, with collagen constituting the bulk of fibers embedded in the proteoglycan/GAG matrix. The vascularity of the scar diminishes. Even though there is a reduction in cellular number, the fibroblasts are very active, exerting change in the shape of the scar. The collagen turnover rate continues to be elevated concurrently with architectural restructuring of the collagen network. Thus the tissue has gradually evolved from being cellular to fibrous, with a well established representation of collagen fibers in the matrix.

The Maturation Phase (Days 60-360)

The connective tissue cell population gradually diminishes after day 60. Collagen turnover remains high until around day 120 then gradually declines. New collagen has replaced about 85% of the original collagen by about day 150 post-injury. The collagen fibers are compact and large, and the scar is relatively devoid of cells and blood vessels (Tillman and Cummings 1992).

   Clinical Implications: The response to physical treatment is poor at this stage. In fact, hypertrophic and keloid scar tissue can respond in a negative manner when stretched at this point.

Effect of Loading on Scar Tissue Repair

As with other connective tissue structures, the mechanical environment to which tendon is exposed is important for the understanding of the mechanism and extent of injury as well as for consideration of repair during a rehabilitation regimen. Mechanical tension and forces of compression play an integral role in scar tissue remodeling processes. Early controlled motion and loading of tendon and ligament repair tissue stimulates collagen synthesis, increases strength and helps align the repair cells

---

Clinical Note

Consolidation Phase:

Implications for Clinical Practice

Because some remodeling activity is still happening, this period remains responsive to physical management. During the first three weeks of wound healing, scar tissue can increase in strength as a result of the increasing bulk of collagen deposited. The breaking strength of the scar tissue is related to the volume of collagen. Subsequent to the first three-week period is another 3-week period during which a high rate of collagen turnover occurs in the newly formed scar. Because of an active remodeling process in which old collagen is degraded and absorbed, the actual volume of scar becomes *less* than predicted. An increase in the strength of the scar occurs during this period without a concurrent increase in scar volume (see Figure 3-13). Finally, collagen bonding becomes more prevalent and more stable with maturation of newly formed collagen fibers, providing a chemical basis for the measurable increase in scar strength. The breaking strength of the scar is therefore related to the increased intermolecular cross-linking pattern ensuring the collagen volume is stabilized.

and collagen fibers whereas lack of tension leaves the repair tissue cells and matrix disoriented (Gelberman et al. 1982; Vailas et al. 1981; and Woo et al. 1982). Immobilization and tension deprivation of ruptured Achilles tendons result in decreased proliferation of connective tissue containing collagen fibers and appear to significantly retard the healing processes (Yasuda et al. 2000). Immobilization negatively affects the ultrastructure (Enwemeka 1991), biochemistry (Kannus et al. 1992) and ultimate strength of the tendon (Murrell et al. 1994). Response to tendon injury has been observed using animal models where (partial) tenotomies have been subjected to either loaded or unloaded conditions (Iwuagwu and McGrouther 1998). In this study, quantitative cell counts were performed on light microscopic cross-sections of tendon substance taken at the tenotomy window recording cell orientation during the acute (days 1, 3, 5, and 7) stages after injury. Loaded tendons demonstrated less cellularity at five days with better longitudinal orientation of cells and matrix than unloaded tendons. While inflammatory cells predominated in early stages (days 1-3), fibroblasts predominated at days 3-7. A low fibroblast count with more matrix interspersed between them in loaded injured tendons suggested a low cell to matrix ratio where fewer fibroblasts were required to produce more matrix relative to the unloaded tendon (Iguagwu and McGrouther 1998). Greater tensile loading appeared to increase collagen matrix earlier. A low cell/matrix ratio at this stage could be interpreted as the result of more effective fibroblast function supporting the need to load tendons early after injury and during initial stages of repair. At days 5-7, the orientation of the fibroblasts and the collagen fibrils in the loaded windows became less random compared with alignment of these cells along the longitudinal axis of the tendon in unloaded windows (Iguagwu and McGrouther 1998).

Mechanical loading and early motion are currently regarded as particularly important in regaining mechanical properties of injured tendon during the healing process. Hence the focus of current clinical research is on the use of early active motion with the intent to minimize adhesions and limit joint stiffness (Elliot et al. 1994; Messina 1992). After surgical repair of the Achilles tendon, functional ankle casting that allowed some degree of movement after injury (allowing 0-20 degrees of plantar flexion) was shown to be of greater benefit in terms of biomechanical parameters than traditional rigid casting (Stehno-Bittel et al. 1998). However, few investigations reveal the mechanism underlying the actual repair process after acute tendon injury. As identified before, the exact mechanism of healing or cellular response of tendon to injury has been controversial (Gelberman et al. 1988; Potenza 1962) and the two concepts, extrinsic and intrinsic, have been considered based on experiments performed on intrasynovial flexor tendons. The extrinsic theory observes the tendon tissue as being fairly inert and considers the adhesions from the flexor sheath to the tendon wound contribute extensively to the repair process (Potenza 1962). The intrinsic theory observes the tendon cells as being capable of replicating and healing tendon injuries. Researchers have suggested that the intrinsic/extrinsic theories may not be exclusive repair processes and that local conditions such as the presence or absence of a synovial sheath may determine which process is utilized (Gelberman et al. 1988). Several studies support that loading (tension) and motion enhance and stimulate the intrinsic healing response of flexor tendons (Kubota et al. 1996), however extensor tendons may differ in their cellular response to injury (Seiler et al. 1993).

The literature indicates that more investigational studies of normal tendons and the effects of age, immobilization, and recovery following injury are required. For instance, the effects of post-repair rehabilitation modalities, such as the dose-response curve for the use of controlled passive motion, or the effect of dynamic splints on the eventual outcome of tendon healing, remain unmeasured.

Changes across the Lifespan: Tendon and Ligament

Growth and Maturation

Developing tendons contain more fibroblasts than the tendons of older animals. These fibroblasts are also very active, and a high rate of synthesis of collagen exists in young animals. Across the lifespan, tendons undergoing repair and regrowth after an injury also demonstrate a relative increase in numbers and activity of fibroblasts.

Clinical Note

Effects of Aging on Tendon and Ligament

Age-related changes may be associated with degenerative changes in the dense nonmineralized fibrous connective tissues such as tendons, ligaments and joint capsules. In fact, significant impairment may result from age-related changes in these dense fibrous connective tissues. Injuries that may occur as a result of these changes include low-energy or spontaneous ruptures of these structures as may be seen in rotator cuff injuries of the shoulder (Brewer 1979), the long head of biceps (Burkhead 1990), the posterior tibial tendon (Noyes and Grood 1976), patellar and Achilles tendons (Hattrup and Johnson 1985) and sprains of joint capsules and ligaments (Woo et al. 1986).

Complaints of aches or soreness in older persons after physical activity may be, in part, attributed to injuries to fibrous components of the muscle-tendon junctions or of tendon, ligament and joint-capsule insertions into bone; these complaints appear similar to the chronic musculoskeletal pain arising from overuse syndromes affecting the same sites (Buckwalter et al. 1993).

A clinical paradox exists in that decreasing levels of vigorous physical activity with increasing age may prevent some injuries to the dense fibrous tissues; however, any decline in physical activity also may have a negative effect on tissue composition and strength. Involvement in lifelong physical activity is clearly important to the health of the musculoskeletal tissues. Clinical interventions in the form of preventive and education programs that display an awareness of lifespan changes in the musculoskeletel system have the potential to modify age-related changes and ultimately impact upon quality of life.

Age-Related Changes

Histologic evidence exists of degenerative change in tendons with increasing age (Kannus and Jozsa 1991). Cellular changes include the flattening and elongation of fibroblasts with attrition of their rough endoplasmic reticulum and Golgi membranes with age (Amiel et al. 1991). In addition to the age-related changes in cell function and morphology, matrix composition and internal organization also have been considered a cause in the decline in mechanical properties seen in the dense connective tissues. Reports, both quantitative (Moore and DeBeaux 1987) and qualitative (Squier and Magnes 1983) indicate that with increased age the tenoblast volume density drops, whereas the relative collagen fiber density increases.

Progressive cross-linking of human tendon collagen has been demonstrated with increased age (Fujimoto 1984). Biochemical analyses have shown that in both tendon and ligaments, collagen and water concentration of the dense fibrous tissues decline with age as the number of reducible collagen cross-links decreases and nonreducible cross-links increases (Amiel et al., 1991). In some animal model studies, alignment of the collagen fibrils and organization of the fiber bundles appear to deteriorate with increasing age (Amiel et al. 1991). Collagen fiber diameter in ligament and tendon increases with age. In locations such as the rotator cuff, the nutrition of dense fibrous tissue cells may decline as a result of decreased vascular perfusion that ultimately leads to tissue degeneration and decrease in tissue strength (Brewer 1979; Lohr and Uhthoff 1990) leading to ultimate impairment at this site.

Ligament: Specific Characteristics

Ligaments are organized structures made of dense regular fibrous connective tissue that physically act to stabilize joints. Specifically, ligaments resist forces of elongation to restrict joint mobility. In addition, ligaments play a role in joint proprioception in that different fibers of the ligament may be recruited according to the position of the joint (Sakane et al., 1996) and when forces to the ligament are increased, more fibers are recruited (Hildebrand and Frank 1998a). Ligaments, for the most part, share a similar structure to tendons with the architecture of ligaments presenting between that of capsules and tendons. In this way, collagen fiber bundles found in ligaments, albeit arranged longitudinally from insertion site to insertion site, may not be as parallel as are found in tendon

(Figures 3-15 and 3-16). This arrangement reflects that while ligaments typically sustain tensile loads in one main direction they also may bear relatively smaller tensile loading in other directions. The integrity of ligaments thus relies upon the independent characteristics of the collagen bundles.

Ultrastructure

Generally, ligaments consist of predominantly water (70%), collagen (25%), proteoglycans and other non-collagenous components (4%), and cells

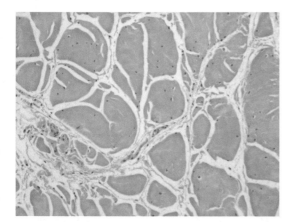

Figure 3-15. Transverse section through the dorsal radial ligament at the trapeziometacarpal joint (magnification X10). (Courtesy Maksim Kovler, BSc[PT], MSc, Toronto, Canada.)

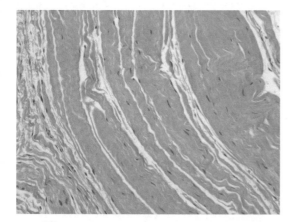

Figure 3-16. Longitudinal section through the dorsal radial ligament at the trapeziometacarpal joint (magnification X10). (Courtesy Maksim Kovler, BSc[PT], MSc, Toronto, Canada.)

(1%), with the proportion of these components depending on the nature and location of the ligament (Figure 3-17). Most ligaments are composed of collagen types I and III, with small proportions of glycosaminoglycans, elastin, actin, and fibronectin (Figure 3-18). Similar to tendon, an important structural feature of ligaments is a periodic wave of collagen known as its *crimp*. Crimp is believed to contribute to the nonlinear mechanical properties of ligament substance. Researchers have suggested that this crimp in collagen arrangement results in a certain degree of elasticity. This allows ligaments to accommodate for large internal stresses during normal joint motion.

Vascular and Nerve Supply

A vascular network and nerve supply is found in the outer (epiligament) layer of ligaments, with these neurovascular units piercing the ligament in a longitudinal fashion (Bray et al. 1996). Ligaments contribute greatly to the neurophysiologic function of joints as they contain receptors that may play a role in the "ligamentomuscular reflex loop" critical to joint proprioception (Frank et al. 1994).

Biomechanical Properties of Ligaments

Skeletal ligaments are highly specialized dynamic dense connective tissues that connect bones, stabilize and guide joint motion. The ligaments of the knee joint, for instance, maintain joint stability by resisting tensile forces that would otherwise result in joint separation, as well as preserve compressive loads that maximize congruity among bones and cartilage in the joint (Hsieh et al. 2000). The mechanical behavior of ligaments is similar to that of other nonlinear viscoelastic soft tissues but with adaptations that allow joints to be flexible yet stable. In the spinal column, the ligaments are required to be somewhat elastic in nature and while collagen is the major extracellular fiber of most ligaments, these ligaments of the spinal column contain mainly elastic fibers and relatively fewer collagen fibers. Factors known to have a major influence on the structural and mechanical properties of ligaments and their insertions are age and stress. During routine activity, length changes in

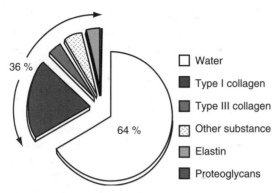

36 %

64 %

- □ Water
- ■ Type I collagen
- ■ Type III collagen
- ▨ Other substance
- ▧ Elastin
- ■ Proteoglycans

Figure 3-17. Approximate biochemical composition of a rabbit ligament. (From Frank C et al. Normal Ligament: Structure, Function, and Composition. In SL-Y Woo, JA Buckwalter (eds), Injury and Repair of the Musculoskeletal Soft Tissues. Rosemont, Ill: (American Academy of Orthopaedic Surgeons, 1988;86.)

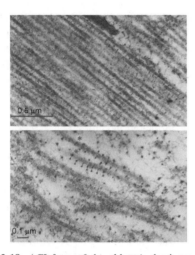

0.5 μm

0.1 μm

Figure 3-18. ACL from a 6-day old rat (ruthenium red). *Top,* Regular interfiber linking filaments (magnification X69,000). *Bottom,* relationship of proteoglycan granules to collagen fibers. A regular association can be seen in the two marked fibers (**). Granules are associated with the C and D bands of the collagen fibers (magnification X103,500). (From Frank C et al. Normal Ligament: Structure, Function, and Composition. In SL-Y Woo, JA Buckwalter (eds), Injury and Repair of the Musculoskeletal Soft Tissues. Rosemont, Ill: American Academy of Orthopaedic Surgeons, 1988;71.)

the ligamentous tissue occur in response to mechanical stresses. As with the other dense connective tissues, the geometric configuration of the constituent collagen fibers and the interaction of collagen fibers with noncollagenous tissue components in ligaments provide the basis of their mechanical behavior (Figure 3-19). Biomechanical

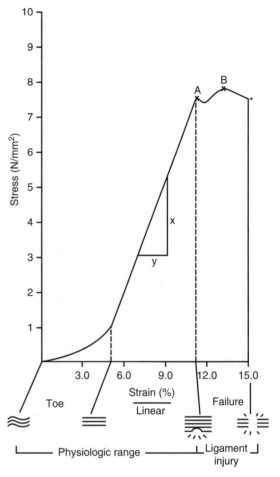

Figure 3-19. Normal stress-strain curve for ligament illustrating toe, elastic and plastic regions. (From Binkley J. Overview of ligament and tendon structure and mechanics: Implications for clinical practice. Physiother Canada 1989;41(1):24-30.)

studies that quantified strains in the anterior cruciate ligament (ACL) and medial collateral ligament (MCL) have shown that these ligaments are routinely subjected to 4% to 5% strains during normal activities and can be strained to as much as 7.7% during external application of loads to the knee joint (Hollis et al. 1991).

Ligaments are often too short to be tested in isolation when seeking information on their individual biomechanical properties (Woo et al. 1982). In addition, because of the complex geometry of ligaments such as the ACL, it is impossible to load all the fiber bundles uniformly during a uniaxial tensile test (Buckwalter et al. 1993; Woo et al. 1991).

The study of tensile testing of the femur-ACL-tibia complex (FATC) has identified two important factors that influence the structural properties of the human FATC: specimen age and orientation (Woo et al. 1991). Testing the FATC along the anatomical axis of the ACL, while maintaining its anatomical angles of insertion to the femur and tibia, allows a greater portion of the ACL to be loaded during tensile testing as opposed to specimens tested in the tibial orientation (tibia aligned vertically). A higher percentage of ligament substance failures occur for the FATCs tested in the anatomical orientation, whereas when FATCs were tested in the tibial orientation a higher incidence of insertion site failures occurred (Woo et al. 1991). Therefore the bone-ligament-bone complex model often is used to give biomechanical information about the tensile properties of the entire structural unit during structural failure tests (Hildebrand and Frank 1998a). However, tensile testing of the ligament may also be examined at stresses (tensile forces) below whole structure failure. These tests are known as stress-relaxation tests (see Chapter 6) where the ligament is elongated and held under a constant stress; the decline in stress over time and the increase in length (creep) with time is evaluated. Ligaments, through application of loading therefore are capable of adjustment in length because of their inherent viscoelastic behavior.

Immobilization and Mechanical Stimulation in the Uninjured Ligament

Many animal models have been developed to examine the biologic effects of mechanical stresses and lack thereof on ligament health. Experiments on the ACL in the rabbit demonstrated that immobilization results in compromised mechanical and ultrastructural properties as well as in changes to the shape and intracellular morphology of its fibroblasts and altered cellular expression of fibronectin and increased expression of $\beta 1$, $\alpha 5$ and α_v integrins (AbiEzzi et al. 1995; AbiEzzi et al. 1997). With immobilization, the suggestion is made that the number of small fibrils diminish in number (Binkley and Peat 1986). An increase in small diameter fibrils has been observed in exercised ligaments of mature ligaments that may be responsible for the decreased elastic stiffness seen in exercised ligaments.

Changes in Length of Ligaments: Effects of Shortened vs. Lengthened Structures

A limited number of studies exist on the mechanisms underlying growth and/or contracture of ligaments even though ligaments and tendons clearly demonstrate the ability to change length during growth or contracture (Nishijima et al. 1994; Muller and Dahners 1988). Evidence exists that collagen fibrils within ligaments are discontinuous and tapered at their ends (Trotter and Wofsy 1989) which may allow the fibrils to slide past one another to produce changes in ligament length during growth or contracture (Wood et al. 1998). In this way, shortening of ligaments can contribute to joint contracture. In contrast, when excessive forces are applied that extend beyond the range of maximal fiber recruitment in a ligament, ultimate failure of collagen fibers occurs, resulting in disruption of ligament structure (e.g., ankle sprain). The sliding of collagen fibers gradually past one another, however, is believed to play an important role in change of ligament length during growth. Furthermore, growth in ligaments from animal models has been shown to be relatively uniform throughout the entire span of the ligament and does not occur at a single localized growth plate (Muller and Dahners 1988; Wood et al. 1998).

Effects of Development, Maturation, and Age

Normal Ligament Growth

Although altered ligament growth may be important in pathologic musculoskeletal conditions, little knowledge is available about the mechanisms underlying these processes. Much work has been directed toward determining whether or not mechanical distraction influences growth. Ligament growth must be coordinated in some sense with the enlargement of the bones beneath the ligament. In adults, ligaments relieved of tension routinely contract (Dahners et al. 1986). Ligaments from growing animals can be induced to lengthen by the application of mechanical distraction, but distraction does not always result in lengthening of ligaments in adult animals. Both developmental and exercise studies suggest the existence of a higher proportion of new collagen fibrils that have small cross-sectional diameters may contribute to both the relative weakness and compliance of newly formed tissues. At maturity, mostly large diameter collagen fibers exist. A strong correlation exists between the size of the collagen fibril and the ultimate load capacity of the ligament (Larson and Parker 1982). In mature ligament tissues, generally a balance exists between collagen synthesis and degradation with the half-life of collagen estimated to be between 300 and 500 days. The mechanical properties of ligament-bone complexes can deteriorate significantly with age (Woo et al. 1986; Noyes and Grood 1976). In one study, a twofold decrease in strength of the ligament-bone complex with age in the human anterior longitudinal ligament was demonstrated as subjects increased in age from 21 to 79 years (Neumann et al. 1994). A progressive decline in tensile stiffness and ultimate load to failure with increasing age was demonstrated in the ACL (Woo et al. 1991). A steep decrease in ultimate load to failure was evident between the third decade (ages 22 to 35 years) and middle age (ages 40 to 50 years). Ligament complexes from older persons (from 60 to 97 years) failed at less than one third the ultimate load to failure compared to younger individuals (Woo et al. 1991). In one study, the site and mechanism of tensile failure in an older individual in whom a ligament complex was taken to failure was identified as resulting from rupture of the ligament substance rather than by avulsion from the bone (Buckwalter et al. 1993). The rate and extent of change in mechanical properties with age may further differ depending upon the nature and location of the ligament. In animal models, medial collateral ligaments have displayed a decline in their mechanical properties with increasing age after skeletal maturity, however the change in anterior cruciate ligament bone complexes appears to occur relatively more rapidly (Woo et al. 1986). Fibroblasts from ligaments have been shown to demonstrate less synthetic activity in response to exercise in older animals, indicating a possible decreased ability to participate in tissue turnover or response to injury (Wang et al. 1990).

The Influence of Hormones on Ligament Metabolism

Estrogen and progesterone receptors have been identified in the human anterior cruciate ligament (Yu et al. 2001). Physiologic changes in fibroblast proliferation in the ACL with changes in hormone levels may provide a biologic explanation for increased ACL injury rates observed in female athletes suggesting the acute cyclical hormonal variations in the female athlete during menstruation may predispose her to ligamentous injury (Yu et al. 2001).

Healing and Repair of the Injured Ligament

Ligaments are designed in such a way that when forces are applied to them, there is an increase in recruited fibers in response to increased physiologic levels of these forces. Beyond this range, progressive failure of collagen fibers is sustained with the potential for full disturbance of the ligament substance. Ligamentous injury induces a healing response of which the hallmark is scar tissue formation created to bridge gaps between the torn ends. The mode of healing in an injured medial collateral ligament appears to be initiated via crucial bridging of the wound by scar tissue composed of type III collagen (Frank et al. 1983a; Frank et al. 1983b). Autonomic nerve supply to ligament structures may alter and regulate blood flow in normal and healing ligaments (McDougall et al. 1997), representing an important mechanism for the repair of injured ligaments. Some ligament injuries, such as in the case of the anterior cruciate ligament, are renowned for the difficulty in establishing satisfactory repair (Zeichen et al. 2000). In fact, the ACL has been the subject of numerous research efforts, mainly because of its inability to heal fully after injury, as opposed to the MCL in the knee that demonstrates high capacity for healing (Hsieh et al. 2000). One study of the effects of cyclic strains on fibroblasts from the healing MCL and ACL showed greater amounts of type I collagen mRNA expressed by fibroblasts at the injury site in the ACL. This may indicate the lack of an intermediary but essential source of type III collagen bridging scar tissue that may contribute to the poor ability of the ACL to heal. In contrast, the healing medial collateral ligament exhibited characteristic increased type III collagen expression (Figure 3-20) and better healing capability after strains (Hsieh et al. 2000). Recall that mechanical stress is essential for tendons and ligaments in health, with

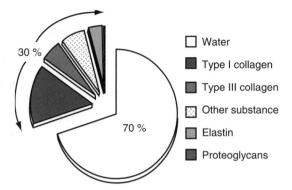

Figure 3-20. Approximate proportions of important biochemical components of rabbit MCL 21 days after surgery. (From Andriacchi T et al. Ligament: Injury and Repair. In SL-Y Woo, JA Buckwalter (eds), Injury and Repair of the Musculoskeletal Soft Tissues. Rosemont, Ill: American Academy of Orthopaedic Surgeons, 1988;116.)

stress deprivation resulting in alteration of the biochemical and biomechanical properties of both. Atrophy of tissue follows immobilization of ligaments as well as tendons and other periarticular connective tissues (Yasuda and Hayashi 1999). Hence mechanical forces play an important role in both ligament and tendon healing after injury to these tissues (Buckwalter 1995; Buckwalter 1996b). The biologic principles underlying the impact of these mechanical forces remain unclear, and mechanisms by which fibroblasts respond to different strains and/or duration of these strains continue to be difficult to ascertain. However, early mobilization of ligament repairs appears to benefit the formation of bridging scar tissue, and a degree of stress of the ligament tissue during normal activities promotes the remodeling processes in ligaments (Hsieh et al. 2000). The response to injury is generally similar among the dense connective tissues, with exceptions relating to the nature of the individual structures. The general response includes fibroblast proliferation, expression of α-smooth muscle actin and revascularization after injury. The ACL however, displays poor healing capacity that is believed to be the result of a lack in bridging scar formation as well as an additional epiligamentous reparative phase (see below) unique to the healing of the ACL in humans. The ACL, however, differs from other intra-articular tissues that also fail to heal, eg. articular cartilage,

in that it exhibits proliferative fibroblastic and angiogenic responses to rupture (Murray et al, 2000).

Response to Microdamage in Ligaments

Remodeling of the ligament tissue also may occur through some type of continuous microhealing process. Small areas of damage to which the ligament may be subjected during normal physiologic use or exercise may require the formation of localized areas of scar tissue that then matures and becomes remodeled (Hsieh et al. 2000). The theoretical mechanisms of effects of mechanical strain on collagenous tissues will be more fully addressed in Chapter 6.

Histological Changes in the Human ACL after Rupture

Histologically, four phases have been described in response to injury of the ruptured human ACL: inflammatory, epiligamentous regeneration, proliferative, and remodeling (Murray et al. 2000). During the epiligamentous repair phase, synovial tissue appears to form that covers the ends of the ruptured ACL; many of the synovial lining cells are myofibroblast-like cells that contain α-smooth muscle actin. Therefore this formation of an α-smooth muscle actin-expressing synovial cell layer on the surface of the ruptured ends, the lack of tissue bridging the rupture site and the presence of an epiligamentous reparative phase lasting eight to 12 weeks distinguishes the healing response of the ACL from other ligaments (Box 3-2) after rupture (Murray et al. 2000). The formation of this layer of the human intraarticular anterior cruciate ligament, within which lie myofibroblast-like cells that contain α-smooth muscle actin which have contractile properties causing retraction, may in fact impede repair of the ligament in contrast to the healing of extraarticular ligaments that heal more readily after injury (Murray et al. 2000).

Changes in Material Properties after Ligamentous Injury

The long-term structural limitations of ligaments after injury healing and repair are evident in the failure of the material properties of the ligament

Box 3-2. Stages of Healing of Ligament (MCL)

Inflammatory Phase (Days 1-5)	**Proliferative/Fibroplastic Phase (Day 5-Week 6)**	**Remodeling/Consolidation Phase (6 Weeks to 12 Months +)**
• Hemostasis • Fibrin clot established • Removal of debris (macrophages) • Recruitment of angiogenic and fibroblastic cells	• Fibroblasts form matrix (collagens type I, III, V and VI: less type I than in normal ligament) • Becoming less cellular, more fibrous	• Few cells • Few vessels • Increase in collagen alignment • Increase in type I collagen, other types decreased to normal levels • Up to 12 months the strength and tissue quality improve with minimal change thereafter

Modified from Frank CB et al. Soft Tissue Healing. In FHFO et al. (eds), Knee Surgery, Baltimore: Williams and Wilkins 1994; 189-229.

scar tissue to return to normal even after a two-year period (Loitz-Ramage et al. 1997). Several possible reasons can be attributed to the inferior material properties in scarred ligaments:

1. Levels of hydroxypyridinium cross-links that normally form mature covalent bonds between collagen molecules are reduced up to one year after injury and this decrease correlates with the inferior material properties of scars (Frank et al. 1995).
2. The presence of Type I collagen in healing ligaments may alter fibril diameters with increased levels of type V collagen related to presence of smaller fibrils (Hildebrand and Frank 1998b).
3. The increased presence of areas of nontensile-bearing tissue such as blood vessels, fat cells, loose and disorganized collagen, and cellular infiltrates (Figure 3-21) may play a role as stress-risers within scar (Hildebrand and Frank 1998b).

Therefore despite the ability to improve with healing, ligaments with gap scars are inferior to controls in terms of their ability to resist creep (static, cyclic and total) at comparable stresses. Collagen cross-link density, proteoglycan content, soft-tissue flaws, and the combined effect of collagen fiber changes may be mechanistic factors involved in increased scar creep behavior and the increase in strain under constant or repetitive stress observed in healing ligaments (medial collateral ligament) compared with controls after 14 weeks of healing (Thornton et al. 2000) (Table 3-2).

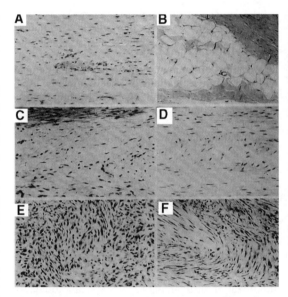

Figure 3-21. Photomicrograph of a healing medial collateral ligament showing flaws in the tissue, consisting of blood vessels (**panel A**), fat cells (**panel B**), loose collagen (**panel C**), disorganized collagen (**panel D**), cellular infiltrate (**panel E**) and combinations of flaws stained with hematoxylin and eosin (**panel F**). (From Hildebrand KA, Frank CB. Biology of Ligament Healing and Repair. In RJ Johnson, E Lombardo (eds), Current Review of Sports Medicine (ed. 2). Philadelphia: Current Medicine, 1998;126.)

The Role of Other Joint Complex Structures in Healing Ligaments

Ligament healing may be improved if other structures in or around the joint can compensate and contribute to the biomechanical stability of the joint complex. In this way, the relatively poorer

Table 3-2. Changes in Properties of Ligament 1 Year After Injury versus Uninjured Tissue (Biomechanics, Biochemical, and Histologic)

Property	Presentation
Biochemistry	• Elevated levels of type V collagen
	• Diminished levels of hydroxypyridinium crosslinks
Histology	• Aberrant levels of matrix blood vessels, fat cells, loose collagen, disorganized collagen, cellular infiltrate (Hildebrand and Frank, 1998b)
	• Altered distribution of collagen fibrils with different diameters
Biomechanics	• Scar tissue is weaker and demonstrates greater creep behavior

Modified from Hildebrand KA, Frank CB. Scar Formation and Ligament Healing. Can J Surg 1998a;41(6): 425-430.

Clinical Note

Methods to Promote Ligament Healing

Physical Measures: **Evidence from animal models demonstrates that biomechanical properties of healing ligaments (particularly where an increase in size of ligament scar exists) can be improved with controlled motion as compared with immobilized joints (Hildebrand and Frank 1998b).**
Surgical Measures: **Bringing the ruptured edges of injured ligament together using surgical suturing methods often is necessary. In one study, while structural strength of repaired ligaments with ends in contact was shown to be significantly greater than that of ligaments with an initial gap between the ruptured edges, scars formed in both groups continued to display an inferior strength tissue compared with normals (Loitz-Ramage et al. 1997).**

---

functional healing response of the injured ACL may be attributed to the few structural options available to protect it during the healing process (Sakane et al. 1996). Where multiple ligament injuries prevail (e.g., MCL and ACL), the MCL healing is reported to be inferior biomechanically where an accompanying ACL injury exists as opposed to when it is injured alone (Hildebrand and Frank 1998b).

Allografts vs. Autografts

Tendon grafts are tissue sources for allografts/autografts in ligament reconstruction surgery. Once in situ, both experience necrosis and cell death followed by revascularization and repopulation with host cells after placement. Graft incorporation is regarded to be somewhat longer for allografts, and in both cases, ligament grafts are weaker when compared with normals in the case of the ACL (Hildebrand and Frank 1998b). In the case in which the central third of the ipsilateral patellar tendon was used to replace

the posterior cruciate ligament in the sheep model, macromolecular components (GAGs and PGs) remained different in the PCL autograft, indicating that the autograft did not completely assume the biochemical properties of the PCL even after two years (Bosch et al. 1998). The bone patella-tendon bone (BTB) autograft procedure has been utilized with beneficial long-term result in the reconstruction of the ACL (Jarvela et al. 1999; Shelbourne and Gray 1997). The optimal timing (in terms of early being less than 6 weeks, or delayed being greater than three months) for the reconstruction procedure remains controversial. While no significant difference in knee stability, pain, functional outcome and isokinetic strength tests between these groups was seen at 9-year follow-up, patients with early reconstruction had fewer degenerative changes observed in the tibio-femoral joint and were able to return to more strenuous athletic activities than those with delayed ACL reconstruction (Jarvela et al. 1999). Accelerated rehabilitation is currently advised after ACL reconstruction, as opposed to bracing and immobilization, to avoid postoperative stiffness and adhesions (Shelbourne and Gray 1997). The most typical long-term problems after an ACL reconstruction with a BTB graft are anterior knee pain and degenerative changes in the patello-femoral joint (Jarvela et al. 1999).

Future Directions

Current research efforts aim to determine the effects of therapeutic agents, including growth factors and gene therapy to improve and accelerate ligament healing. Improved understanding of origins of pain from chronic ligament and tendon disorders is required. Advances in the understanding of mechanisms underlying the adaptation or failure to adapt to mechanical stresses of both ligaments and tendons has the potential to create better methods aimed at preventing or managing degenerative disorders as well as injury and repair processes in these dense connective tissues.

Joint Capsule

Collagen fibrils of joint capsules (Figures 3-22 and 3-23) assume an approximately parallel arrangement, with some fibrils interspersed in a nonparallel order (Kennedy et al. 1976). The internal composition of shoulder capsule from patients with shoulder instability identified that more stable and reducible collagen crosslinks, significantly greater mean collagen fibril diameter, more cysteine and higher density of elastin staining prevailed compared to controls. Repeated capsular deformation to which patients with shoulder instability are subjected may result in changes in the capsule that increase its strength and resistance to stretching (Rodeo et al. 1998).

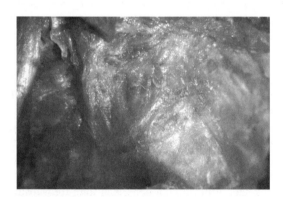

Figure 3-22. Voloradial aspect of trapeziometacarpal joint capsule (magnification X6.5). (Courtesy Maksim Kovler, BSc[PT], MSc, Toronto, Canada.)

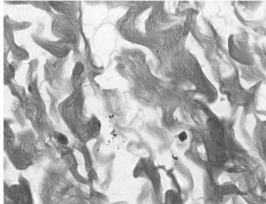

Figure 3-23. Longitudinal section through the trapeziometacarpal joint capsule (magnification X40). (Courtesy Mr. Maksim Kovler, BSc[PT], MSc, Toronto, Canada.)

Clinical Note

Adhesive Capsulitis

Adhesive capsulitis is a common but poorly understood syndrome of painful shoulder stiffness (Griggs et al. 2000). "Frozen shoulder," or idiopathic adhesive capsulitis, is defined as a condition of unknown etiology and pathogenesis characterized by substantial restriction of both active and passive shoulder range of motion that occurs in the absence of a known intrinsic shoulder disorder.

Presentation: The classic description of adhesive capsulitis encompasses three clinical phases: a *painful* phase, a phase of *progressive stiffness*, and a *thawing* phase (Murnaghan 1988). In one study, adhesive capsulitis was reported to have a mean duration of 18 to 24 months (Grey 1978). Adhesive capsulitis affects women more frequently than men and typically presents during the fifth to seventh decades. The presentation is insidious in nature with increasing generalized aching around the shoulder, which can radiate to the elbow and that may or may not be accompanied by nonspecific neck discomfort. Loss in glenohumeral range of motion eventually occurs as the shoulder progressively stiffens with significant loss in external rotation and, to a lesser extent, abduction and internal rotation (Brukner and Nye 1981). Wiley and Older (1980) reported no obliteration of the infraglenoid recess in patients with adhesive capsulitis who were observed using arthroscopic procedures. Discomfort may be experienced at the end of available range of motion at the affected shoulder; however, patients with primary adhesive capsulitis do not have pain on the resisted use of specific muscle groups about the shoulder (Murnaghan 1988). Impairment of function is demonstrated with the loss in ability to dress (e.g., putting on a coat) or to reach above shoulder level (e.g., brushing or washing hair).

Other conditions that may mimic components of adhesive capsulitis include posterior glenohumeral dislocation with marked restriction of external rotation, tendinitis, subacromial impingement, degenerative osteoarthritis of the acromioclavicular joint, and shoulder-hand syndrome (Murnaghan 1988).

Treatment: The condition of adhesive capsulitis is considered to be self-limiting, but the search for best practice measures to expedite the resumption of range of motion has been subject to much investigation. Of these measures benign neglect (Grey 1978), manipulation (Polkinghorn 1995), injection of corticosteroids (Rizk et al. 1991), physical therapy exercises and modalities (Lee et al.1973; Miller et al. 1988), manipulation under anaesthesia (Hill and Bogumill 1988), and arthroscopic (Ogilvie-Harris et al. 1995) and open releases of the contracture (Neviaser and Neviaser, 1987) have been attempted with controversial results about which of these available treatments is best. Based on the results of a recent study that evaluated the effect of shoulder-stretching exercises on functional outcome of nonoperative treatment of idiopathic adhesive capsulitis, researchers recommended that phase-II idiopathic adhesive capsulitis (progressive stiffness phase) should be treated with a four-direction shoulder-stretching regime that includes passive forward elevation, passive external rotation, passive internal rotation, and passive horizontal adduction, and should be continued for at least three months before more aggressive or invasive management is considered (Griggs et al. 2000).

Summary

Tendinous tissue is composed of dense fibers of connective tissue. The collagen fibers within tendons assume a largely longitudinal but also transverse and horizontal arrangement that allows the tendon to cope with potentially high uniaxial tensile loading as well as transverse and rotational forces during activity. In this way tendons are prepared to withstand and recover from direct contusions and pressures and act as a unit to prevent disruption of individual fibers. Type I collagen is the major collagen found in tendon, with its major contributing function to provide tensile strength. However, tendons are an example of a type of connective tissue that responds or adapts to mechanical stresses with its ultrastructure reflecting this phenomenon at specific sites along the structure. Because of tendon matrix composition and organization both great tensile stiffness and strength offered by the tendon in the majority of regions exists, whereas in a few locations fibrocartilagenous appearance occurs where tendon is subjected to repeated compressive forces.

Ligaments are composed of dense fibrous tissue that is organized to stabilize joints and contribute to joint proprioception. Ligaments consist of predominantly water (70%), collagen (25%), proteoglycans and other noncollagenous components (4%), and cells (1%). Most ligaments are composed of collagen types I and III, with small proportions of glycosaminoglycans, elastin, actin, and fibronectin. An important structural feature of tendon and ligament is a periodic wave of collagen known as its *crimp*. Crimp is believed to contribute to the nonlinear mechanical properties of both tendon and ligament substance, and results in a certain degree of tissue elasticity. This allows ligaments, in particular, to accommodate for large internal stresses during normal joint motion. Collagen fibrils of joint capsules assume an approximately parallel arrangement, with some fibrils interspersed in a nonparallel order. The hallmark of dense connective tissue healing such as is experienced in ligament or tendon is a scar that manifests in an ultimately inferior tissue quality with altered biochemical, ultrastructural, and decreased material properties.

References

AbiEzzi SS et al. Increased expression of the β1, α5, and αv integrins adhesion receptor subunits occurs coincident with remodeling of stress-deprived rabbit anterior cruciate and medial collateral ligaments. J Orthop Res 1995;13:594-601.

AbiEzzi SS et al. Decrease in fibronectin occurs coincident with the increased expression of its integrin receptor α5,β1 in stress-deprived ligaments. Iowa Orthop J 1997;17:102-109.

Abrahams M. Mechanical behaviour of tendon in vitro. Med and Biol Engrg 1967;5:433-443.

Aggeler J et al. Changes in cell shape correlate with collagenase gene expression in rabbit synovial fibroblasts. J Cell Biol 1984;98:1662-7.

Alfredson H et al. Heavy-load eccentric calf muscle training for the treatment of chronic Achilles tendinosis. Am J Sports Med 1998;26:360-366.

Alfredson H. In situ microdialysis in tendon tissue: high levels of glutamate, but not prostaglandin E2 in chronic Achilles tendon pain. Knee Surg Sports Traumatol Arthrosc 1999;7:378-381.

Alfredson H, Lorentzon R. Chronic Achilles tendinosis-recommendations for treatment and prevention. J Sports Med 2000;29(2):135-146.

Amiel D et al. Age-related properties of medial collateral ligament and anterior cruciate ligament: a morphologic and collagen maturation study in the rabbit. J Gerontol 1991;46:B159-B165.

Banes AJ et al. Mechanoreception at the cellular level: the detection, interpretation and diversity of responses to mechanical signals. Biochem Cell Biol 1995;73:349-365.

Bell E et al. Production of a tissue-like structure by contraction of collagen lattice by human fibroblasts of different proliferative potential in vitro. Proc Natl Acad Sci USA 1979;187:1274-1278.

Benjamin M, Ralphs JR. Functional and Developmental Anatomy of Tendons and Ligaments. In SL Gordon et al (eds). Repetitive Motion Disorders of the Upper Extremity. Rosemont, Ill: American Academy of Orthopedic Surgeons, 1995;185-203.

Bershadsky AD et al. Destruction of microfilament bundles in mouse embryo fibroblasts treated with inhibitors of energy metabolism. Exp Cell Res 1980;127:421-489.

Betsch D, Baer E. Structure and mechanical properties of rat tail tendon. Biorheology 1980;7:83-94.

Binkley J. Overview of ligament and tendon structure and mechanics: implications for clinical practice. Physiotherapy Canada 1989;41(1):24-30.

Binkley J, Peat M. The effect of immobilization on the ultrastructure and mechanical properties of the rat medial collateral ligament. Clin Orthopaed 1986;203:301-308.

Birk DE et al. Collagen fibrillogenesis in vitro: Interaction of types I and V collagen regulates fibril diameter. J Cell Sci 1990; 95:649-657.

Bosch U et al. Alterations of glycosaminoglycans during patellar tendon autograft healing after posterior cruciate ligament replacement: a biochemical study in a sheep model. Am J Sports Med 1998;26(1):103-108.

Bray RC et al. 1996. Normal and healing ligament vascularity: a quantitative histological assessment in the adult rabbit medial collateral ligament. J Anatomy 1996;188:87-95.

Brewer BJ. Aging of the rotator cuff. Am J Sports Med 1979;7:102-110.

Brukner FF, Nye CJS. A prospective study of adhesive capsulitis of the shoulder in a high-risk population. Q J Med 1981;198:191-204.

Buckwalter JA. Fine Structural Studies of Human Intervertebral disc. In AA White, SL Gordon (eds), Proceedings of the Workshop on Idiopathic Low Back Pain. St. Louis: Mosby, 1982;108-143.

Buckwalter JA et al. Proteoglycans of human infant intervertebral disc. Electron microscopic and biochemical studies. J Bone Joint Surg Am 1985;67:284-294.

Buckwalter JA, Cruess R. Healing of musculoskeletal tissues. In CA Rockwood Jr et al. (eds), Fractures (3rd ed). Philadelphia: JB Lippincott, 1991;181-222.

Buckwalter JA et al. Soft-tissue aging and musculoskeletal function. J Bone Joint Surgery 1993;75A(10):1533-1548.

Buckwalter JA et al. Age-related changes in cartilage proteoglycans: quantitative electron microscopic studies. Microscopy Res Tech 1994;28:398-408.

Buckwalter JA. Activity vs. rest in the treatment of bone, soft tissue and joint injuries. Iowa Orthop J 1995;15:29-42.

Buckwalter JA et al. Healing of the Musculoskeletal Tissues. In CA Rockwood Jr et al. (eds), Fractures (4th ed). Philadelphia: Lippincott-Raven, 1996;261-304.

Buckwalter JA. Effects of early motion on healing of musculoskeletal tissues. Hand Clin 1996b;12:13-24.

Burgeson R, Nimni M. Collagen types: molecular structure and tissue distribution. Clin Orthopaed Rel Res 1992;282:250-272.

Burkhead WZ. The Biceps Tendon. In CA Rockwood, FA Matsen (eds), The Shoulder. WB Saunders: Philadelphia, 1990;791-836.

Butler D et al. Biomechanics of ligaments and tendons. Exer Sport Sci Rev 1978;6:125-181.

Chazal J et al. Biomechanical properties of spinal ligaments and a histological study of the supraspinal ligament in traction. J Biomech 1985;18:167-176.

Clement DB et al. Achilles tendonitis and peritendonitis: Etiology and treatment. Am J Sports Med 1984;12:179-184.

Couchman JR et al. Adhesion, growth and matrix production by fibroblasts on laminin substrates. J Cell Biol 1983;96:177-183.

Curwin S. Biomechanics of tendon and the effects of immobilization. Foot Ankle Clin 1997;2:371-389.

Dahners LE et al. The relationship of actin to ligament contraction. Clin Orthopaed 1986;210:246-251.

DeKlerk AJ, Jonck LM. Tendon response to trauma and its possible clinical application. S African Med J 1991; 80(2):444-449.

Diament J et al. Collagen: ultrastructure and its relation to mechanical properties as a function of aging. Proceed Royal Soc London 1972;180:293-315.

Elliott DH. Structure and function of mammalian tendon. Biol Rev 1965;40:392-421.

Elliott D et al. The rupture rate of acute flexor tendon repairs mobilized by the controlled active motion regimen. J Hand Surg Br 1994;19:607.

Enwemeka CS. Ultrastructural changes induced by cast immobilization in the isolated soleus tendon. APTA Annual Conference Abstract R-123, Anaheim, Calif, June 24-28, 1990;65.

Enwemeka CS. Membrane-bound intracytoplasmic collagen fibrils in fibroblasts and myofibroblasts of regenerating rabbit calcaneal tendons. Tissue Cell 1991;23:173-190.

Eyre DR, Muir H. Quantitative analysis of types I and II collagens in human intervertebral discs at various ages. Biochem Biophys Acta 1977;492:29-42.

Fleischmajer R et al. Type I and type III collagen interactions during fibrillogenesis. Ann NY Acad Sci 1990;580:161-175.

Folkman J, Klagsburn M. Angiogenic factors. Science 1987;235:4442-4446.

Forslund C, Aspenberg P. Tendon healing stimulated by injected CDMP-2. Med Sci Sports Exer 2001;33(5):685-687.

Frank C et al. Natural history of healing in the repaired medial collateral ligament. J Orthop Res 1983a;1:179-188.

Frank C et al. Medial collateral ligament healing: a multidisciplinary assessment in rabbits. Am J Sports Med 1983b;11:379-389.

Frank C et al. Normal Ligament: Structure, Function and Composition. In SL-Y Woo, JA Buckwalter (eds.), Injury and Repair of the Musculoskeletal Soft Tissues. Park Ridge, Ill: American Academy of Orthopaedic Surgeons, 1988;45-101.

Frank CB et al. Soft tissue healing. In FH Fu et al. (eds). Knee Surgery. Baltimore: Williams and Wilkins, 1994;189-229.

Frank CB et al. Rabbit medial collateral ligament scar weakness is associated with decreased collagen pyridinoline cross-link density. J Orthop Res 1995;13:157-165.

Fujimoto D. Human tendon collagen: aging and crosslinking. Biomed Res 1984;5:279-282.

Galou M et al. The importance of intermediate filaments in the adaptation of tissues to mechanical stress: evidence from gene knockout studies. Biol Cell, 1997;89(2): 85-97.

Gardner D. Aging of Articular Cartilage and Joints. In Textbook of Geriatric Medicine and Gerontology (3rd ed). New York: Churchill Livingstone, 1991;792-812.

Gathercole LJ, Keller A. Early development of crimping in rat tail tendon. Micron 1968;9:83-89.

Gelberman RH et al. Effects of early intermittent passive mobilization on healing canine flexor tendons. J Hand Surg 1982;7A:170-175.

Gelberman R et al. Tendon. In SL-Y Woo and JA Buckwalter (eds), Injury and Repair of the Musculoskeletal Soft Tissues. Rosemont, Ill. American Academy of Orthopedic Surgeons 1988;5-40.

Geneser F (1986). Textbook of Histology. Philadelphia: Lea & Febiger, 1986;157-184, 219-257.

Giori NJ et al. Cellular shape and pressure may mediate mechanical control of tissue composition in tendons. J Orthop Res 1993;11:581-591.

Grey RG. The natural history of "idiopathic" frozen shoulder. J Bone Joint Surg 1978;60-A:564.

Griggs SM et al. Idiopathic adhesive capsulitis. A prospective funcional outcome study of nonoperative treatment. J Bone Joint Surg 2000;82-A(10):1398-1407.

Hamerman D. Aging and osteoarthritis: basic mechanisms. JAGS, 1993;41(7):760-770.

Harris AK et al. Fibroblast traction as a mechanism for collagen morphogenesis. Nature 1981;290:249-251.

Harwood FL, Amiel, D. Differential metabolic responses of periarticular ligaments and tendon to joint immobilization. J Appl Physiol 1992;72:1687-1691.

Hattrup SJ, Johnson KA. A review of ruptures of the Achilles tendon. Foot Ankle 1985;6:34-38.

Hayashi K. Biomechanical studies of the remodeling of knee joint tendons and ligaments. J Biomech 1996;29:707-716.

Hembry RM et al. Immunolocalization of tissue inhibitor of metalloproteinases (TIMP) in human cells. J Cell Sci 1985;73:105-119.

Henderson B, Edwards JCW (eds). The Synovial Lining. London: Chapman and Hall 1997.

Hildebrand KA, Frank CB. Scar formation and ligament healing. Canad J Surg 1998a;41(6):425-430.

Hildebrand KA, Frank CB. Biology of Ligament Injury and Repair. In R Johnson, J Lombardo. (eds), Current Review of Sports Medicine (2nd ed). Philadelphia: Current Medicine, 1998b;121-131.

Hill JJ, Bogumill H. Manipulation in the treatment of frozen shoulder. Orthopedics 1988;11:1255-1260.

Hollis JM et al. The effects of knee motion and external loading on the length of the anterior cruciate ligament (ACL): a kinematic study. J Biomech Eng. 1991;113:208-214.

Hsieh AH et al. Time-dependent increases in type-III collagen gene expression in medial collateral ligament fibroblasts under cyclic strains. J Orthopaed Res 2000;18:220-227.

Ippolito E et al. Morphological, immunochemical and biochemical study of rabbit Achilles tendon at various ages. J Bone Joint Surg Am 1980;62:583-592.

Iwuagwu FC, McGrouther DA. Early cellular response in tendon injury: the effect of loading. J Plast Reconstr Surg 1998;102(6):2064-2071.

Jackson D, Bentley J. Collagen-Glycosaminoglycan Interactions. In Ramachandran GN (ed), Treatise on Collagen V2A. London: Academic Press, 1968;300-321.

Jarvela T et al. Bone-patellar tendon-bone reconstruction of the anterior cruciate ligament. Internat Orthopaed (SICOT) 1999;23:227-231.

Jozsa L et al. Alterations in dry mass content of collagen fibers in degenerative tendinopathy and tendon-rupture. Matrix 1989;9:140-146.

Jozsa L et al. Three-dimensional ultrastructure of human tendons. Acta Anat 1991;142:306-312.

Jozsa L, Kannus P. Human Tendons. Anatomy, Physiology and Pathology. Champaign, Ill: Human Kinetics, 1997;47-104.

Kannus P, Jozsa L. Histopathological changes preceding spontaneous rupture of a tendon. A controlled study of 891 patients. J Bone Joint Surg 1991;73-A: 1507-1525.

Kannus P et al. The effect of immobilization on myotendinous junction: an ultrastructural, histochemical, and immunohistochemical study. Acta Physio Scand 1992;144:387-394.

Kannus P. Structure of the tendon connective tissue. Scand J Med Sci Sports 2000;10:312-320.

Kellett J. Acute soft tissue injuries: a review of the literature. Med Sci Sports Exerc 1986;8:489-500.

Kennedy J et al. Tension studies of human knee ligaments. J Bone Joint Surg 1976;58-A: 350-355.

Khan KM et al. Where is the pain coming from in tendinopathy? It may be biochemical, not only structural, in origin. Br J Sports Med 1998;34(2):81-83.

Khan KM et al. Histopathology of common overuse tendon conditions: update and implications for clinical management. Sports Med 1999;27:393-408.

Khan U et al. Differences in proliferative rate and collagen lattice contraction between endotenon and synovial fibroblasts. J Hand Surg 1998;23A:266-273.

Kivirikko KI. Collagens and their abnormalities in a wide spectrum of diseases. Annals Med, 1993;25:113-126.

Kivirikko K, Kulvaniemi H. Posttranslational Modifications of Collagen and their Alterations in Heritable Diseases. In J Uitto, A Perejda (eds), Connective Tissue Disease. Molecular Pathology of the Extracellular Matrix. New York: Marcel Dekker, 1987;263-292.

Kivirikko K et al. Hydroxylation of Proline and Lysine Residues in Collagens and other Animal and Plant Proteins. In JJ Harding, M Crabbe (eds), Post-Translational Modifications of Proteins. Boca Raton: CRC Press, 1992;1-51.

Kubota H et al. Effect of motion and tension on injured flexor tendons in chickens. J Hand Surg Am 1996;21:456.

Kvist H, Kvist M. The operative treatment of chronic calcaneal paratendonitis. J Bone Joint Surg 1980;62B:353-357.

Kvist M. Achilles tendon injuries in athletes. Sports Med 1994;18:173-201.

Kvist M. Achilles Tendon Overuse Injuries. Academic Dissertation. Turku, Finland: University of Turku, 1991.

Langberg H et al. Age-related blood flow around the Achilles tendon during exercise in humans. Europ J Appl Physiol 2001;84(3):246-248.

Larsen AI et al. Low-dose heparin in the treatment of calcaneal peritendinitis. Scand J Rheumatol 1987;16:47-51.

Larson N, Parker WW. Physical Activity and Its Influence on the Strength and Elastic Stiffness of Knee Ligaments. In ML Howell, AW Parker (eds), Sports Medicine: Medical and Scientific Aspects of Elitism in Sport (8th vol). Brisbane, Aust: Australian Sports Medicine Federation 1982;63-73.

Leach RE et al. Achilles tendonitis. Am J Sports Med 1981;9:93-98.

Leadbetter WB. Anti-inflammatory therapy in sports injury: the role of nonsteroidal drugs and corticosteroid injection. Clin Sports Med 1995;14:353-410.

Lee M et al. Periarthritis of the shoulder: a controlled trial of physiotherapy. Physiotherapy 1973;59:312-315.

Little B et al. The effect of strenuous versus moderate exercise on the metabolism of proteoglycans in articular cartilage from different weight-bearing regions of the equine 3rd carpal bone. Osteoarthr Cartilage, 1997;5(3): 161-172.

Lohr JF, Uhthoff HK. The microvascular pattern of the supraspinatus tendon. Clin Orthop 1990;254:35-38.

Loitz-Ramage BJ et al. Injury size affects long term strength of the rabbit medial collateral ligament. Clin Orthop 1997;337:272-280.

Madden JW, Peacock EE. Dynamic metabolism of scar collagen and remodeling of dermal wounds. Annals Surg 1971;174:511-520.

Manske PR, Lesker PA. Biochemical evidence of flexor tendon participation in the repair process-an in vitro study. J Hand Surg 1984;9B:117-120.

Martin G et al. The genetically distinct collagens. TIBS July 1985;285-288.

McDougall JJ et al. Sympathetically-mediated constrictor responses in normal and ACL-deficient rabbit knees. Proceedings of the 31st Annual Meeting of the Canadian Orthopaedic Research Society, Hamilton, Ont, 1997;51.

Messina A. The double armed suture: tendon repair with immediate mobilization of the fingers. J Hand Surg 1992;17A:137-142.

Mehr D et al. Tenascin-C in tendon regions subjected to compression. J Orthop Res 2000;18:537-545.

Merriless MJ, Flint MH. Ultrastructural study of tension and pressure zones in a rabbit flexor tendon. Am J Anat 1980;157:87-106.

Messina A. The double-armed suture: tendon repair with immediate mobilization of the fingers. J Hand Surg Am 1992;17:137.

Miller MD et al. Thawing the frozen shoulder: the "patient" patient. Orthopedics 1988;11:849-853.

Moore MJ, DeBeaux A. A quantitative ultrastructural study of rat tendon from birth to maturity. J Anat 1987;153:163.

Morgan CJ, Pledger WJ. Fibroblast Proliferation. In KI Cohen et al (eds), Wound Healing. Philadelphia: WB Saunders, 1992;63-76.

Mow VC et al. Biomechanics of Articular Cartilage. In M Nordin, VH Frankel (eds), Basic Biomechanics of the Musculoskeletal System. Philadelphia: Lea & Febiger, 1989;31-57.

Muller P, Dahners LE. A study of ligamentous growth. Clin Orthop 1988;229:274-277.

Murnaghan, JP. Adhesive capsulitis of the shoulder: current concepts and treatment. Orthopedics 1988;11(1):153-158.

Murray MM et al. Histological changes in the human anterior cruciate ligament after injury. J Bone Joint Surg 2000;82-A(10):1387-1397.

Murrell G et al. Effects of immobilization on Achilles tendon healing in a rat model. J Orthop Res 1994;12:582-591.

Nakatsuji N, Johnson KE. Experimental manipulation of a contact guidance system in amphibian gastrulation by mechanical tension. Nature 1984;307:453-455.

Neumann P et al. Aging, vertebral density and disc degeneration alter the tensile stress-strain characteristics of the human anterior longitudinal ligament. J Orthop Res 1994;12:103-112.

Neviaser RJ, Neviaser TJ. The frozen shoulder. Diagnosis and management. Clin Orthop 1987;223:59-64.

Newton PO et al. Ultrastructural changes in knee ligaments following immobilization. Matrix 1990;10:314-319.

Newton PO et al. Immobilization of the knee joint alters the mechanical and ultrastructural properties of the rabbit anterior cruciate ligament. J Orthop Res 1995;13:191-200.

Nimni M. Collagen: Structure, function, and metabolism in normal and fibrotic tissues. Sem Arthr Rheum 1983;11(1):1-66.

Noyes FR, Grood ES. The strength of the anterior cruciate ligament in humans and rhesus monkeys. Age-related and species-related changes. J Bone Joint Surg 1976;58-A:1074-1082.

Nishijima N et al. Flexor tendon growth in chickens. J Orthop Res 1994;12:576-581.

Ogilvie-Harris D et al. The resistant frozen shoulder: manipulation versus arthroscopic release. Clin Orthop 1995;319:238-248.

Orava S et al. Operative treatment of typical overuse injuries in sports. Am Chir Cyanaecol 1991;80:208-211.

Paavola M et al. Long-term prognosis of patients with Achilles tendinopathy. Am J Sports Medicine 2000;28(5):634-642.

Peterson WW. Effect of various methods of restoring flexor sheath integrity on the formation of adhesions after tendon injury. J Hand Surg 1990;15A:48-56.

Polkinghorn BS. Chiropractic treatment of frozen shoulder (adhesive capsulitis) utilizing mechanical force, manually assisted short lever adjusting procedures. J Manip Physiol Therapeut 1995;18:105-115.

Poole AR. Proteoglycans in health and disease: Structures and functions. Biochem J 1986;236:1-14.

Pope MH. Structure and Function of the Lower Spine. Occupational Low Back Pain: Assessment, Treatment, and Prevention. St. Louis: Mosby, 1991;562.

Potenza AD. Tendon healing within the flexor digital sheath in the dog. J Bone Joint Surg 1962;44A:49-64.

Prockop D, Kivirikko K. Heritable diseases of collagen. New Engl J Med 1984;311:376-386

Prockup D et al. The biosynthesis of collagen and its disorders. New Engl J Med 1979;301:13-23.

Reeves B. The natural history of the frozen shoulder syndrome. Scand J Rheumatol 4:193-196.

Rigby BJ et al. The mechanical behaviour of rat tail tendon. J Gen Physiol 1959;43:265-283.

Rizk TE et al. Corticosteroid injections in adhesive capsulitis: an investigation of their value and site. Arch Phys Med and Rehab 1991;72:20-22.

Roberts AB, Sporn MB. Growth factors. Science 1993;8:1-9.

Rodeo SA et al. Analysis of collagen and elastic fibers in shoulder capsule in patients with shoulder instability. Am J Sports Med 1998;26(5):634-643.

Rowe RWD. The structure of rat tail tendon fascicles. Connect Tissue Res 1985;14:21-30.

Sakane M et al. The contribution of the anterior cruciate ligament to knee joint kinematics: evaluation of in situ forces using a robot/universal force-moment sensor test system. J Orthop Sci 1996;1:335-347.

Seiler JG III et al. Autogenous flexor-tendon grafts: A biochemical and morphological study in dogs. J Bone Joint Surg Am 1993;75:1004.

Shelbourne KD, Gray T. Anterior cruciate ligament reconstruction with autogenous patellar tendon graft followed by accelerated rehabilitation, a 2- to 9-year follow-up. Am J Sports Med 1997;25:786-795.

Shyy JYJ, Chien S. Role of integrins in cellular-responses to mechanical stress and adhesion. Curr Opin Cell Biol 1997;9(5):707-713.

Spadara JA. The distribution of trace metal metal ions in bone and tendon. Calcif Tissue Res 1970;6:49-54.

Stehno-Bittel L et al. Biochemistry and biomechanics of healing tendons: Part I. Effects of rigid plaster casts and functional casts. Medicine and Science in Sports and Exercise 1998;788-793.

Squier CA, Magnes C. Spatial relationships between fibroblasts during the growth of rat-tail tendon. Cell Tissue Res. 1983;234:17.

Strickland JW. Flexor tendon injuries: flexor tendon repair. Orthop Rev 1986;15:49-68.

Sutker BD. Cyclic strain stimulates DNA and collagen synthesis in fibroblasts cultured from rat medial collateral ligaments. Trans Orthop Res Soc 1990;15:130.

Tillman LJ, Cummings GS. Biologic Mechanisms of Connective Tissue Mutability. In D Currier, R Nelson (eds), Dynamics of Human Biologic Tissues. Philadelphia: FA Davis, 1992;1-44.

Thornton GM. Early medial collateral ligament scars have inferior creep behaviour. J Orthop Res 2000;18:238-246.

Trotter JA. Wofsy C. The length of collagen fibrils in tendon. Trans Orthop Res Soc 1989; 14:180.

Tuderman L, Kivirikko K. Immunoreactive prolyl hydroxylase in human skin, serum and synovial fluid: changes in the content and components with age. Europ J Clin Invest 1997;7:295-299.

Vailas AC. Physical activity and its influence on the repair process of medial collateral ligaments. Connect Tissue Res 1981;9:25-31.

Vogel KG, Heinegard, D. Characterization of proteoglycans from adult bovine tendon. J Biol Chem 1985; 260:9298-9306.

Vogel KG, Koob TJ. Structural specialization in tendons under compression. Int Rev Cytol 1989;115:267-293.

Vogel JG et al. Specific inhibition of type I and type II collagen fibrillogenesis by the small proteoglycans of tendon. Biochem J 1984;223:587-597.

Vogel KG et al. Aggrecan in bovine tendon. Matrix Biol 1994;14:171-179.

Waggett AD et al. Characterization of collagens and proteoglycans at the insertion of the human Achilles tendon. Matrix Biol 1998;16:457-470.

Wang CW et al. Lifelong exercise and aging effects on the canine medial collateral ligament. Orthop Trans 1990;14:488-489.

Warren CG et al. Elongation of rat tail tendon: effect of load and temperature. Arch Phys Med Rehabil 1971;50: 481-487.

Wess TJ et al. Molecular packing of type I collagen in tendon. J Molec Biol 1998;275:255-267.

Wight TN et al. Proteoglycans. Structure and Function. In ED Hay (ed), Cell Biology of the Extracellular Matrix. New York: Plenum Press, 1991;45-78.

Wiley AM, Older MW. Shoulder arthroscopy. Am J Sports Med 1980;8:31-38.

Williams JGP. Achilles tendon lesions in sport. Sports Med 1986;3:114-135.

Wiltse LL. The effect of common anomalies of the lumbar spine upon disc degeneration and low back pain. Orthop Clin North Am 1971;2:569-582.

Witonski D, Wagrowska-Danielewicz M. Distribution of substance-P nerve fibres in the knee joint in patients with anterior knee pain syndrome. A preliminary report. Knee Surg Sports Traumatolo Arthrosc 1999;7:177-183.

Woo SL-Y et al. Connective tissue response to immobility. Arthr Rheumatol 1975;18:257-264.

Woo SL-Y. The effect of immobilization and exercise on the strength characteristics of bone-medial collateral ligament-bone complex. Biomech Symp 1979;67-71.

Woo SL-Y et al. The effects of exercise on the biomechanical and biochemical properties of swine digital flexor tendons. J Biomech Eng Trans ASME 1981;103:51-56.

Woo SL-Y et al. Mechanical properties of tendons and ligaments. I and II. The relationships of immobilization and exercise on tissue remodeling. Biorheology 1982;19:385-408.

Woo SL-Y et al. Tensile properties of the medial collateral ligament as a function of age. J Orthop Res 1986;4: 133-141.

Woo SL-Y et al. The biomechanical and morphological changes in the medial collateral ligament of the rabbit after immobilization and remobilization. J Bone Joint Surg 1987;69-A:1200-1211.

Woo SL-Y et al. Tensile properties of the human femuranterior cruciate ligament-tibia complex. The effects of specimen age and orientation. Am J Sports Med 1991;19(3):217-225.

Wood ML et al. Collagen fiber sliding during ligament growth and contracture. J Orthopaed Res 1998;16: 438-444.

Wren TAL et al. Tendon and ligament adaptation to exercise, immobilization and remobilization. J Rehabil Res Dev 2000;37(2):217-224.

Wren TAL, Carter DR. A microstructural model for the tensile constitutive and failure behaviour of soft skeletal connective tissues. J Biomech Eng 1998;120:55-61.

Yasuda K, Hayashi K. Changes in biomechanical properties of tendons and ligaments from joint disuse. Osteoarthr Cartilage 1999;7:122-129.

Yasuda T et al. Unfavourable effect of knee immobilization on Achilles tendon healing in rabbits. Acta Orthop Scandinavica 2000;71(1):69-73.

Young RG et al. Use of mesenchymal stem-cells in a collagen matrix for Achilles-tendon repair. J Orthopaed Res 2000;16(4):406-413.

Yu WD et al. Combined effects of estrogen and progesterone on the anterior cruciate ligament. Clin Orthopaed Rel Res 2001;383:268-281.

Zeichen J et al. The proliferative response to isolated human tendon fibroblasts to cyclic biaxial mechanical strain. Am J Sports Med 2000;28(6);888-892.

Chapter 4

The Nature of the Dense Connective Tissues of the Musculoskeletal System: Structure, Function, and Biomechanics of Articular Cartilage and Meniscus

Harpal K. Gahunia

Articular Cartilage Structure and Biochemistry

Articular cartilage (AC), also referred to as *hyaline cartilage,* is a highly specialized connective tissue with biophysical properties consistent with its ability to withstand high compressive forces. Its smooth, lubricated surface allows bones to glide over one another with minimal friction. The synovial fluid plays an important role in joint lubrication and wear resistance (Kuettner et al. 1991). Adult cartilage is typically avascular, alymphatic, and aneural (Ghadially 1978). Nourishment is provided primarily through long-range diffusion of the synovial fluid (Ogata and Whiteside 1979). In addition, cartilage canals that connect the cartilage and subchondral bone are thought to contribute to the cartilage nourishment. During growth and development, these cartilage canals extend as branches of the blood vessels to the articular-epiphyseal cartilage complexes, epiphyseal centers of ossification, and growth plates (Visco et al. 1989, Clark 1990). Although cartilage canals are abundant in young cartilage, with increasing age the cartilage canal distribution changes and their numbers decrease (Visco et al. 1989). Immature cartilage is traversed by blood vessels, therefore cartilage nourishment also is provided through diffusion of nutrients from blood.

AC, a highly hydrated tissue, is composed of cells called the *chondrocytes* (2% to 5% of cartilage volume) and the extracellular matrix (ECM) (95% of cartilage volume), which is secreted and maintained by the chondrocytes. The ECM of cartilage is a resilient gel comprising 60% to 80% (cartilage wet weight) tissue fluid with a complex macromolecular organization. The ECM macromolecules consist mainly of type II collagen and proteoglycans (PGs), which in humans represents approximately 55% and 35% of the cartilage dry weight, respectively.

Chondrocytes and Chondrons

Chondrons are the microanatomical, micromechanical, and metabolically active functional units of AC that play an important role in maintaining the homeostasis of the AC. Anatomically, a chondron comprises of the chondrocyte and its pericellular microenvironment (Muir 1995). A transparent pericellular glycocalyx is present on the chondrocyte surface, which is enclosed by a collagenous fibrillar capsule.

Throughout life, AC undergoes continual internal remodeling. Chondrocytes can synthesize and secrete the major macromolecular components of the ECM, and they also can degrade the matrix by releasing degradative enzymes, such as collagenase, and other metalloproteinases, including stromelysin. During growth and development, synthesis outweighs the degradation process. In adults, matrix synthesis is finely balanced by controlled matrix degradation (Poole 1992; Poole et al. 1993). Hence chondrocytes continually replace the matrix macromolecules lost during normal degradation. However, disruption to the normal balance of synthesis and degradation can lead to variation in the intrinsic characteristics of cartilage matrix. This can lead to a gradual degeneration of the ECM that is responsible for the development of clinically recognizable disease(s) (Poole et al. 1993; Venn and Maroudas 1977).

Proteoglycans

The PG molecules are strongly hydrophilic, and this property is important in the lubrication of the weightbearing surfaces. PGs are composed of a protein core onto which one or more glycosaminoglycan (GAG) chains are covalently bonded. The heterogeneity of PG structure and function is a reflection of the variation not only in protein core but also in the type and size of the GAG chains and the position of GAG sulphation. The GAG molecules are unbranched chains of repeating disaccharides, which confer negative charge to the cartilage matrix. The concentration of the negative charge is known as fixed charge density (FCD) and is of great importance in maintaining the compressive properties of AC. The GAG groups present in the cartilage PGs are primarily chondroitin sulphate (87%) (CS) chains, which exist both as chondroitin-4-sulphate (C4S) and chondroitin-6-sulphate (C6S). Other GAGs present in AC are keratan sulphate (KS) (6%) and hyaluronic acid (HA) (Table 4-1). The CS chains are covalently attached to the protein core through a xylose residue linkage to specific serine residues, whereas KS chains are attached to protein via N- and O-

linked glycosidic linkages to asparagine or serine/threonine, respectively. HA is a nonsulphated, large polyanionic molecule that can have a molecular weight up to 6,000 kDa. HA is the only GAG that is not bound to a core protein.

In AC, PGs are present as PG monomers or PG aggregates. The large aggregating PGs (aggrecan and versican) form 50% to 58% of the total PGs, whereas nonaggregating PGs form 40% of the total PG content (Ratcliffe and Mow 1996). Aggrecan is a large PG molecule consisting of more than 100 CS chains, 20 to 40 KS chains, and approximately 40 O- and N-linked oligosaccharides. Aggrecans have the ability to bind with HA through their HA-binding region, and the link protein stabilizes the interaction between aggrecan and HA.

Collagen and Collagen Cross-links

Collagen is the major structural protein that maintains cartilage integrity by providing tensile strength and resilience to cartilage matrix (Akizuki et al. 1986; Mayne 1989). These mechanical properties of the collagen fibers are dependent on the formation of the molecular cross-links (see Chapter 2). Collagen is secreted as a procollagen molecule and is processed further in the ECM by the enzymatic cleavage of the C- and N-propeptides (Uitto et al. 1979). Although propeptide removal is required for fibrils to grow normally (Prockop et al. 1979), partially processed N-procollagen also can assemble into thin collagen fibrils (Yang et al. 1995). In the ECM, the collagen molecules co-polymerize to

Table 4-1. Proteoglycans in Articular Cartilage

Proteoglycan Type	Disaccharide Repeating Units	Molecular Weight (KiloDaltons)
Proteoglycan aggregate	NA	3×10^3 to 3×10^6
Hyaluronic acid (hyaluronan)	N-acetylglucosamine glucuronate linkage 1–3	4–6000
Proteoglycan monomer (PGM) (aggrecan)	NA	1×10^3 to 3×10^3
Protein core	NA	200–250
Keratan sulphate (KS)	N-acetylglucosamine galactose linkage 1–4	4–19
Chondroitin-4-sulphate (C4S) (chondroitin sulphate A)	N-acetylgalactosamine glucuronate linkage 1–3	5–50
Chondroitin-6-sulphate (C6S) (chondroitin sulphate C)	N-acetylgalactosamine glucuronate linkage 1–3	5–50

form a fibrillar framework and are stabilized by covalent crosslinks formed between adjacent collagen chains (intramolecular cross-link) and adjacent collagen molecules (intermolecular cross-link). Crosslinking of collagen fibrils is initiated extracellularly through lysyl oxidase, a 30 kDa copperrequiring enzyme (Pokharna et al. 1995). This enzyme catalyzes the oxidative deamination of certain $^-NH_2$ groups in collagen and acts on specific lysine or hydroxylysine residues in the telopeptide region at each end of the collagen molecule, eventually resulting in the formation of mature hydroxypyridinium crosslinks (Frazer 1998; Knott and Bailey 1998).

Of the five genetically distinct collagen types known to exist in AC (Table 4-2), three are cartilage-specific collagen: types II, IX, and XI. Type II collagen, the principal fibrillar macromolecule that provides the structural integrity to AC, represents 90% to 95% of the total collagen in AC (Eyre et al. 1992, 1987). Type IX collagen represents 1% to 2% of collagen in adult cartilage and at least 10% in fetal cartilage. Type IX collagen is located on the outside of the type II collagen fibril, to which it is covalently crosslinked (Wu and Eyre 1984, 1989), and also is distributed in ECM without association with type II collagen (Wu et al. 1992). Type IX collagen also has been considered a PG because its α-2 (IX) chain contains CS or dermatan sulphate (DS) GAG chains (Bruckner et al. 1985). The GAG chains in type IX collagen are thought to stabilize type II collagen fibril structure (Olsen 1997). Type XI collagen, a fibril-forming collagen, contributes to about 2% to 3% of the total collagen and is incorporated in the type II collagen fiber in a ratio of about 1:30 in mature tissues (Eyre et al. 1987). Type XI collagen is thought to mediate

physical interactions between collagen fibrils and PGs in cartilage and to regulate the size of the type II collagen fibers (Cremer et al. 1998; Mendler et al. 1989; Wu and Eyre 1995). Two cartilage nonspecific and nonfibrillar collagens also have been detected in the cartilage matrix, namely types VI collagen and X collagen. Type VI collagen, a short-helix molecule concentrated pericellularly, represents 1% to 2% of the total collagen (Hambach et al. 1998). Type VI collagen mediates the attachment of chondrocytes to the macromolecular framework of the matrix. Type X collagen (1%), a short nonfibrillar collagen, is present in the calcified cartilage lamina (Gannon et al. 1991). Synthesized and deposited largely by chondrocytes of hypertrophic cartilage, type X collagen is thought to play an important role in the development of the growth plate and cartilage calcification (Nerlich et al. 1992).

Two types of pyridinium collagen crosslinks have been identified in mature AC, namely, the pyridinoline (Pyd) and deoxypyridinoline (Dpyd). Pyd, first isolated from rat tail tendon (Fujimoto 1977; Fujimoto et al. 1978), is present in collagen-containing tissues such as cartilage, synovial membrane, meniscus, bone, and ligament. Pyd is far more abundant in cartilage than in bone, and its concentration remains relatively constant in adult cartilage with age (Eyre et al. 1988). However, Dpyd content is more abundant in bone compared with AC. Yet another crosslinking molecule, pentosidine, was isolated from senescent human AC. Pentosidine was first identified in dura mater and characterized by Sell and Monnier (1989). Pentosidine, a condensation product of arginine, lysine, and ribose, is an end result of advanced glycosylation (Grandhee and Monnier 1991).

Table 4-2. Collagen Types in Articular Cartilage

Collagen Type	Molecular Organization	Molecular Weight (KiloDaltons)
Fibril Constituents of Collagen		
type II	α1 (II)$_3$	290
type IX	α1 (IX), α2 (IX), α3 (IX)	250
type XI	α1 (XI), α2 (XI), α3 (XI)	300
Nonfibril Constituents of Collagen		
type VI	α1 (VI), α2 (VI), α3 (VI)	500–550
type X	α1 (X)$_3$	170

Noncollagenous Proteins

Small, noncollagenous proteins and glycoproteins (Table 4-3) are present in the cartilage ECM, which are thought to be crucial for modulating several fibril properties (Hagg et al. 1998; Paulsson and Heinegard 1984). Although glycoproteins form a small fraction (2% to 5%) of the cartilage ECM, they play an important role in matrix assembly and/or regulation of matrix metabolism. The matrix glycoproteins contain distinct and functionally active peptide domains that allow interactions with chondrocyte surface receptors and other ECM molecules.

Cartilage oligomeric matrix protein (COMP), a 524 kDa glycoprotein, is found in cartilage during chondrogenesis and is preferentially localized in the territorial matrix surrounding the chondrocytes (Hedbom et al. 1992; Newton et al. 1994). Human cartilage glycoprotein (HC gp-39), also termed *YKL-40*, is a 40 kDa glycoprotein (De Ceuninck et al. 1998; Hakala et al. 1993; Harvey et al. 1998; Johansen et al. 1993, 1996). HC gp-39 is a major secretary glycoprotein of human chondrocytes and synovial fibroblasts.

Transforming growth factor-beta (TGF-β) is the prototype of a large family of signaling molecules, which also includes bone morphogenic protein (BMP), growth factors, activins, and inhibins. Members of the TGF-β superfamily are important regulators of embryogenesis, and they are also critical in postnatal development, tissue homeostasis, and repair processes. TGF-β, the major growth factor expressed by chondrocytes, plays an important role during endochondral ossification, affecting the proliferation, growth, and maturation of the growth plate and during cartilage repair.

Biglycan, decorin, and fibromodulin are members of a family of structurally related PGs called the *small CS/DS PGs*. These molecules play significant roles in matrix assembly and stabilization as well as the metabolic regulation of AC, such as collagen fibrillogenesis and binding of matrix molecules (e.g. fibronectin and growth factors) (Scott 1993). Fibronectin (FN) is an ECM glycoprotein thought to affect cell adhesion, morphology, migration, differentiation, and matrix assembly (Burton-Wurster and Lust 1986; Clark 1990; Couchman et al. 1990). FN plays a significant role in the adhesion of chondrocytes to ECM and during tissue repair (Piperno et al. 1998). Tenascin is an oligomeric glycoprotein that functions in processes such as wound repair and formation of bone and cartilage. Tenascin is involved in the assembly of the chondrocyte matrix and is thought to influence interactions between the chondrocytes and the matrix.

Other noncollagenous proteins in cartilage ECM include cartilage matrix glycoprotein, matrix Gla protein, anchorin CII, chondronectin, and laminin. These molecules are known to mediate the attachment of chondrocytes to type II collagen or aggrecan, thus stabilizing the cartilage matrix (Agraves et al. 1987; Carsons and Horn 1988; Durr et al. 1996;

Table 4-3. Non-Collagenous Proteins in Articular Cartilage

Glycoprotein/Protein	Molecular Weight (Kda)	Anatomic Location
Cartilage oligomeric matrix protein (COMP)	524	Territorial matrix
Human cartilage glycoprotein (HC gp-39); also called YKL-40 and chondrex	40	ECM*
Biglycan	100	Pericellular matrix
Decorin	74	Interterritorial matrix, superficial lamina, ECM*
Fibromodulin	59	Superficial lamina
Fibronectin	440	ECM*
Tenascin (two size variants)	220 and 320	Territorial matrix
Cartilage matrix glycoprotein (CMP)	54	ECM*
Matrix gla protein (MGP)	10	ECM*
Anchorin CII (cartilage annexin V)	31	Chondrocyte membrane
Chondronectin	180	ECM*
Link protein	45	ECM*

*ECM, extracellular matrix; compartment not specified.

Kuhne et al. 1998; Mollenhauer et al. 1999, 1984; Muller et al. 1998; Tondravi et al. 1993).

Articular Cartilage Heterogeneity

AC has several morphologically distinct components, uncalcified or calcified, which are involved in its attachment to the bone and the formation of an articulating surface and a compression-resistant core in the cartilage (Figure 4-1). The uncalcified AC is attached to the subchondral bone plate via a narrow layer of calcified cartilage. This interface between uncalcified and calcified cartilage is demarcated by a 2- to 5-mm thick, densely basophilic and calcified line called the *tidemark* (Havelka et al. 1984; Redler et al. 1975). The calcified cartilage lamina functions in distributing the cartilage stress during locomotion and increased levels of physical activity (Anderson et al. 1993).

Articular Cartilage Lamina

The heterogeneous uncalcified cartilage can be distinguished histologically, biochemically, and mechanically as three compartments, or laminae, which are parallel to and extend from the articular surface to the tidemark. The differences between the three laminae are based on chondrocyte morphology and distribution, collagen and PG composition and concentration, collagen architecture and fiber diameter, and water content.

The lamina closest to the cartilage surface is called *superficial lamina, tangential lamina,* or *lamina splendens*. The superficial lamina (about 200 μm thick) is characterized by small ellipsoid chondrocytes with their long axis parallel to the cartilage surface. The middle lamina, known as *transitional lamina,* consists of large, round, and more randomly distributed chondrocytes than those in the superficial lamina. The third lamina, called *deep* or *radial lamina*, is superficial to the calcified cartilage. The deep chondrocytes are largest and arranged in longitudinal columns that orient themselves perpendicular to the tidemark. These deep chondrocytes synthesize alkaline phosphatase that is likely involved in the calcification of the adjacent calcified lamina (Xu et al. 1994). The calcified lamina is characterized by small chondrocytes embedded in a heavily calcified matrix (Hunziker 1992).

Polarized light, transmission electron, and scanning electron microscopic studies revealed the spatial orientation and fibril diameter of collagen in the various laminae of adult human AC (Benninghoff 1925; Jeffery et al. 1991; Muir et al. 1970). The architectural concept of cartilage collagen is based on the three-dimensional orientation of collagen within the various observable laminae. Accordingly, the superficial lamina is thought to be 10% to 20%, the transitional lamina is 40% to 60%, and the deep lamina constitute about 20% to 30% of the total uncalcified cartilage thickness. Comosso et al (1962) observed that in bovine cartilage less than 2 years old, the tangential collagen fibers in the superficial lamina extended up to 50%

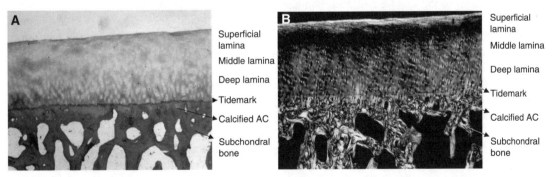

Figure 4-1. Photomicrograph of normal articular cartilage of rhesus macaque knee joint showing the smooth articular surface, uncalcified and calcified cartilage. **A,** Haematoxylin and Eosin stained. Note the division of cartilage to calcified and uncalcified laminae and the prominent tidemark. **B,** Picro-sirius stained cartilage observed under Polarized light. Note gothic arrangement of collagen fibers.

of the total cartilage thickness, whereas in mature animals it constituted only about 10% of the tissue. The collagen fibril diameter is thin in the superficial cartilage lamina where the fibrils are densely packed and lie parallel to the plane of the cartilage surface (Figure 4-1). The fibril diameter increases from the superficial toward the deep cartilage laminae. Collagen fibers in the middle lamina form gothic-arcadelike architecture, whereas the deep lamina collagen is more loosely packed and oriented perpendicular to the tidemark (Benninghoff 1925; Hukins et al. 1984).

Biochemical variations in the tissue fluid, collagen, and PG content in the AC laminae have been reported (Maroudas et al. 1977; Venn et al. 1977). In adult human hip cartilage, the water content decreases from 74% in the superficial lamina to 67% in the deep lamina (Maroudas et al. 1977). The collagen type II content is highest in the superficial lamina and lowest in the middle lamina (Lipshitz et al. 1976; Muir et al. 1970). In immature cartilage, PG content is least in the middle lamina; however, in mature cartilage, PG content is lowest in the superficial lamina (Maroudas et al. 1969; Stockwell 1979.) During development, cellularity is considerably reduced, especially in the deep lamina. The variations in the depth-dependent structure and biochemical composition of cartilage could explain the varied cartilage function in processes such as aging, repair, and degeneration.

Articular Cartilage Compartmentalization

Matrix compartmentalization studies revealed a clear subdivision of the middle and deep laminae into pericellular, territorial, and interterritorial matrices (Poole et al. 1984, 1985). Each chondrocyte membrane is immediately surrounded by pericellular (or lacunar) matrix composed of a mixture of HA (Mason 1981); sulphated PGs; biglycan (Miosge et al. 1994); glycoproteins; fibronectin (Glant et al. 1985); laminin (Durr et al. 1996); and collagen types VI and IX (Poole 1998; Poole et al. 1997). Encapsulating the pericellular matrix is the territorial (or capsular) matrix, characterized by a fine network of fibrillar collagen (Poole et al. 1984, 1985). The chondrocytes establish contact with these collagen fibrils by extending fine cytoplasmic processes. Adjacent to the territorial matrix is the outermost and largest ECM compartment called the *interterritorial matrix* that lies in space between various territorial regions. The interterritorial matrix is characterized by cross-banded collagen fibers running in parallel and varying concentration of PGs depending on the laminae in which the chondrocytes lie (Poole et al. 1985).

Articular Cartilage Function and Biomechanics

Arthrodial joints are functional units that transmit mechanical loads between contacting bones during normal daily or specialized activities (e.g., sports). During daily activities such as walking and running, the joint complex is loaded dynamically, and all its components, namely, AC, bone, muscles, ligaments, tendons, and nerves, participate in load transmission. AC has unique material properties that enable it to perform its physiological functions over a lifetime and under a wide range of loading conditions. Mechanical stress is an important environmental factor in maintaining the differential function of the cartilage (Carter et al. 1987; Wong and Carter 1988; Yutani et al. 1994).

The primary functions of normal AC are to absorb shock, bear load, and provide articulating surfaces for arthrodial joints. These unique biologic and mechanical properties of AC depend on the complex cartilage structure as well as the interactions of its biochemical constituents, mainly water, electrolytes, collagen, and PG, and the chondrocytes (Cohen et al. 1998; Huber et al. 2000). The deformation behavior and mechanical properties of articular chondrocytes are believed to play an important role in their response to the mechanical loading of ECM. The viscoelastic properties of cartilage, primarily caused by fluid flow through the ECM, can explain much of these deformational responses observed under many loading conditions. The effects of load on AC are complex. Within the normal physiologic range of pressure, the cartilage matrix is intrinsically incompressible when loaded (Bachrach et al. 1998). The mechanical changes of degenerated human cartilage include decreased stiffness during compression, tension, shear, and increased permeability caused by fluid flow (Mow et al. 1998).

Dynamic loading of cartilage is associated with slight cell and tissue deformation as well as cyclical fluctuations in the hydrostatic pressure of cartilage and in fluid movement (Wilkins et al. 2000). However, static loading results in release of fluid from the tissue, therefore concentrating the matrix macromolecules, increasing the concentrations of cations, reducing extracellular pH and increasing extracellular osmolarity. Each of these alterations is implicated in regulating the synthetic response of chondrocytes to load.

Mechanical forces have great influence on the synthesis and rate of turnover of cartilage molecules (Arokoski et al. 2000). *In vitro* experiments show that both static and dynamic compressive stress decreases the PG biosynthesis (range 25% to 85%); this inhibition is proportional to the applied stress but independent of loading time (Torzilli et al. 1997). Regular cyclic loading of the joint enhances PG synthesis and augments cartilage stiffness. Several *in vitro* studies using cartilage or osteochondral explants have been aimed at investigating the effects of load magnitude, frequency, and duration on the macromolecular biosynthesis, chondrocyte viability, as well as loss, and structural deformation. The results from these studies corroborate in that an increased duration and intensity of loading stimulated the inhibition of PG biosynthesis, whereas PG loss is only modulated by increasing the magnitude and duration of loading (Steinmeyer et al. 1997, 1999). The stiffness of the collagen network limits hydration in normal cartilage, thus ensuring a high PG concentration in the matrix, which is essential for effective load bearing (Basser et al. 1998).

The interactions between PG aggregates and collagen fibers (Hammerman et al. 1970; Matthews 1965; Smith et al. 1967) determine the biochemical and biomechanical properties of cartilage. The intrinsic physical properties of a collagen fiber network impart high tensile strength (Falcovitz et al. 2001; Hayes et al. 1978; Mow et al. 1998), whereas the high fixed negatively charged GAG constituent of PG molecules interact with tissue fluid to provide compressive resilience to cartilage through negative electrostatic repulsion forces (Mankin et al. 1994; Maroudas 1979; Mow et al. 1997, 1998). The compressive property of AC therefore is a function of the balance between the osmotic swelling, generated by water bound to the

sulphate and carboxylate groups of the PG, and the tension developed in the collagen network surrounding the PGs (Maroudas et al. 1976, 1977, 1980, 1981).

Various mammalian species show topographical variation in the biomechanical properties of AC in different joint areas (Jurvelin et al. 2000) and as a function of age and depth from the articular surface (Schinagl et al. 1997). The biomechanical properties (i.e., the intrinsic tensile stiffness and strength of collagen fibers) of the three cartilage laminae are responsible for the superior mechanical response in tension of immature compared with mature tissue. The fixed charge density of GAG molecules and collagen fibril orientation of the middle and deep lamina are functionally important components during compressive loading. Roth et al. (1980) noted that the tensile strength properties and stiffness of the middle and deep laminae increased in immature cartilage and decreased in mature specimens, whereas the tensile strength properties were comparable in the superficial lamina of both age groups. Kaab et al (2000) reported that high force and long duration loading exhibited high deformation of the collagen fibers in the middle and upper deep cartilage laminae with increased thickness of the layer of collagen fibers oriented almost parallel to the surface and a 54% reduction in cartilage thickness. The compressive modulus of collagen fibers significantly increases with depth from the articular surface (Schinagl et al. 1997). The relatively low moduli and the compression-induced stiffening of the superficial lamina could affect the biomechanical behavior of cartilage.

Articular Cartilage Formation, Growth, and Remodeling

During embryonic development, external to the early mesodermal limb bud is a specialized region called the *apical ectodermal ridge* that plays an important role in limb bud growth (Solursh 1984). Within the limb bud is a vascular-rich myogenic region and a central chondrogenic core surrounded by a perichondrium (Solursh 1989). The embryonic mesenchymal cells aggregate in the shape of the bone-to-be and, because of the avascular environment, differentiate into chondroblasts. The chondroblasts then secrete ECM and enlarge (length and width) through the process of interstitial and appositional growth. Once surrounded by the matrix, the cells are referred to as *chondrocytes*. With continued growth of this cartilage model, the chondrocytes in its midsection hypertrophy (enlarge), mature, and start depositing insoluble calcium salts. These events result in chondronecrosis, or disintegration of calcified cartilage, followed by vascular invasion, formation of primary and secondary centres of ossification, and the progressive replacement of cartilage by bone through the process of endochondral ossification. During bone growth, the epiphysis of the growing bone is capped with articular-epiphysial cartilage, also retaining the growth plate. However, in adults, only the AC remains in the arthrodial joints. At skeletal maturity, although the AC thickness is relatively stabilized, several studies have shown that endochondral ossification at the cartilage and subchondral interface remains active throughout life and is responsible for the gradual changes in joint shape that occur with aging (Green et al. 1970; Lane and Bullough 1980).

During skeletal development and postnatal growth, the biochemical composition of AC, particularly the PG, collagen, and Pyd cross-links per tissue volume increases (Eyre et al. 1988; Pal et al. 1981; Thonar and Sweet 1981). Mechanical forces strongly influence skeletal morphogenesis, growth, and development, beginning at a very early stage (Wong and Carter 1988). Among the mechanobiological factors, the intermittent hydrostatic pressure and shear stresses play an important role in modulating cartilage development and maintenance, as well as cartilage degeneration (Beaupre et al. 2000; Stevens et al. 1999). The intermittent hydrostatic pressure regulates the distribution of cartilage thickness within the joint and maintains a stable AC. On the other hand, shear stress (or strain energy) encourages cartilage destruction and ossification, eventually contributing to the cartilage degeneration and progression of osteoarthritis. In nonfunctional, immobilized or nonload-bearing mature joints, the absence or reduction of intermittent hydrostatic pressure in the AC is conducive to cartilage degeneration and the progressive advancement of the ossification front toward the joint surface until the AC has been ossified (Carter et al. 1987). Sustained "creep" loading intensifies the stress concentrations within AC, which in turn

reduces its water content (Adams et al. 1999). In humans, AC thickness tends to be greatest in joints that experience high forces and high joint contact pressures (Carter et al. 1987). Furthermore, regular joint loading in youth may assist in the establishment and strengthening of the cartilage collagen network (Helminen et al. 2000). Investigation of the cartilage thickness of cadaveric lower limb joints revealed an inverse relation between the mean cartilage thickness and mean compressive modulus in each of the joints examined (Shepherd and Seedhom 1999). Additionally, a direct correlation was noted between the cartilage thickness and donor weight. Animal studies (Kirviranta et al. 1988; Smith et al. 1992) have shown that increased physical activity correlates with increased cartilage thickness and PG content, whereas reduced physical activity from immobilization leads to cartilage thinning. Takada et al. (1999) reported that the superficial cartilage lamina acts as a membrane barrier against substances that invade from the bursa through this cartilage lamina. The development period of the superficial lamina coincide with the initiation of weight bearing, and joint pressure changes could further promote maturation.

Interactions between the matrix molecules and chondrocytes are responsible for the biological and mechanical properties of AC. Throughout life, AC undergoes continual internal remodeling and serves as a load-bearing elastic material that is responsible for the frictionless gliding movement of the surfaces of articulating joints (Huber et al. 2000). Cartilage homeostasis reflects a delicate balance between synthesis (anabolism) and degradation (catabolism) of matrix components, which is in part mediated by endogenous chondrocytes. Chondrocytes can synthesize and secrete the major macromolecular components of the ECM, and they can also degrade these matrix molecules by releasing degradative enzymes such as collagenase and other metalloproteinases, including stromelysin. During growth and development, synthesis outweighs the degradation. In adults, matrix synthesis is finely balanced by controlled matrix degradation (Poole 1992; Poole et al. 1993). Hence chondrocytes continually replace the matrix macromolecules lost during normal degradation. However, disruption to the normal balance of synthesis and degradation that occur with age and as a consequence of cartilage related diseases can lead to variation in the intrinsic biochemical and biomechanical properties of cartilage. This can lead to a gradual degeneration of the ECM that is responsible for the development of clinically recognizable disease(s) such as osteoarthritis and rheumatoid arthritis (Poole et al. 1993; Venn and Maroudas 1977).

Age-related Changes in Articular Cartilage

Aging implies changes in joint components over time that contribute later in life to an increasing frequency of clinical complaints, including pain, and impairments in function and mobility. Aging appears to modify the cartilage, subchondral bone, muscle, soft tissues, synovium, and synovial fluid. Whether the changes in aging inevitably progress through an intermediary phase of "degenerated cartilage" to the fibrillated state of osteoarthritis is not clear. The tensile stiffness and strength of adult AC decreases markedly during aging (Kempson 1982). However, the molecular basis for this change is unknown. The relative concentration of GAGs varies markedly with age. In immature cartilage, a preponderance of C4S and little KS is evident. With advancing age, an appreciable increase in KS content and a corresponding fall in C4S (Inerot et al. 1978) occurs. One of the prominent age-related changes in AC matrix is the presence of advanced glycosylation end-product cross-links such as pentosidine (Pokharna and Pottenger 1997). Studies have shown that in human cartilage, pentosidine levels increase exponentially with age (Bank et al. 1998; Uchiyama et al. 1991). Age-associated accumulation of senescent crosslinks could result in changes in the cartilage collagen network and mechanical properties (Mow et al. 1997).

Articular Cartilage Degradation and Related Diseases

Failure in any of the joint components can compromise the normal joint function, which in turn may lead to pathological aberrations in other arthrodial structures. Degenerative processes involving damage of cartilage structure is reflected in the breakdown of the normal mechanical

function of cartilage. Several factors may lead to the cartilage mechanical breakdown such as direct trauma to the cartilage, obesity, immobilization, and excessive repetitive loading of the cartilage. Although sports activity, without traumatic injury, does not appear to be a risk factor for the cartilage degradation in the normal joint, such activity may be harmful to an abnormal joint and could lead to and/or accelerate cartilage degradation. Cartilage shear stresses, particularly within the deep lamina, increase in response to the thinning of the AC, and this is associated with tidemark advancement and reduplication as well as thickening of calcified cartilage/subchondral plate (Anderson et al. 1993). These events are associated with the attempt of AC and bone to repair the inflicted injury. Furthermore, tensile stress may initiate or propagate the splits and cracks observed in diseased cartilage (Kelly and O'Connor 1996). Also, proteolytic mediated degradation of cartilage could occur through the action of proteinases or free radicals (Roughley et al. 1993). During normal metabolic processes and in disease states, cartilage-specific compounds are released into the synovial fluid of the joint capsule, which could be used as diagnostic markers to monitor the status of cartilage (Lohmander 1990; Lohmander et al. 1992). Consequently, the identification of biological markers can be extremely valuable for clinical diagnosis of cartilage diseases.

Osteoarthritis: Etiologic Factors, Histology, and Biochemistry

Osteoarthritis (OA) is an extremely common, slowly progressive, and often debilitating form of degenerative arthritis (Setton et al. 1993). The clinical manifestation of OA includes joint pain, stiffness, and limitations in activity, and the prevalence of OA increases with age (Buckwalter and Mankin 1998; Lawrence et al. 1998; Praemer et al. 1992). Although the lifelong moderate use of normal joints does not increase the risk of OA, high-impact and torsional loads may increase the risk of degeneration of normal joints. Individuals who have an abnormal joint anatomy, joint instability, disturbances of joint or muscle innervation, or inadequate muscle strength or endurance have a high risk of degenerative joint disease and the associated cartilage degradation.

Despite its clinical prevalence, OA remains difficult to define, characterize, or assess (Pritzker, 1994). OA can be viewed as the clinical and pathological outcome of a range of disorders that results in structural and functional failure of diarthrodial joints that occurs when the dynamic equilibrium between the breakdown and repair of joint tissues is overwhelmed. The pathogenesis of OA is thought to be multifactorial, involving environmental factors such as the influence of occupation, body weight, trauma, recreational activities, surgical manipulations, and genetic factors such as collagen gene mutations (Nuki 1999). OA is associated with defective integrity of AC and intraarticular inflammation, in addition to related reactive changes in the underlying trabecular and cortical bone and at the joint margin, particularly the synovium (Altman et al. 1986; Oegema et al. 1997). Structural failure of AC could result from abnormal mechanical strains on pathologically impaired cartilage. Although OA is viewed primarily (Ghosh and Cheras 2001) as a disorder of cartilage with reactive subchondral changes, the primary role of a subchondral problem with secondary changes in the articular cartilage also has been documented (Imhof et al. 1997; Radin and Rose 1986; Radin et al. 1984). Imhof et al (1999) reported that the repetitive overloading in OA leads primarily to lesions in the subchondral region (including blood vessels), which is more stress sensitive than cartilage, that in turn impede

flow of nutrition to articular cartilage. The early subchondral changes include redistribution of vascular supply with marrow edema and micronecrosis along with specific architectural changes in the subchondral trabecular bone (Imhof et al. 1997, Burr 1998). Whether the bony changes precedes the cartilage degeneration remains unproven but may best be considered necessary for progression of the disease.

Osteoarthritis: Histology, Biochemistry, and Biomechanics

Gross macroscopic observations show that with the progression of OA, the normally whitish-blue translucent cartilage takes on an opaque yellowish appearance (Figure 4-2). An extensively ulcerated area leading to partial or full cartilage thickness erosion follows surface irregularities, caused by fissuring and pitting. These erosions, which are initially focal, become confluent and progress to large denuded areas, particularly in the load-bearing area (Dieppe 1995). Biochemically, OA is associated with a loss of the normal balance between synthesis and degradation of the macromolecules that provide AC with its structural, functional, and mechanical properties (Lohmander et al. 1997; Poole 1992; Poole et al. 1993). OA starts from the cartilage surface through cartilage edema and PG

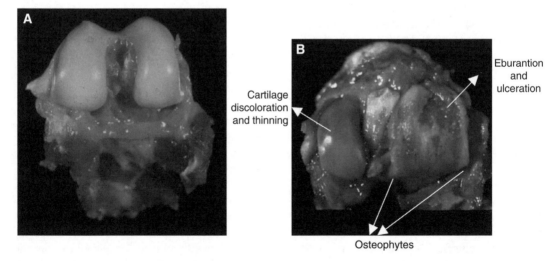

Figure 4-2. Gross pathologic macrographs of the femoral condyles of rhesus macaque. **A,** Normal. Note smooth glossy cartilage surface. **B,** Severe osteoarthritis. Note the extent of irregularity in the cartilage surface and various cartilage lesions.

depletion followed by fibrillation of the superficial collagen network.

Biomechanically, OA cartilage has decreased modulus or stiffness when placed in tension, compression and shear loading, which in turn increases its propensity to swell when compared with healthy cartilage. Deterioration of the collagen-PG solid network appears to be focused at the articular surface. However, whether the initial disruption of the cartilage surface is a direct result of mechanical forces or a product of altered chondrocyte activity is unclear. Continuous compression of the cartilage diminishes PG synthesis and causes damage of the tissue through necrosis. This further creates an altered stress pattern on joint surfaces, eventually leading to frank cartilage structural damage, and ultimately, its mechanical failure. Early subchondral changes include redistribution of blood supply with marrow hypertension, edema, and regions of micronecrosis (Imhof et al. 1997). Differences in the viscoelastic properties of cartilage, reflected by alterations in the structure and composition of the chondrocyte cytoskeleton, have also been associated with OA (Tricky et al. 2000).

The mechanisms for the onset and progression of OA, though not fully understood, involve a combination of biomechanical and biochemical factors. Elevated metabolic activity in human OA cartilage is an early event, which also is characterized by increased tissue fluid (Mankin and Thrasher 1975; Venn and Maroudas 1977). The microstructural alterations, rather than compositional changes, of the collagen-PG solid network, which appears to be focused at the cartilage surface, are responsible for the early increase of hydration (Setton et al. 1993, 1999). This structural change promotes the deterioration of biomechanical properties of AC. Although PG synthesis is markedly increased in OA cartilage compared with normal cartilage, the rate of PG turnover also is increased, resulting in a decrease in total PG and GAG content, which is directly proportional to the OA severity (Maroudas et al. 1973). Compared with normal cartilage, the PGs synthesized by OA cartilage chondrocytes are also structurally different with shorter GAGs, increased number of PG fragments, decreased size of its subunits with diminished and/or defective aggregation, increased C4S compared with C6S, and an increased CS/KS ratio. Increased levels of aggrecan, decorin, biglycan, fibromodulin, link protein (Cs-Szabo

et al. 1997), anchorin CII (annexin V epitopes) (Mollenhauer et al. 1999), and tenascin (Chevalier et al. 1996; Salter 1993) have been reported in human OA cartilage (compared with age matched controls). Furthermore, several studies have documented an increased pentosidine level in the cartilage and body fluids of arthritic patients (Chen et al. 1998; Takahashi et al. 1994).

Although the total collagen content of OA cartilage varies little (Lane and Weiss 1975), levels of type I, III, VI, and X collagens often increase (Aigner et al. 1993; Girkontaite et al. 1996; Pullig et al. 1999). Collagen fiber diameter and orientation also may show considerable variation from normal (Weiss 1973). A switch to type I collagen synthesis with a decrease in the synthesis of type II collagen is observed in OA cartilage. Under physiological conditions, type II collagen fibrils contain more water than type I fibrils (Grynpas et al. 1980; Studer et al. 1996). Therefore an increased type I collagen and decreased type II collagen could account for decreased water content in severe OA tissue. An enhanced deposition of fibronectin and tenascin in human OA cartilage has been reported (Chevalier 1993; Homandberg et al. 1998; Jones et al. 1987; Pfander et al. 1999). von der Mark et al. (1992, 1995) documented increased synthesis of type X collagen by OA chondrocytes.

Osteoarthritis: Animal Models

OA can be induced, or the disease may occur spontaneously in animals (Bendele and Hulman 1998; Chateauvert et al. 1990; Pritzker et al. 1989; Tulamo et al. 1996;). Thus OA may result from mechanical disturbances resulting from surgical procedures (e.g., meniscectomy or transection of the medial collateral or cruciate ligaments) or from the administration of single major or multiple impact of the joints. Intraarticular injection of chymopapain or human recombinant interleukin-1 into the joint cavity and response to vitamin A or hormones such as corticosteroids or testosterone can also induce OA (Fife and Brandt 1989; Masse et al. 1997; Panula et al. 1998; Ratcliffe et al. 1993 and 1994; Williams et al. 1988). The advantages in studying the induced OA models include the enhanced evolution of the disease and more importantly, the ability to study the early stages of OA.

Osteoarthritis Versus Aging

A strong correlation exists between increasing age and the prevalence of osteoarthritis. Recent report of important age-related changes in the function of chondrocytes suggest that age-related changes in AC can contribute to the development and progression of OA, which was once believed to be "a disease of the elderly." OA is now regarded as distinct from and superimposed on aging processes. OA itself may not be a consequence of aging, but age-related changes in the function of chondrocytes may contribute to the initiation and progression of the disease. Therefore aging could alter the matrix composition and accelerate the degradation of the cartilage. Both bone density and the incidence of OA are known to vary with age in humans (Sokoloff 1969). Mitrovic et al (1983) documented age-related decrease in cell density in all laminae of the human femoral condyle AC, although more markedly in superficial lamina. Vascularity of the calcified cartilage lamina (a sign of remodeling) is well developed after 55 to 65 years of age. Lane et al. (1977) observed an age-related decline in calcified cartilage thickness in human femoral condyles with attenuated number of tidemarks after the sixth decade. These findings suggest that remodeling of the bone appears to decrease with increasing age. Reduction in the water content from 70% to 80% (normal wet weight) to 50% to 65% (wet weight) accompanies the aging process especially in the deeper cartilage lamina (Venn 1978).

Other Joint Arthropathies

Rheumatoid arthritis (RA) is a chronic systemic inflammatory disorder that mainly affects the joint tissues. Although RA is of unknown etiology, autoimmunity plays a pivotal role in its chronicity and progression (Harris 1990; Mitchell 1985). The initial pathologic event in RA appears to be activation and/or injury of synovial microvascular endothelial cells. As the disease progresses to more chronic stages, the synovium becomes massively hypertrophic and edematous, and the chondrocytes synthesize excessive amounts of collagenase and stromelysin, which degrades the matrix type II collagen and PG. In addition, a decreased synthesis of collagen and PGs has been reported (Mitchell

1985). A variety of acute and chronic joint disorders are associated with crystal deposits. Endogenous crystals such as monosodium urate, calcium pyrophosphate dihydrate, calcium pyrophosphate (CPPD) crystals, and basic calcium phosphate (hydroxyapatite) have been shown to be pathogenic. These endogenous crystals produce disease by triggering the cascade that results in cytokine-mediated cartilage destruction. The two common crystal arthropathies are gout, caused by urates, and pseudogout, associated with CPPD crystals. Gout involves urate crystal deposition on the cartilage surface and in the synovial fluid, leading to synovial hyperplasia, fibrosis, and pannus formation, which in turn destroys the underlying cartilage. CPPD crystal deposition can occur in tendons, ligaments, synovium, and AC (Ryan and McCarty 1993).

Articular Cartilage Visualization in Health and Disease

The ability to diagnose and monitor early changes in AC is crucial in the assessment of effective drug treatments used to halt or slow the progression of cartilage lesions. Imaging techniques commonly used to assess AC lesions are based on x-ray radiography, arthrography, computed tomography (CT), ultrasound imaging, magnetic resonance imaging (MRI), and arthroscopy (Blackburn et al. 1996; Hodler 1996). Plain radiographs are the simplest and most readily employable means of joint evaluation, and now, microfocal radiographs have been developed, which magnify the radiograph and help portray the joint space more accurately. However, radiography, nuclear medicine scans, arthrography, and CT scans are limited in their use in joint imaging because they are unable to detect early stages of cartilage abnormalities. Because of the inability to visualize uncalcified AC, the diagnosis of uncalcified cartilage lesion is based on the extent of narrowing of the joint space (Figure 4-3).

Recent advances in the ultrasonic imaging technology of AC is focused toward measuring cartilage thickness and evaluating the subsurface characteristics of normal and OA cartilage (Figure 4-4). High frequency ultrasound, in the range of 50 to 100 MHz, provides a sensitive technique for the analysis of cartilage structure and properties

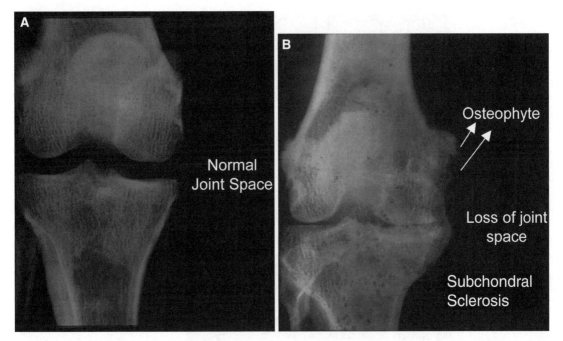

Figure 4-3. Plain radiographs of rhesus macaque knee joint. **A,** Normal. Note the presence of joint space. **B,** Severe osteoarthritis. Note the presence of subchondral sclerosis, osteophytes and decrease or lack of knee joint space.

(Foster et al. 2000; Kim et al. 1995; Myers et al. 1995; Saied et al. 1997). Thus ultrasound imaging has the potential to be used for intraarticular quantitative imaging and assessment of early changes in bone and cartilage structure associated with cartilage degeneration. Studies (Agemura and O'Brien 1990) have shown that the ultrasonic propagation in the cartilage sample is primarily sensitive to the amount of collagen, collagen architecture, and degree of cross-linking. Although lesser in extent compared with collagen, PGs also influence the acoustic propagation in cartilage. The limitation in the use of ultrasound is that subchondral bone cannot be readily imaged because of the soundwave scattering, which occurs at the cartilage/bone interface. As such, the depth of acoustic penetration is compromised in high-resolution, high frequency ultrasound systems.

MRI is the preferred modality for assessing AC lesions because of its advantages of direct visualization of AC, multiplanar capability, superior soft tissue contrast, and noninvasiveness (Figure 4-5). Numerous experimental and clinical studies have evaluated different MR pulse sequences to achieve high signal-to-noise ratio, obtain high-resolution magnetic resonance images, delineate AC from the adjacent soft tissue/synovial fluid, and/or determine the extent of lesions within AC itself. Improved magnetic resonance pulse sequences have significantly enhanced AC visualization to the microscopic level and have increased its sensitivity to detect AC structural changes, e.g., cartilage fissures and small surface defects. Cartilage is characterized on proton-density weighted MRI as a trilaminar structure with superficial high, middle-low, and deep-high signal intensity. The width of each magnetic resonance laminae varies with age (Babyn et al. 1996 and 1998; Gahunia et al. 1995; Fry et al. 1991; Hutton et al. 1992; Lehner et al. 1989; Modl 1991). Studies pertaining to the Rhesus Macaque model for spontaneous degenerative arthritis showed that MRI is effective in the detection and assessment of AC lesions with greater capability of detecting early stages of cartilage lesions than other available diagnostic modalities (Gahunia et al. 1993, 1995). MRI of patients who have undergone autologous chondrocyte implantation (ACI) of the knee for deep cartilage defects proved useful in assessing the morphologic features of ACI grafts, including volume of graft filling the defect, restoration of surface contour, and status of the subchondral

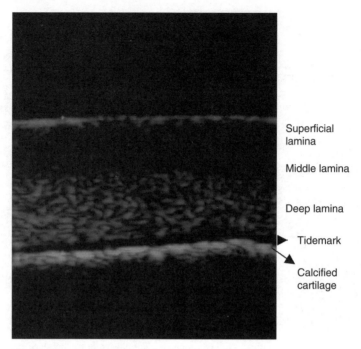

Figure 4-4. Ultrasound backscatter micrograph of porcine articular cartilage with the use of a 50 MHz transducer. Note the location of various laminae and hyperechoic subchondral bone surface.

bone plate (Alparslan et al 2001). MRI can reliably detect graft hypertrophy, especially when the repair tissue has overgrown the native cartilage (edge overgrowth type) and can also identify partial and complete graft delamination, with or without the use of contrast-enhanced magnetic resonance arthrography. MRI often detects edema-like signals in the marrow underlying the ACI repair tissue. However, although MRI is useful in determining the morphology of the ACI repair tissue the specific tissue type cannot be identified. The meaning of signal changes in studies involving osteochondral repair remains a topic of active research.

In a study involving qualitative assessment of intracartilagenous morphology, Lang et al. (2000) reported that the MR signal can delineate margins of cartilage defects showing the potential of MRI to detect early lesions. Quantitative magnetic resonance techniques can produce two- and three-dimensional maps of cartilage thickness, a technique that may prove useful in surgical planning and treatment strategies. As such, magnetic resonance is a useful diagnostic tool in the preoperative assessment of osteochondral defect and other intraarticular

pathology as well as the post-mosaic plasty assessment of osteochondral plugs and cartilage coverage.

Arthroscopy, a sensitive technique for assessing superficial articular abnormalities, is another diagnostic tool that provides an appreciation of the extent of cartilage lesions associated with joint injuries. Arthroscopy uses small-bore arthroscopes to assess joint damage in conscious, nonsedated patients. As such, arthroscopic techniques have reduced the morbidity of treatment methods for cartilage repair and enable early detection of chondral defects of the knee. Curl and colleagues (1997) documented the prevalence rate of chondral lesions as 63% in 31,516 knee arthroscopies. However, arthroscopy faces some limitations in that it cannot detect deep AC and subchondral bone lesions. Although usually well tolerated by the patient, arthroscopy is inherently associated with risks and discomforts of any invasive technique.

A challenge faced by the imaging industry is its limited ability to diagnose and assess initial structural changes of AC and bone developed at the early stage of degenerative diseases. Further development in imaging technology to improve visualization of cartilage integrity at the early stages of degeneration

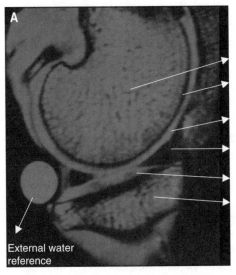
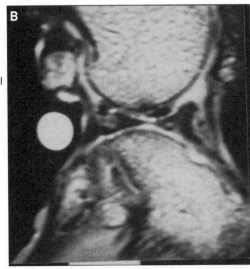

Femoral
condyle

Subchondral
bone

Articular
cartilage

Meniscus

Articular
cartilage

Tibial
plateau

External water
reference

Figure 4-5. Sagittal proton-density weighted magnetic resonance image of intact right knee joint of rhesus macaque. **A,** Normal. Note the smooth cartilage contour. **B,** Severe osteoarthritis. Note the high- and low-signal intensity in the articular cartilage, subchondral bone, and bone marrow.

will enhance the evaluation of cartilage changes resulting from interventions (e.g., therapies) in culture studies, tissue-engineered systems, animal models, and *in vivo* studies in humans. These new techniques have the potential as powerful diagnostic tools to detect and characterize pathologic load distributions across AC.

Articular Cartilage Repair

Current Treatment Method

AC is a complex structure that allows smooth, gliding movement of joints during skeletal mobility. However, cartilage is vulnerable to injuries and degenerative diseases over time. Joint pain caused by cartilage degeneration is a serious problem, affecting people of all ages (Buckwalter et al. 1998). Unlike the situation with other musculoskeletal tissues, the healing process, i.e., capacity to replenish its ECM in injured cartilage, is poor because of the avascular nature of AC and small chondrocyte population (Buckwalter et al. 1993). Moreover, the intrinsic healing response to cartilage injury decreases markedly with skeletal maturation. Hence, when disease or trauma affects the health of AC, an inevitable degenerative process occurs (Convery et al. 1972).

Cartilage repair (Bobic 1999; Bobic and Noble 2000) refers to the healing of injured cartilage or its replacement through cell proliferation and synthesis of new ECM. *Regeneration,* on the other hand, refers to the formation of an entirely new surface that essentially duplicates the native AC. Although full-thickness cartilage defects are capable of stimulating a repair response, the fibrous- or fibrocartilagenous repair tissue is morphologically, biochemically, and mechanically different from normal AC (Hasler et al. 1999, Mooney and Ferguson 1966). Therefore the repair tissue, which generally fails to replicate and/or maintain the structure, composition, and function of normal AC, is inferior and cannot withstand long-term, repetitive use. Although chondrocytes from the adjacent native cartilage have the capability for limited migration at the damaged site, they are not able to proliferate and secrete the essential macromolecules of ECM (Frenkel and Di Cesare 1999). Furthermore, from a macroscopic viewpoint, the complete repair of an AC defect requires good integration of repair tissue with the surrounding host cartilage and bone (Ahsan and Sah 1999; Peretti et al. 1999). However, these criteria are usually lacking or poorly represented in repaired tissue.

Recent advances in biology and materials science have pushed tissue engineering to the forefront of new cartilage repair techniques. Many procedures, often invasive, are currently employed to treat the dilemma of AC repair and regeneration, but none have had complete success. For a successful cartilage repair and regeneration program, the cartilage structure-function symbiotic relationship, how cartilage homeostasis is maintained, the relationship between mechanical loading of the cells/ECM and their corresponding biological responses, and how cartilage responds to the ever-changing mechanical environment must all be properly understood. Young and middle-aged patients typically have higher activity levels than older patients, and the implant-bearing material may wear because of higher physical activity over time. Total joint replacement is an adequate procedure for treating severely pathologic or traumatic lesions of AC in many patients, although generally short-lived and thus an unsuitable approach in young and middle-age patients. As such, localized resurfacing at the site of cartilage defect is a more desirable procedure. Current research efforts for cartilage repair in osteochondral defects includes transplantation of chondrocytes and mesenchymal stem cells; use of periosteal and perichondrial grafts; use of biological repair enhancers such as growth factors; and use of biocompatible/biodegradable synthetic or biological implant matrices (Buckwalter and Mankin 1998; Lee et al. 2000, 2001).

Lavage and Debridement

Lavage and débridement are basic arthroscopic techniques used to treat AC damage in the knee. The short-term benefits of "washing out" the loose cartilage fragments, catabolic enzymes, loose bodies, and flaps of damaged cartilage have been demonstrated (Johnson 1986; Dandy 1991). Currently, orthopaedic surgeons often débride joints, penetrate subchondral bone, and perform osteotomies with the intent of decreasing the clinical symptoms and restoring or maintaining a functional cartilage surface.

Clinical reports (Baumgartner et al. 1990; Jackson et al. 1988; Messner and Maletius 1996) on lavage and débridement procedures document initial improvement in clinical symptoms; however the long-term effect may be observed only in a few patients. Biopsy results of the repaired tissue from

patients having undergone this procedure were predominantly fibrous and fibrocartilagenous (Johnson 1991; Ogilvie-Harris and Fitsialos 1991), which do not exhibit the same structural, mechanical, or functional properties of AC. The failure of repair tissue, unable to withstand the load demands of the knee, led to recurrence of symptoms and enlargement of the defect. Factors associated with poor outcome also included creation of defects larger than the critical size of 1 cm and increased impact-loading activity (Dandy 1991). Several studies reported that the condition of patients treated with the above methods steadily deteriorated over a short period postoperatively (Baumgartner et al. 1990; Dzioba 1988; Gibson JN et al. 1992; Rand 1991). In one study (N=137), Jackson (1988) reported that 88% of patients experienced some initial improvement following this procedure. However, after a period of 3 years, the percent of patients with improvement decreased to 68%. Baumgartner (1990) also documented that 52% of 44 patients with OA demonstrated improvement after arthroscopic débridement; however, only 40% continued to benefit from the procedure at 33 months.

Abrasion, Drilling, and Microfracture

In an attempt to improve the long-term results of débridement and lavage, repair mechanisms have been directed toward bone marrow stimulation so that the nutrients and cells from the marrow blood can be brought to the chondral or osteochondral defect site. The blood elements that form a fibrin clot in the defect differentiate and remodel, resulting in a predominantly fibrocartilagenous repair tissue. The essential cells provided by the marrow blood are mesenchymal stem cells, which are pluripotential in nature and can differentiate into various tissue types: cartilage, fibrocartilage, fibrovascular, fibrous, and/or bone. The outcome depends on the biologic and mechanical environment in AC and the status of underlying bone of the knee joint.

Current methods used for bone marrow stimulation include arthroscopic abrasion, drilling, and microfracture (Bert and Maschka 1989; Buckwalter et al. 1994; Johnson 1986; Rodrigo et al. 1994). Each of these techniques includes débridement of the damaged AC remnants and any fibrous tissue within the defect to expose subchondral bone, thus allowing the clot to bind to the margins of the adjacent native cartilage. Abrasion arthroplasty involves the abrasion of the exposed subchondral bone surface with an arthroscopic burr to create a bleeding osteal surface. Arthroscopic drilling relies on multiple drill holes through the exposed subchondral bone to provide access to the marrow blood elements and formation of a clot in the defect. The microfracture technique, developed by Steadman et al (1999), involves surgical perforations through subchondral bone (every 3 to 4 mm) using sharp, awl-shaped picks. With this technique, small holes are created that penetrate the subchondral bone and provide access to the vascular channels of the bone.

To date, inconsistent results from abrasion arthroplasty have been reported. Johnson (1991) noted poor results in an older population of almost 400 patients (average age of 60 years). Postoperatively, 66% of these patients continued to have pain, and only 12% became symptom-free. Almost all of the patients had restriction in activity levels. Some independent clinical studies (Bert 1989; Friedman 1984; Rand 1991) demonstrated only 50% to 60% satisfactory results at 3- to 5-year follow-up using arthroscopic abrasion arthroplasty with better results occurring in younger patients. In a model for cartilage repair, Steadman et al. (1999) monitored and compared the healing of full-thickness AC defects in 12 horses treated with either abrasion arthroplasty or microfracture and evaluated the repair tissue at 2, 4, 6, and 8 weeks postoperatively. Histologic analysis confirmed that more repair tissue and a better quality tissue with good integration at the defect margin in microfractured lesions compared with lesions treated with abrasion arthroplasty. Before 6 weeks, collagen type I predominated, and at 6 weeks, collagen type II was first detected in microfractured lesions. At 8 weeks, aggrecan was predominant in the microfractured lesions. Clinically, arthroscopic microfracture of subchondral bone proved to be safe and effective for treating grade IV chondral lesions of the knee joint with a significant improvement (over 2 to 3 years) in functional outcomes and decreased pain in most patients. Rodrigo et al. (1994) reported the benefit of using continuous passive motion (CPM) after performing the microfracture technique. Arthroscopically, a significant improvement in the quality of the repair tissue (based on tissue morphology) in the CPM group versus the non-CPM group was noted.

Biologic Agents

Experimental models, both *in situ* and *in vitro*, have been developed to investigate the influence of biological agents, primarily growth factors, on cartilage repair. Several growth factors in cartilage and bone have potential to induce both chondrogenesis and osteogenesis. Bone growth factors have a role in the preservation of the cartilage matrix. The most common agents include bone morphogenetic proteins (BMPs), insulin-like growth factors (IGF-I), hepatocyte growth factor (HGF), basic fibroblast growth factor (FGF), and TGF-β (O'Connor et al. 2000). IGF-I is a polypeptide that is anabolic and mitogenic for cartilage. Research involving gene transfer, for example nonviral lipid-mediated gene, OP-1 gene, and human IGF-I cDNA have shown beneficial effects on cartilage repair (Madry et al. 2000, 2001; Matsumoto et al. 2001). The experiments involving the application of gene delivery to the tissue engineering of cartilage indicates that this technology has the potential to enhance the cartilage structural and functional properties.

Cell-seeded Approach

Another arena for cartilage repair involves the transplantation of osteochondral autologous grafts and allografts as well as autologous chondrocyte or mesenchymal implantation. In an attempt to improve the results of patients with full-thickness chondral defects, Homminga et al. (1990) used autologous perichondral grafts obtained from rib cartilage to repair grades III and IV chondral defects in the knees of 25 patients. Eighteen of the 25 patients showed marked functional improvement at 1 year. In another long-term study (8-year follow-up), 20% of the grafts had developed endochondral ossification at the repair site, and failure of procedure was evident in 60% of the patients (Homminga 1997). Similarly, late endochondral ossification and delamination of the perichondral grafts was noted by Minas (1997) and failure of 6 to 10 grafts was determined at 4 years. On the other hand, Kwan et al (1989) and Woo et al (1987) demonstrated that perichondrium autografts implanted in full-thickness cartilage defects in the rabbit femoral condyle produced hyaline-like cartilage. Furthermore, based on histology and biomechanical properties, they reported that intermittent passive motion did not produce better repair tissue than cast immobilization except within the initial 6-week period.

Autologous chondrocyte implantation involves excising and culturing chondrocytes originally harvested from the patient and their *in vivo* implantation after 3 to 4 weeks in culture. Another vehicle for placing autologous chondrocytes into the osteochondral defect is aided by an engineered, biologic or synthetic, scaffolds including agarose gel, alginate gel, collagen type I, collagen type II, or polyglycolic acid (PGA), and polylactic acid (PLLA) with other synthetic scaffolds. Chondrocytes impregnated in agarose and alginate gels or a highly porous scaffold fabricated from bovine tendon type I collagen and shark chondroitin-6-sulfate (CS) respond to dynamic mechanical stimulation or short-term compressive loading by upregulating collagen and PG synthesis (Buschman et al. 1995; Lee et al. 2001; Ragan et al. 2000; Sah et al. 1989). In rabbits with 3 mm–diameter osteochondral defects, a satisfactory cartilage healing response was reported in which allograft chondrocytes (Freed et al. 1984) or mesenchymal stem cells (Grande et al. 1995) were delivered using a PGA scaffold. Tissue-engineered cartilage constructs have also been created *in vitro* from isolated chondrocytes cultured on biomaterial scaffolds in bioreactors (Freed et al. 1999; Vunjak-Novakovic et al. 1999).

Noncell-seeded/Biosynthetic Approach

Orthopaedic industries are attempting to develop a product that has the potential to regenerate hyaline cartilage in focal lesions with a technology that is arthroscopically implantable, hence eliminating the need for radical surgery involving joint removal and replacement. Several implants, based on a non-cell-seeded approach are being developed for the repair of AC defects. An essential element of most cartilage tissue engineering strategies is a suitable, biocompatible, biodegradable, and bioabsorbable material that is inhomogeneous with optimal

porosity to allow permeation of cells and nutrients and to withstand confined compression. Such materials are able to significantly change the mechanical and electrochemical events within the ECM and thus the environments around chondrocytes. Oka et al. (1990) attempted to develop an artificial AC on the basis of a new viewpoint of joint biomechanics in which lubrication and load-bearing mechanisms of natural and artificial joints were compared. The application of dynamic deformational loading at physiological strain levels enhanced chondrocyte matrix elaboration in cell-seeded agarose scaffolds to produce a more functional engineered tissue construct than in free swelling controls. Sulfated GAG content and hydroxyproline content were found to be greater in dynamically loaded disks compared with free swelling controls at day 21 (Mauck et al. 2000). Another implant material, a rubberlike biocompatible gel called *Poly(vinyl alcohol)-hydrogel (PVA-H)*, showed favorable response (no inflammatory or degenerative changes) on cartilage repair and surrounding tissue (Oka 2001).

Future Prospects for Articular Cartilage Repair

Despite a variety of techniques aimed at cartilage repair (Buckwalter and Lohmander 1994; Dandy 1991; Johnson 1991; Ogilvie-Harris and Fitsialos 1991), no method has been successful at generating a cartilage matrix with the characteristics of normal hyaline cartilage that can withstand the demands placed on the chondral surfaces within the knee. Because of the deficiencies of various traditional repair techniques, current research is focused on developing a more durable repair tissue that displays the morphology and biologic and mechanical functions of hyaline cartilage, i.e., a repair tissue that will withstand high compressive forces and stress. In the future, the goal for treating joint degeneration is cartilage regeneration rather than prosthetic replacement. To achieve this goal, one must comprehend how structure and function and metabolic, biochemical, and biomechanical performance of AC can be restored. When cartilage is pressed, a mechanoelectrical transduction is believed to modulate the cellular activity of chondrocytes, which is fundamental for tissue repair. Clinical and experimental work has shown the important influence of loading and motion on the healing of AC and joints. Salter (1994, 1996, 1989) and O'Driscoll et al. (1984, 1986) investigated the effects of CPM on the repair process of tibial periosteal grafts implanted in rabbit knee joints. Histologic and biochemical analyses showed significantly superior cartilage healing with CPM than with immobilization or intermittent active motion. In all patients, regardless of the method used, the impact of rehabilitative procedures on the integrity and health of AC should be a consideration since unloading and overloading are detrimental to AC (Walker 1998).

The successful treatment of focal full-thickness articular defects of the knee has continued to present a great challenge, and to date no treatment method has provided consistent acceptable, long-term clinical results. Because of its avascular nature, AC exhibits a very limited capacity to regenerate and repair (Buckwalter et al. 1998). Although much of the tissue-engineered cartilage in existence is focused on mimicking the morphologic and biochemical constitutes of hyaline cartilage, these tissues are generally mechanically inferior compared with native cartilage with respect to their wear-resistant and weight-bearing functions. Patients with significant chondral defects often have persistent joint pain, swelling, and knee joint incongruency. In contrast to marrow stimulation and treatment techniques such as abrasion arthroplasty, drilling, or microfracture, all of which populate the defect with pluripotential stem cells, the use of cultured autologous chondrocytes fills the defect with cells of a committed pathway to develop hyaline-like cartilage. This hyaline-like cartilage more closely recreates the characteristics and durability of normal hyaline cartilage than the fibrous or fibrocartilage repair tissue formed by pluripotential stem cells. Another challenge in the orthopaedic field is the search for biomaterials suitable as artificial AC in joint restoration. Because AC plays a fundamental role in joint function, the biomaterial aims to mimic the behavior of the natural healthy surface.

The repair of cartilage defects by transplantation of chondrocytes or cell-seed matrices is promising but variable in effectiveness. The expression of exogenous growth factor genes in engineered cartilage may have the potential to modulate chondrogenesis. Gene transfer of growth factors into

cartilage might be used to enhance cartilage repair or to modulate the progression of cartilage degeneration, if a suitable delivery system could be identified. Gravitational forces were found to affect the initial localization of transplanted chondrocytes in articular defects. Further, static compression associated with tightness of the implant fit inhibited proliferation and matrix synthesis. Thus the mechanical environment was identified as a major regulatory factor of transplanted chondrocytes in cartilage repair therapies. Numerous surgical approaches that involve penetration of subchondral bone offer short-term to moderate-term relief of symptoms, whereas other approaches have seen significant improvement through transplantation of osteochondral and periosteal tissue and implantation of autologous chondrocytes. Furthermore, improvements in biochemical and molecular biologic techniques may allow advances in the understanding of chondrocyte and cartilage biology and may provide innovative and novel approaches to stimulating the repair of AC through biologic means.

Meniscal Anatomy

The menisci, originally referred to as *semilunar cartilage,* are wedge-shaped or C-shaped tissues located between the femoral condyle and tibial plateau. When viewed on their axial plane, the concave proximal surfaces of the menisci are in contact with the femoral condyle and the flat distal surfaces rest on the tibia. The medial meniscus is approximately semicircular whereas the lateral meniscus is somewhat circular (Figure 4-6). The menisci are attached to the joint capsule through their thick, convex peripheral borders, which are lined by the synovial membrane, whereas their thin inner borders taper into free edges. The vascular supply within the meniscus varies with age and anatomic location. An infant's meniscus is fully vascularized, whereas an adult meniscus is vascularized in the outer peripheral rim at one third to two thirds of the tissue adjacent to the joint capsule and is avascular towards the inner free edge (Arnoczky and Warren 1982; Ghadially et al. 1983; Petersen and Tillmann 1999). Blood vessels enter the meniscus from the adjacent joint capsule.

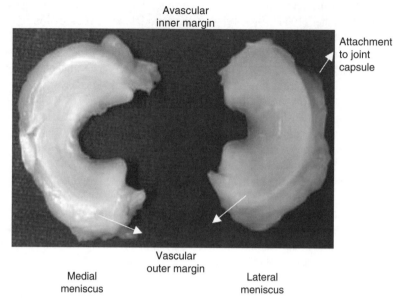

Figure 4-6. Excised menisci of the sheep knee joint. Note the semicircular medial meniscus, somewhat circular lateral meniscus, and the thick lateral margin.

Meniscal Structure

Gross examination of the meniscus reveals a white, glossy, and smooth tissue (Ghadially et al. 1978). Histologically, the meniscus is a dense, fibrocartilagenous connective tissue composed of an interlacing network of collagen fibers interposed with cells. The cells of the meniscus are responsible for synthesizing and maintaining the ECM. Whether the meniscal cells are specialized fibroblasts, chondrocytes, or a mixture of both cell types is unclear. Toward the surface layers, fusiform cells resembling fibroblasts have been identified. On the other hand, ovoid cells resembling chondrocytes, in that they are surrounded by territorial matrix with PG molecules, are more commonly found in the body of the meniscus. Because of its dual morphology and function, these cells have been appropriately referred to as *fibrochondrocytes* (Ghadially 1978; Ghadially et al. 1983).

The meniscus ECM is composed of a collagen fiber framework (65% to 70% by dry weight) interspersed with GAG molecules, matrix glycoproteins, and elastin (Ingman et al. 1974). The predominant collagen in meniscus is type I collagen (90%) with variable amounts of types II, III, IV, V, and VI (Eyre et al. 1983). Light and scanning electron microscopy revealed a three-dimensional array of collagen fibers in a cross-section of a meniscus (Aspden et al. 1985; Yasui 1978). A network of thin collagen fibrils lines the tibial and femoral surfaces of the menisci. Beneath the superficial network is a layer of irregularly aligned collagen bundles that intersect at various angles. The central part of the meniscus is predominantly composed of bundles of thick, coarser collagen fibers, which are primarily oriented in a parallel and circumferential manner. Although collagen fibers are arranged predominantly in the circumferential direction in the knee meniscus, evidence of radially oriented fibers within human menisci exists. Polarized light microscopy showed that the distribution of radial fibers varied greatly among the anterior, central, and posterior regions.

The GAG content of adult meniscus, ranging from 1% to 25% by dry weight varies with age and anatomic location. Various studies (McNicol and Roughley 1980; Roughley et al. 1981) reported the presence of C4S (10% to 20%), C6S (40%), DS (20% to 30%), and KS (15%) with traces of HS and HA. Matrix glycoproteins such as the link proteins, which stabilize the PG-HA aggregates, have been identified within the meniscal matrix (Fife 1985), along with traces of fibronectin (McDevitt and Webber 1990) and thrombospondin (Miller and McDevitt 1991).

Openings with canal-like structures were observed on the surface of the menisci. Their characteristic distribution indicated that they aid in nutrient transport from the synovial fluid to the normal avascular areas of the menisci (Neurath and Stofft 1992).

Meniscal Function and Biomechanics

Menisci are crucial structures within the human knee with clinical importance to joint biomechanics. They maintain knee joint stability and congruity and resist capsular/synovial impingement during locomotion (King 1936). They ensure functional joint congruence guided by the cruciate ligaments, and by achieving functional congruity, they create stability. The menisci contribute to energy/shock absorption during dynamic loading, transmit load in the knee joint, distribute stresses over a large cartilage contact area, and assist in joint lubrication in the contact area between the tibia and femur (Arnoczky et al. 1988; Hoshino and Wallace 1987; Walker and Erkman 1975; Radin et al. 1984). Menisci "elastically" limit rotation and translation movements. Depending on the knee flexion angle, femoral translation and rotation, a mobile meniscus can transmit 50% to 90% of load over the knee joint (Aagaard and Verdonk 1999). Biomechanical studies have demonstrated that at least 50% of the compressive load of the knee joint is transmitted through the meniscus in extension and about 85% of the load is transmitted in 90 degrees of flexion (Ahmed et al. 1992). These meniscal functions enhance the ability of AC to provide a smooth, near-frictionless articulation and to distribute loads evenly to the underlying bone of the femur and tibia.

The ability of menisci to perform the various biomechanical functions is based on their intrinsic material property, anatomic structure, and tissue attachments (Fithian et al. 1990). The material properties of the meniscus are determined by their biochemical composition and concentration, the collagen architecture and interactions of major tissue constituents, namely tissue fluid, PGs, and collagens. Fluid pressurization of the meniscus is an important mechanism for load support and distribution in the knee joint (Mow 1992). The hydraulic permeability is an important parameter governing fluid pressurization and flow-dependent mechanical effects in the meniscus. The meniscal structure and function allows it to adapt to all physiological loading conditions thereby providing knee joint stability. The shape of the menisci and the variability of the collagen fibril diameters and their characteristic orientation are optimal for weight bearing and shock absorption. Meniscal tissue exhibits intrinsic viscoelastic behavior in shear that depends on frequency, shear strain, and compressive strain. The anisotropic shear properties of the meniscus are related to its collagen fiber orientation (Zhu et al. 1994; Spilker et al. 1992). The coarse, circumferential type I collagen fiber bundles of the middle layer provide the meniscus with high tensile stiffness (within a range of 100 to 300 megapascals) and strength, contributes to its capability to resist tensile forces and functions as a transmitter of load across the knee joint (Aspden et al. 1985; Fithian et al. 1990; Yasui 1978). On the other hand, the radial collagen fibers provide structural rigidity and help resist longitudinal splitting of the menisci resulting from undue compression by altering the radial tensile properties of the meniscus (Skaggs et al. 1994). *In vitro* experiments (Zhu et al. 1994) have shown that at low compressive strains (less than or equal to 10%), the circumferentially oriented specimens are stiffer in shear than the axially and radially oriented specimens. However, statistically significant differences between the circumferentially and axially oriented specimens were not observed at high compressive strains (greater than 10%). Leslie et al. (2000) investigated the response of human meniscus to axial, radial, and circumferential compressive forces at physiologically relevant levels of load. They reported that the meniscus was significantly stiffer in response to axial compressive forces than to radial or circumferential forces.

Interactions among the important constituents of the ECM enhances the meniscal strength and allows the meniscus to behave as a fiber-reinforced, porous, permeable composite material similar to AC, in which frictional drag caused by fluid flow determines its response to dynamic loading (Fithian et al. 1990). Energy dissipation or shock absorption by the menisci, the consequence of high frictional drag caused by low permeability of the matrix, is about one-sixth as permeable as that of AC. The meniscal dynamic shear modulus is only one fourth to one sixth as great as that of AC. The menisci are one-half as stiff in compression and dissipate more energy under dynamic loading in comparison to AC. The menisci of the knee joint enlarge the area of support to more than twice the surface of AC contact.

Meniscal Degradation

The menisci play an integral part in the complex biomechanics of the knee joint. Loss of meniscal structure or function eventually leads to progressive degenerative joint disease of the knees and the deterioration of the AC. Mechanical injury to the knee joint results in cell death in the form of apoptosis. Clinically, significant apoptosis in meniscus is usually obtained either through traumatic meniscal tears or degenerative processes. Meniscal apoptosis has been observed from human osteoarthritic knees and in the meniscus from rabbit knees with a transected anterior cruciate ligament (Rodkey 2000).

Several experimental models of meniscectomy have been used to study degeneration of the joint tissues in various animal species (Berjon et al. 1991; Ghosh et al. 1990; Hoch et al. 1983; King 1936; Lindhorst et al. 2000; Little et al. 1996; Lutfi 1975; LeRoux et al. 2000; Mayor and Moskowitz 1974; Moskowitz et al. 1973). Partial or total meniscectomy results in altered joint kinematics, decreased contact area, and associated increases in the magnitude and gradient of contact stresses (Ahmed 1992). In canine studies (King 1936; Cox et al 1977), the development of arthritis, i.e., extent of degenerative changes, was proportional to the amount of meniscus excised. Resection of as little as 15% to 34% of the meniscus increased contact pressures (load per unit area) by more than 350%, resulting in AC damage (Seedhom and Hargreaves 1979). Voloshin et al. (1983) reported that the shock-absorbing capacity of the normal knee is almost 20% higher than that of meniscectomized knees.

Radiological and pathological aberrations of meniscectomized knees include osteophyte formation, joint space narrowing, and condylar flattening. LeRoux et al. (2000) reported that meniscectomy leads to abnormal mechanical function of AC. The decreased concentration of the sulfated GAGs positively correlated with the equilibrium compressive modulus, whereas the shear properties of cartilage directly correlated with collagen fibrillar organization measured at the superficial lamina of corresponding sites. Other changes in cartilage biochemical composition and metabolism after partial or complete meniscectomy include altered PG structure, increased collagen and PG biosynthesis, and elevated synovial fluid biomarkers. Without the meniscus, stress concentration occurs in the knee in conjunction with abnormal joint mechanics, and premature development of arthritic changes from collagen stress occurs. The circular arrangement of collagen fibrils in the central portion of the meniscus provides a functional explanation for the longitudinal orientation of the majority of tears in the meniscus (Petersen 1998). *In vitro* experiments (Fink et al. 2001) have shown that dynamic mechanical stress influences the biological activity of meniscal cells and that the nitric oxide production in vivo could be, in part, regulated by mechanical stress acting upon the menisci. Further, meniscal fibrochondrocytes also respond to environmental mediators such as growth factors and cytokines.

Meniscal Repair

Traumatic meniscal injury is one of the significant factors leading to secondary OA. This has been attributed to structural damage leading to alteration in load transfer across the knee. Treatment of injured or diseased menisci has generally been by surgical repair, transplantation, and excision. The goal of meniscus surgery is to relieve the symptoms associated with the tear and to preserve the meniscal function as much as possible. Minimal partial meniscectomy performed arthroscopically or meniscal repair when practical have become the standard treatments. Therefore great efforts have been directed toward preserving as much of the meniscus as possible.

Allografting or meniscal transplantation is one method of replacement, which has been executed both in dogs and humans. Replacement of an injured meniscus in an otherwise healthy joint can prevent arthritic changes and stabilize the joint. In diseased joints, replacement of the meniscus can reduce the progression of the disease process and provide pain relief. However, the transplantation approach has been only partially successful over the long term because of the host's immunological response to the graft, to failures in the cryopreservation process, and to failures of the attachment sites.

Clinical studies have shown that early mobilization while minimizing loading of healing tissues can prevent complications of prolonged immobilization after knee surgery. Sommerlath (1991) and Lynch et al. (1983) reported that meniscal repair results in a significantly lower incidence of arthritis compared with partial or total meniscectomy. Anderson et al. (1993) documented that by preventing weight bearing while permitting limited mobility of the knee prevents or minimizes detrimental effect on the tensile properties of the meniscus in the circumferential direction (Anderson et al. 1993).

In a study on the canine meniscus, King (1936) was the first to document healing of meniscus. He reported that the meniscal tears that extended into the highly vascularized meniscosynovial junction showed a healing response. Meniscus is capable of self repair when exposed to bleeding tissues; however, the intrinsic ability of meniscus to heal itself is limited only to the vascular region of the tissue. The potential of meniscal repair is determined by the vascular supply of the meniscus and the ability of the peripheral blood supply to support the inflammatory response associated with the process of wound healing (Arnoczky et al. 1982). Repair of meniscal tears occurs mostly in the region of the capsular attachment. The farther the tear from the site of capsular attachment, the less the vascularity and the healing response. Studies (Roeddecker et al. 1993) have shown that meniscal fibrochondrocytes have the ability to migrate into a defect filled with a fibrin clot and to form fibrocartilagenous tissue similar to that of normal meniscal tissue. Meniscal cells in tissue culture are capable of cell division and matrix synthesis. LeRoux et al. (2001) provided insight into the significance of fluid pressurization and suggested that a low permeability to fluid flow is an important characteristic to emulate in meniscal repair.

Current meniscal repair techniques employ sutures, staples, or biological adhesives. The adhesives have the theoretical advantage of minimizing the gap and providing full contact of the bonded surfaces, which may in turn aid repair.

Recent trends in meniscal repair and regeneration also include the implant of commercially available resorbable or nonresorbable scaffolds. Menisci have also been replaced with prostheses constructed from artificial resilient materials such as plastic, silicone rubber or Teflon coating, with reinforcing materials of stainless steel or nylon strands. These prostheses are designed to withstand the high and repeated loads encountered within the knee and to minimize the possibility of an immunological response. Prostheses composed of a single or composite macromolecule of the meniscus ECM not considered to be immunogenic to the body, such as type I collagen scaffold, is under investigation. Generally, the replacement of meniscal tissue with structures consisting of artificial materials has been unsuccessful because the opposing AC cannot withstand abrasive interfaces caused by the implant.

The most common meniscal lesion in young patients is the longitudinal bucket-handle lesion, which is usually located in the avascular region of the meniscus and is incapable of repair. A technique creating an access channel to the avascular region for tissue ingrowth, originating from the synovial lining has been described (Arnoczky and Warren 1983). Klompmaker et al. (1996) created longitudinal lesions in the avascular part of the dog's meniscus and implanted porous polyurethane in a full-thickness defect to connect the synovial tissue with the central rim of the meniscus. They reported fibrocartilagenous ingrowth into the porous polymer and better healing compared with the empty defects. Van Tienen et al. (2001) reported the repair characteristics of longitudinal lesions in lateral menisci after implantation of a porous polymer. At 6 months, the implant integrated well with the native meniscal tissue and induced formation of fibrocartilage, whereas the controls with empty defects had poor margin integration filled with a fibrous defect. Furthermore, implantation of a polymer induced less cartilage degeneration. A degrading porous polymer is a promising biocompatible scaffold that enables a vascular repair tissue to reach lesions in the avascular zone and to rapidly restore the fibrocartilage in the created defect.

Efforts must be continued to find better techniques to manage meniscal injuries. In the future, availability of better repair techniques and the option of meniscal replacement with allograft or prosthetic menisci are expected to improve outcomes. This in turn will help minimize the instability of the joint, decrease pain associated with loss of the meniscus, minimize or prevent degenerative joint changes, and obviate the need for multiple surgical procedures. Specific targets should include improved methods of meniscectomy, new and better techniques of repair for meniscus tears, methods to enhance the cellular response for healing of meniscus tissue, and, finally, new ways to regenerate lost or damaged tissue.

Summary

To understand the repair mechanisms of cartilage and meniscus, a detailed knowledge of their structure and function, their relationship, and the intricate balance between matrix synthesis and degradation is required. External stimuli that induce an internal stress field in these arthrodial soft tissues are known to play an important role in their biomechanical properties. Current clinical and research interest in orthopaedics lie in the concepts and mechanisms of cartilage and meniscal repair and regeneration.

Normal adult cartilage is an avascular, alymphatic and aneural dense connective tissue. AC depends on long-range diffusion of the nutrient-filled synovial fluid to provide nourishment to its cells and ECM. Cartilage canals also contribute to the cartilage nourishment, which are more abundant in immature AC compared with mature AC. The tissue fluid along with the biochemical composition and interaction of various molecules within cartilage determine the biomechanical properties of the cartilage. The functional integrity of AC is dependent on (1) the low hydraulic permeability and high swelling pressure of the highly sulfated proteoglycan moiety and (2) the entrapment and confinement of the PGs caused by the tensile strength and swelling-resistant nature of the collagen fiber network within various cartilage laminae. The structurally and functionally differentiated lamina and matrices of cartilage act synergistically to provide an integrated biological hydroelastic suspension system capable of absorbing, redistributing, and transmitting functional compressive forces across articulating joints. The efficacy of this system is primarily dependent on the variation in stiffness, compliance, and compressibility of the collagen and PG components within each matrix component and the metabolic response of the chondrocyte to mechanical, physiochemical, and osmotic changes induced in the AC matrix during physiological function. The menisci are fibrocartilagenous connective tissue composed of interlacing thick collagen fibers that are of clinical significance to joint biomechanics. They play a crucial role in knee joint stability and congruity and contribute to shock absorption and transmission during locomotion.

The mechanical forces to which AC and meniscus are normally exposed *in vivo* are insufficient to destroy these tissues directly. However, biochemical/enzymatic attack, gene mutations, or abnormal biomechanical impact compromises the chemical integrity of the matrix, resulting in cartilage degradation, which eventually leads to conditions such as spontaneous degenerative arthritis. Mechanical forces are more likely to destroy cartilage indirectly through insults to the subchondral bone, synovium, meniscus or chondrocytes. Damage to the meniscus results in abnormal mechanical function of AC, inevitably leading to cartilage degeneration. Although excessive forces lead to loss of cartilage, removal of all mechanical stimulation leads to atrophy. Some intermediate level and frequency of loading maintain normal cartilage structure and function. Current research activities in the field of musculoskeletal sciences and orthopaedics focus on various strategies involved in the repair and regeneration of cartilage and meniscal tissues.

References

Aagaard H, Verdonk R. Function of the normal meniscus and consequences of meniscal resection. Scand J Med Sci Sports 1999;9(3):134-140.

Adams MA et al. Experimental determination of stress distributions in articular cartilage before and after sustained loading. Clin Biomech 1999;14(2):88-96.

Agemura DH, O'Brien WD. Ultrasonic propagation properties of articular cartilage at 100 MHz. J Acoust Soc Am 1990;87(4):1786-1791.

Agraves SW et al. Structural features of cartilage matrix protein deduced from cDNA. Proc Natl Acad Sci USA 1987;84:464-468.

Ahmed AM. The Load-bearing Role of the Knee Menisci. In VC Mow et al. (eds), Knee Meniscus: Basic and Clinical Foundations. New York: Raven Press, 1992:59-73.

Ahsan T, Sah RL. Biomechanics of integrative cartilage repair. Osteoarthr Cartilage 1999;7(1):29-40.

Aigner T et al. Independent expression of fibril-forming collagens I, II, and III in chondrocytes of human osteoarthritic cartilage. J Clin Invest 1993;91:829-837.

Akizuki S et al. Tensile properties of human knee joint cartilage: I. Influence of ionic conditions, weight bearing, and fibrillation on the tensile modulus. J Orthop Res 1986;4(4):379-392.

Alparslan L et al. Magnetic resonance imaging of autologous chondrocyte implantation. Semin Ultrasound CT MR 2001;22(4):341-351.

Altman R et al. Development of criteria for the classification and reporting of osteoarthritis. Arthritis Rheum 1986;29:1039-1049.

Anderson DD et al. The influence of basal cartilage calcification on dynamic juxtaarticular stress transmission. Clin Orthop 1993;(286):298-307.

Anderson DR et al. The effects of non-weight-bearing and limited motion on the tensile properties of the meniscus. Arthroscopy 1993;9(4):440-445.

Arnoczky SP et al. Meniscal repair using an exogenous fibrin clot: An experimental study in dogs. J Bone Joint Surg Am 1988;70(8):1209-1217.

Arnoczky SP, Warren RF. The microvasculature of the meniscus and its response to injury: An experimental study in the dog. Am J Sport Med 1983;11(3):131-141.

Arnoczky SP, Warren RF. Microvasculature of the human meniscus. Am J Sport Med 1982;10:90-95.

Arokoski JP et al. Normal and pathological adaptations of articular cartilage to joint loading. Scand J Med Sci Sport 2000;10(4):186-198.

Aspden RM et al. Collagen orientations in the meniscus of the knee joint. J Anat 1985;140:371-380.

Babyn PS et al. High-resolution magnetic resonance imaging of normal porcine cartilaginous epiphyseal maturation. J Magn Reson Imaging 1996;6(1):172-179.

Babyn PS et al. MRI of the cartilaginous epiphysis of the femoral head in the piglet hip after ischemic damage. J Magn Reson Imaging 1998;8(3):717-723.

Bachrach NM et al. Incompressibility of the solid matrix of articular cartilage under high hydrostatic pressures. J Biomech 1998;31(5):445-451.

Bank RA et al. Ageing and zonal variation in post-translational modification of collagen in normal human articular cartilage. The age-related increase in non-enzymatic glycation affects biomechanical properties of cartilage. Biochem J 1998;330(Pt 1):345-351.

Basser PJ et al. Mechanical properties of the collagen network in human articular cartilage as measured by osmotic stress technique. Arch Biochem Biophys 1998;351(2):207-219.

Baumgartner MR et al. Arthroscopic debridement of the arthritic knee. Clin Orthop 1990;253;197-202.

Beaupre GS et al. Mechanobiology in the development, maintenance, and degeneration of articular cartilage. J Rehabil Res Dev 2000;37(2):145-151.

Bendele AM, Hulman JF. Spontaneous cartilage degeneration in guinea pigs. Arthritis Rheum 1998;31:561-565.

Benninghoff A. Form und bau der gelenkknorpel in ihren beziehungen zur funktion. Zweiter teil: Der aufbau des gelenkknorpels in seinin beziehungen zur funktion. Zeitschrift fuer Anatomie und Entwicklungsgeschichte (English Translation). 1925;76(1):43-63.

Berjon JJ et al. Degenerative lesions in the articular cartilage after meniscectomy. Preliminary experimental study in dogs. J Trauma 1991;31:342-350.

Bert JM, Maschka K. The arthroscopic treatment of unicompartmental gonarthrosis: a five-year follow-up study of abrasion arthroplasty plus arthroscopic debridement and arthroscopic debridement alone. Arthroscopy 1989;5:25-32.

Blackburn WD Jr et al. Cartilage imaging in osteoarthritis. Semin Arthritis Rheum 1996;25(4):273-281.

Bobic V. The Utilization of Osteochondral Autografts in the Treatment of Articular Cartilage Lesions. International Society of Arthroscopy, Knee Surgery and Orthopaedic Sports Medicine. Anaheim, Danville (CA, USA) Feb 5 1999:1-4.

Bobic V, Noble J. Articular cartilage—to repair or not to repair. J Bone Joint Surg Br 2000;82(2):165-166.

Brama PA et al. Influence of site and age on biochemical characteristics of the collagen network of equine articular cartilage. Am J Vet Res 1999;60:341-345.

Bruckner P et al. Type IX collagen from sternal cartilage of chicken embryo contains covalently bound glycosaminoglycans. Proc Natl Acad Sci USA 1985;82:2608-2612.

Buckwalter JA, Mankin HJ. Articular cartilage: degeneration and osteoarthritis, repair, regeneration, and transplantation. Instr Course Lect 1998;47:487-504.

Buckwalter JA, Mankin HJ. Articular cartilage repair and transplantation. Arthritis Rheum 1998;41(8):1331-1342.

Buckwalter J et al. Soft tissue aging and musculoskeletal function. J Bone Joint Surg 1993;75(10):1533-1548.

Buckwalter JA, Lohmander S. Operative treatment of osteoarthritis. J Bone Joint Surg Am 1994;76:1405-1418.

Burr DB. The importance of subchondral bone in osteoarthrosis. Curr Opin Rheumatol 1998;10(3):256-262.

Burton-Wurster N, Lust G. Fibronectin and water content of articular cartilage explants after partial depletion of proteoglycans. J Orthop Res 1986;4:437-445.

Buschmann MD et al. Mechanical compression modulates matrix biosynthesis in chondrocytes/agarose culture. J Cell Sci 1995;108(Pt 4):1497-1508.

Camosso ME, Marotti G. The mechanical behaviour of articular cartilage under compressive stress. J Bone Joint Surg 1962;44(A):699-709.

Carsons S, Horn VJ. Chondronectin in human synovial fluid. Ann Rheum Dis 1988;47:797-800.

Carter DR et al. Influences of mechanical stress on prenatal and postnatal skeletal development. Clin Orthop 1987;(219):237-250.

Chateauvert JM et al. Spontaneous osteoarthritis in rhesus macaques. II. Characterization of disease and morphometric studies. J Rheumatol 1990;17(1):73-83.

Chen JR et al. Pentosidine in synovial fluid in osteoarthritis and rheumatoid arthritis: relationship with disease activity in rheumatoid arthritis. J Rheumatol 1998;25:2440-2444.

Chevalier X. Fibronectin, cartilage, and osteoarthritis. Semin Arthritis Rheum 1993;22:307-317.

Chevalier X et al. Influence of interleukin 1 beta on tenascin distribution in human normal and osteoarthritic cartilage: A quantitative immunohistochemical study. Ann Rheum Dis 1996;55:772-775.

Clark JM. The structure of vascular channels in the subchondral plate. J Anat 1990;171:105-115.

Clark RAF. Fibronectin matrix deposition and fibronectin receptor expression in healing and normal skin. J Invest Dermatol 1990;94:128S-134S.

Cohen NP et al. Composition and dynamics of articular cartilage: structure, function, and maintaining healthy state. J Orthop Sport Phys Ther 1998;28(4):203-215.

Convery F et al. The repair of large osteochondral defects: An experimental study in horses. Clin Orthop 1972;82:253-262.

Couchman JR et al. Fibronectin-Cell interactions. J Invest Dermatol 1990;94:7S-14S.

Cox JS, Cordell LD. The degenerative effects of medial meniscus tears in dogs' knees. Clin Orthop 1977;125:236-242.

Cremer MA et al. The cartilage collagens: a review of their structure, organization, and role in the pathogenesis of experimental arthritis in animals and in human rheumatic disease. J Mol Med 1998;76:275-288.

Cs-Szabo G et al. Changes in messenger RNA and protein levels of proteoglycans and link protein in human osteoarthritic cartilage samples. Arthritis Rheum 1997;40:1037-1045.

Curl WW et al. Cartilage injuries: a review of 31,516 knee arthroscopies. Arthroscopy 1997;13(4):456-460.

Dandy DJ. Arthroscopic debridement of the knee for osteoarthritis (editorial). J Bone Joint Surg Br 1991;73:877-888.

De Ceuninck F et al. Purification of guinea pig YKL 40 and modulation of its secretion by cultured articular chondrocytes. J Cell Biochem 1998;69:414-424.

Dieppe P. Recommended methodology for assessing the progression of OA of the hip and knee joints. Osteoarthr Cartilage 1995;3:73-77.

Dzioba R. The classification and treatment of acute articular cartilage lesions. Arthroscopy 1988;4:72-80.

Durr J et al. Identification and immunolocalization of laminin in cartilage. Exp Cell Res 1996;22:225-233.

Eyre DR et al. Collagen cross-linking in human bone and articular cartilage. Age-related changes in the content of mature hydroxypyridinium residues. Biochem J 1988;252(2):495-500.

Eyre DR, Wu JJ. Collagen of fibrocartilage: A distinctive molecular phenotype in bovine meniscus. FEBS Lett 1983;158(2):265-270.

Eyre DR et al. Cartilage-Specific Collagens. Structural Studies. In K. Keuttner et al (eds), Articular Cartilage and Osteoarthritis. Raven: New York, 1992;119-131.

Eyre D, Wu JJ. Type XI or 1, 2, 3 Collagen. In R Mayne and RE Burgeson (eds): Structure and Function of Collagen Types. Orlando: Academic Press, 1987:261-281.

Eyre DR et al. A growing family of collagens in articular cartilage: Identification of 5 genetically distinct types. J Rheumatol 1987;14:25-27.

Falcovitz YH et al. Compressive properties of normal human articular cartilage:age, depth and compositional dependencies (Abstr). 47th Annual Meeting, San Francisco: Orthopaedic Research Society, Feb. 25-28, 2001;26:58.

Fife RS. Identification of link proteins and a 116,000-Dalton matrix protein in canine meniscus. Arch Biochem Biophys 1985;240:682-688.

Fife RS, Brandt KD. Cartilage matrix glycoprotein is present in serum in experimental canine osteoarthritis. J Clin Invest 1989;84:1432-1439.

Fink C et al. The effect of dynamic mechanical compression on nitric oxide production in the meniscus. Osteoarthr Cartilage 2001;9(5):481-487.

Fithian DC et al. Material properties and structure-function relationships in the menisci. Clin Orthop 1990;252: 19-31.

Foster FS et al. Advances in ultrasound biomicroscopy. Ultrasound Med Biol 2000;26(1):1-27.

Frazer WD. The collagen crosslinks pyridinoline and deoxypyridinoline: A review of their biochemistry, physiology, measurement, and clinical applications. J Clin Ligand Assay 1998;21:102-110.

Freed LE et al. Joint resurfacing using allograft chondrocytes and synthetic biodegradable polymer scaffolds. J Biomed Mater Res 1984;28:891-899.

Freed et al. Frontiers in tissue engineering: In vitro modulation of chondrogenesis. Clin Orthop (Suppl) 1999;367:S46-S58.

Frenkel SR, Di Cesare PE. Degradation and repair of articular cartilage. Front Biosci 1999;4:D671-D685.

Friedman MJ et al. Preliminary results with abrasion arthroplasty in the osteoarthritic knee. Clin Orthop 1984;182:200-205.

Fry ME et al. High-resolution magnetic resonance imaging of the interphalangeal joints of the hand. Skeletal Radiol 1991;20:273-277.

Fujimoto D. Isolation and characterization of a fluorescent material in bovine Achilles tendon collagen. Biochem Biophys Res Commun 1977;76:1124-1129.

Fujimoto D et al. The structure of pyridinoline, a collagen crosslink. Biochem Biophys Res Commun 1978;84: 52-57.

Gahunia HK et al. Osteoarthritis in Rhesus Macaques: Assessment of Cartilage Matrix Quality by Quantitative Magnetic Resonance Imaging. In WB van den Berg et al. (eds): Joint Destruction in Arthritis and Osteoarthritis (Agents and Actions Supplements, Vol 39). Basel: Birkhäuser, 1993:255-259.

Gahunia HK et al. Osteoarthritis staging: comparison between magnetic resonance imaging, gross pathology and histopathology in the rhesus macaque. Osteoarthr Cartilage. 1995;3(3):169-180.

Gahunia HK et al. Osteoarthritis in rhesus macaque knee joint: quantitative magnetic resonance imaging tissue characterization of articular cartilage. Osteoarthr Cartilage 1995;22:1747-1756.

Gannon JM et al. Localization of type X collagen in canine growth plate and adult canine articular cartilage. J Orthop Res 1991;9:485-494.

Ghadially FN. Fine Structure of Joints. In L Sokoloff (ed): The Joints and Synovial Fluid (Vol 1). New York: Academic Press, 1978;105-176.

Ghadially FN. Fine Structure of Synovial Joints. In FN Ghadially (ed): A Text and Atlas of the Ultrastructure of Normal and Pathological Articular Tissues. London: Butterworth, 1983:103-144.

Ghadially FN et al. Ultrastructure of normal and torn menisci of the human knee joint. J Anat 1983;136 (Pt 4):773-791.

Ghadially FN et al. Ultrastructure of rabbit semilunar cartilages. J Anat 1978;125:499-517.

Ghosh P, Cheras PA. Vascular mechanisms in osteoarthritis. Best Pract Res Clin Rheumatol 2001;15(5):693-709.

Ghosh P et al. The influence of weight-bearing exercise on articular cartilage of meniscectomized joints: an experimental study in sheep. Clin Orthop 1990;252:101-113.

Gibson JN et al. Arthroscopic lavage and debridement for osteoarthritis of the knee. J Bone Joint Surg Br 1992;74:534-537.

Girkontaite I et al. Immunolocalization of type X collagen in normal fetal and adult osteoarthritic cartilage with monoclonal antibodies. Matrix Biol 1996;15:231-238.

Glant TT et al. Appearance and persistence of fibronectin in cartilage. Specific interaction of fibronectin with collagen type II. Histochemistry 1985;82:149-158.

Grande DA et al. Repair of articular cartilage defects using mesenchymal stem cells. Tissue Eng 1995;1(4):345-353.

Grandhee SK, Monnier VM. Mechanism of formation of the Maillard protein cross-link pentosidine. J Biol Chem 1991;266:11649-11653.

Green WT et al. Microradiographic study of the calcified layer of articular cartilage. Arch Pathol 1970;90(2):151-158.

Grynpas MD et al. Collagen type II differs from type I in native molecular packing. Biochim Biophys Acta 1980;626:346-355.

Hagg R et al. Cartilage fibrils of mammals are biochemically heterogeneous: differential distribution of decorin and collagen IX. J Cell Biol 1998;142:285-294.

Hakala BE et al. Human cartilage gp-39, a major secretory product of articular chondrocytes and synovial cells, is a mammalian member of a chitinase protein family. J Biol Chem 1993;268:25803-25810.

Hambach L et al. Severe disturbances of the distribution and expression of type VI collagen chains in osteoarthritic articular cartilage. Arthritis Rheum 1998;41:986-996.

Hammerman D et al. Diarthrodial joints revisited. J Bone Joint Surg 1970;52-A:725-744.

Harris ED Jr. Mechanisms of disease: Rheumatoid arthritis-pathophysiology and implications for therapy. N Engl J Med 1990;322:1277-1289.

Harvey S et al. Chondrex: new marker of joint disease. Clin Chem 1998;44:509-516.

Hasler EM et al. Articular cartilage biomechanics: theoretical models, material properties, and biosynthetic response. Crit Rev Biomed Eng 1999;27(6):415-488.

Havelka S et al. The calcified-noncalcified cartilage interface: the tidemark. Acta Biol Hung 1984;35(2-4):271-279.

Hayes WC, Bodine AJ. Flow-independent viscoelastic properties of articular cartilage matrix. J Biomech 1978;11:407-419.

Hedbom E et al. Cartilage matrix proteins. An acidic oligomeric protein (COMP) detected only in cartilage. J Biol Chem 1992;267:6132-6136.

Helminen HJ et al. Regular joint loading in youth assists in the establishment and strengthening of the collagen network of articular cartilage and contributes to the prevention of osteoarthrosis later in life: a hypothesis. J Bone Miner Metab 2000;18(5):245-257.

Hoch DH et al. Early changes in material properties of rabbit articular cartilage after meniscectomy. J Orthop Res 1983;1:4-12.

Hodler J, Resnik D. Current status of imaging of articular cartilage. Skeletal Radiol 1996;25:703-709.

Homandberg GA et al. Cartilage damaging activities of fibronectin fragments derived from cartilage and synovial fluid. Osteoarthr Cartilage 1998;6:231-244.

Homminga GN. Long-term follow-up of perichondral grafting for cartilage lesions of the knee. Bermuda: Cartilage Repair Symposium, August 1997.

Homminga GN et al. Perichondral grafting for cartilage lesions of the knee. J Bone Joint Surg Br 1990;72:1003-1007.

Hoshino A, Wallace WA. Impact-absorbing properties of the human knee. J Bone Joint Surg Br 1987;69(5):807-811.

Huber M et al. Anatomy, biochemistry, and physiology of articular cartilage. Invest Radiol 2000;35(10):573-580.

Hukins DW et al. Fiber reinforcement and mechanical stability in articular cartilage. Eng Med 1984;13(3):153-156.

Hunziker EB. Articular Cartilage Structure in Humans and Experimental Animals. In K Kuetter et al. Articular Cartilage and Osteoarthritis (Ed). New York: Raven Press, 1992:183-199.

Hutton CW et al. Magnetic resonance imaging of cartilage microstructure in normal and osteoarthritic interphalangeal joints. 11th Annual Scientific Meeting. Proceedings of Society of Magnetic Resonance in Medicine. (Abstract) 1992:416.

Inerot S et al. Articular cartilage proteoglycans in ageing and osteoarthritis. Biochem J 1978;169:143-156.

Imhof H et al. Degenerative joint disease: cartilage or vascular disease? Degenerative joint disease: cartilage or vascular disease? Skeletal Radiol 1997;26(7):398-403.

Imhof H et al. Importance of subchondral bone to articular cartilage in health and disease. Top Magn Reson Imaging 1999;10(3):180-92.

Ingman AM et al. Variation of collagenous and non-collagenous proteins of human knee joint menisci with age and degeneration. Gerontology 1974;20:212-223.

Jackson RW et al. Arthroscopic debridement versus arthroplasty in the osteoarthritic knee. J Arthroplasty 1997;12(4):465-469.

Jeffery AK et al. Three-dimensional collagen architecture in bovine articular cartilage. J Bone Joint Surg Br 1991;73(B):795-801.

Johansen JS et al. A new biochemical marker for joint injury. Analysis of YKL-40 in serum and synovial fluid. Br J Rheumatol 1993;32:949-955.

Johansen JS et al. Serum YKL-40 levels on healthy children and adults. Comparison with serum and synovial fluid levels of YKL-40 in patients with osteoarthritis or trauma of the knee joint. Br J Rheumatol 1996; 35:553-559.

Johnson LL. Arthroscopic Abrasion Arthroplasty. In JB McGinty (ed): Operative Arthroscopy. New York: Raven Press, 1991:341-360.

Jones Kl et al. An immunohistochemical study of fibronectin in human osteoarthritic and disease free articular cartilage. Ann Rheum Dis 1987;46:809-815.

Jurvelin JS et al. Topographical variation of the elastic properties of articular cartilage in the canine knee. J Biomech 2000;33(6):669-675.

Kaab MJ et al. Effect of mechanical load on articular cartilage collagen structure: a scanning electron-microscopic study. Cells Tissues Organs 2000;167(2-3):106-120.

Kelly PA, O'Connor JJ. Transmission of rapidly applied loads through articular cartilage. Part 1: Uncracked cartilage. Proc Inst Mech Eng [H] 1996;210(1):27-37.

Kelly PA, O'Connor JJ. Transmission of rapidly applied loads through articular cartilage. Part 2: Cracked cartilage. Proc Inst Mech Eng [H] 1996;210(1):39-49.

Kempson GE. Relationship between the tensile properties of articular cartilage from the human knee and age. Ann Rheum Dis 1982;41(5):508-511.

Kim HKW et al. Imaging of immature articular cartilage using ultrasound backscatter microcopy at 50 MHz. J Orthop Res 1995;13:963-970.

King D. The healing of semilunar cartilages. J Bone Joint Surg 1936;18:333-342.

King D. The function of semilunar cartilages. J Bone Joint Surg 1936;18:1069-1076.

Kirviranta I et al. Moderate running exercise augments glycosaminoglycans and thickness of articular cartilage in the knee joint of young beagle dogs. J Orthop Res 1988;6(2):188-195.

Klompmaker J et al. Meniscal repair by fibrocartilage in the dog: characterization of the repair tissue and the role of vascularity. Biomaterials 1996;17(17):1685-1691.

Knott L, Bailey AJ. Collagen cross-links in mineralizing tissues: a review of their chemistry, function, and clinical relevance. Bone 1998;22:181-187.

Kuettner KE et al. Articular cartilage matrix and structure: A minireview. J Rheumatol 1991;18:4-48.

Kuhne SA et al. Persistent high serum levels of cartilage oligomeric matrix protein in a subgroup of patients with traumatic knee injury. Rheumatol Int 1998;18:21-25.

Kwan MK et al. Morphological and biomechanical evaluations of neocartilage from the repair of full-thickness articular cartilage defects using rib perichondrium autografts: A long-term study. J Biomech 1989;22(8-9): 921-930.

Lane LB, Bullough PG. Age-related changes in the thickness of the calcified zone and the number of tidemarks in adult human articular cartilage. J Bone Joint Surg Br 1980;62(3):372-375.

Lane LB et al. The vascularity and remodelling of subchondral bone and calcified cartilage in adult human femoral and humeral heads. J Bone Joint Surg 1977;59B:272-278.

Lane JM, Weiss C. Current comment: Review of articular cartilage collagen research. Arthritis Rheum 1975;18:553-559.

Lang P et al. Magnetic resonance tomography (MRI) of joint cartilage. Current status of knowledge and new developments. Radiologe 2000;40(12):1141-1148.

Lawrence RC et al. Estimates of the prevalence of arthritis and selected musculoskeletal disorders in the United States. Arthritis Rheum 1998;41(5):778-799.

Lee C et al. Effects of short term dynamic loading on adult canine chondrocytes seeded into porous collagen-glycosaminoglycan scaffolds (Abstr). 47th Annual Meeting, San Francisco: Orthopaedic Research Society, Feb. 25-28, 2001;26:53.

Lee CR et al. Effects of harvest and selected cartilage repair procedures on the physical and biochemical properties of articular cartilage in the canine knee. J Orthop Res 2000;18(5):790-799.

Lehner KB et al. Structure, function and degeneration of bovine hyaline cartilage: Assessment with MR imaging in vitro. Radiology 1989;170:495-499.

LeRoux MA et al. Simultaneous changes in the mechanical properties, quantitative collagen organization, and proteoglycan concentration of articular cartilage following canine meniscectomy. J Orthop Res 2000;18:383-392.

LeRoux MA et al. Effects of collagen fiber anisotropy on the hydraulic permeability of the meniscus. (Abstr). 47th Annual Meeting, San Francisco: Orthopaedic Research Society, Feb. 25-28, 2001;26:45.

Leslie BW et al. Anisotropic response of the human knee joint meniscus to unconfined compression. Proc Inst Mech Eng [H] 2000;214(6):631-635.

Lindhorst E et al. Longitudinal characterization of synovial fluid biomarkers in the canine meniscectomy model of osteoarthritis. J Orthop Res 2000;18:269-280.

Lipshitz H et al. Changes in the hexosamine content and swelling ratio of articular cartilage as functions of depth from the surface. J Bone Joint Surg 1976;58(A): 1149-1153.

Little CB et al. Topographic variation in biglycan and decoring synthesis by articular cartilage in the early stages of osteoarthritis: an experimental study in sheep. J Orthop Res 1996;14:433-444.

Lohmander LS, Felson DT. Defining the role of molecular markers to monitor disease, intervention, and cartilage breakdown in osteoarthritis. J Rheumatol 1997;24(4):782-785.

Lohmander LS. Cartilage Markers in Joint Fluid in Human Osteoarthritis. In K Brandt (ed): Cartilage Changes in Osteoarthritis. Indianapolis: Indiana University School of Medicine Press, 1990:98-104.

Lohmander LS et al. Cartilage matrix metabolism in osteoarthritis: markers in synovial fluid, serum, and urine. Clin Biochem 1992;25:167-174.

Lutfi AM. Morphological changes in the articular cartilage after meniscectomy: An experimental study in the monkey. J Bone Joint Surg Br 1975;57:525-528.

Lynch, MA et al. Knee joint surface changes: long-term follow-up meniscus tear treatment in stable anterior cruciate ligament reconstruction. Clin Orthop 1983;172:148-153.

Madry H et al. Tissue engineering of cartilage enhanced by the transfer of a human insulin-like growth factor-I gene. (Abstr). 47th Annual Meeting, San Francisco: Orthopaedic Research Society, Feb. 25-28, 2001;26:53.

Madry H, Trippel SB. Efficient lipid-mediated gene transfer to articular chondrocytes. Gene Ther 2000;7(4):286-291.

Mankin HJ et al. Form and Function of Articular Cartilage. In SR Simon (ed): Orthopaedic Basic Science. Rosemont, Illinois, Am Acad Orthop Surg 1994:2-44.

Mankin HJ, Thrasher AZ. Water content and binding in normal and osteoarthritic human cartilage. J Bone Joint Surg 1975;57-A:76-80.

Maroudas A et al. Cartilage of the hip joint: topographical variation of glycosaminoglycan content in normal and fibrillated tissue. Ann Rheum Dis 1973;32:1-9.

Maroudas A. Physicochemical properties of articular cartilage. In MAR Freeman (ed): Adult Articular Cartilage. Bath, Great Britain: Pitman Medical (2nd ed), 1979:215-290.

Maroudas A. Balance between pressure and collagen tension in normal and degenerate cartilage. Nature 1976;260(5554):808-809.

Maroudas A, Bannon C. Measurement of swelling pressure in cartilage and comparison with the osmotic pressure of constituent proteoglycans. Biorheology 1981;18 (3-6):619-632.

Maroudas A et al. Further studies on the composition of human femoral head cartilage. Ann Rheum Dis 1980;39(5):514-523.

Maroudas A et al. The correlation of fixed negative charge with glycosaminoglycan content of human articular cartilage. Biochim Biophys Acta 1969;177(3):492-500.

Maroudas A, Venn M. Chemical composition and swelling of normal and osteoarthritic femoral head cartilage: II. Swelling. Ann Rheum Dis 1977;36:399-406.

Mason RM. Recent Advances in the Biochemistry of Hyaluronic Acid in Cartilage. In Z Deyl, M Adam (eds): Connective Tissue Research: Chemistry, Biology and Physiology. New York: Alan R Liss, 1981:87-112.

Masse PG et al. Loss of decoring from the surface zone of articular cartilage in a chick model of osteoarthritis. Acta Histochem 1997;99:431-444.

Matsumoto T et al. Transfer of osteogenic protein-1 gene by gene gun system promotes matrix synthesis in bovine intervertebral disc and articular cartilage cells (Abstr). 47th Annual Meeting, San Francisco: Orthopaedic Research Society, Feb. 25-28, 2001;26:30.

Matthews MB. The interaction of collagen and acid mucopolysaccharides. A model for connective tissue. J Biochem 1965;96:710-716.

Mauck RL et al. Functional tissue engineering of articular cartilage through dynamic loading of chondrocyte-seeded agarose gels. J Biomech Eng 2000;122(3): 252-260.

Mayne R. Cartilage collagens: What is their function, and are they involved in articular disease? Arthritis Rheum 1989;32:241-246.

Mayor MB, Moskowitz RW. Metabolic studies in experimentally- induced degenerative joint disease in the rabbit. J Rheumatol 1974;1:17-23.

McDevitt CA, Webber RJ. The ultrastructure and biochemistry of meniscal cartilage. Clin Orthop 1990;252:8-18.

McNicol D, Roughley PJ. Extraction and characterization of proteoglycan from human meniscus. Biochem J 1980;185:705-713.

Mendler M et al. Cartilage contains mixed fibrils of collagen types II, IX and XI. J Cell Biol 1989;108:191-197.

Messner K, Maletius W. The long-term prognosis for severe damage to weight-bearing cartilage in the knee. Acta Orthop Scand 1996;67:65-68.

Miller RR, McDevitt CA. Thrombospondin in ligament, meniscus and intervertebral disc. Biochim Biophys Acta 1991;1115:85-88.

Minas T, Nehrer S. Current concepts in the treatment of articular cartilage defects. Orthopedics. 1997;20(6): 525-538.

Miosge N et al. Light and electron microscopical immuno-histochemical localisation of the small proteoglycan core proteins, decorin and biglycan in human knee joint cartilage. Histochem J 1994;26:939-945.

Mitchell DM. Epidemiology. In PD Utsinger et al. (eds): Rheumatoid Arthritis: Etiology, Diagnosis and Treatment. Philadelphia: JB Lippincott, 1985:133-150.

Mitrovic D et al. Cell density of adult human femoral condylar articular cartilage: joints with normal and fibrillated surfaces. Lab Invest 1983;49:309-316.

Modl JM et al. Articular Cartilage: correlation of histologic laminas with signal intensity at MR imaging. Radiology 1991;181:853-855.

Mollenhauer J et al. Expression of anchorin CII (cartilage annexin V) in human young, normal adult, and osteoarthritic cartilage. J Histochem Cytochem 1999;47:209-220.

Mollenhauer J et al. Role of anchorin CII, a 31,000-mol-wt membrane protein, in the interaction of chondrocytes with type II collagen. J Cell Biol 1984;98:1572-1579.

Mooney V, Ferguson AB. The influence of immobilization and motion on the formation of fibrocartilage in the repair granuloma after joint resection in the rabbit. J Bone Joint Surg 1966;48A:1145.

Moskowitz RW et al. Experimentally induced degenerative joint lesions following partial meniscectomy in the rabbit. Arthritis Rheum 1973;16:397-405.

Mow VC. In VC Mow, WC Hayes (eds): Basic Orthopaedic Biomechanics. Philadelphia: Lippincott-Raven (2nd ed), 1997:113.

Mow VC. In VC Mow et al (eds): Knee Meniscus: Basic and Clinical Foundations. New York: Raven Press, 1992:37-57.

Mow VC, Setton LA. Mechanical Properties of Normal and Osteoarthritis Articular Cartilage. In KD Brandt et al. (eds): Osteoarthritis. Oxford, Oxford University Press, 1998:108-122.

Muller G et al. COMP (Cartilage Oligomeric Matrix Protein) is synthesized in ligament, tendon, meniscus, and articular cartilage. Connect Tissue Res 1998;39:233-244.

Muir H et al. The distribution of collagen in human articular cartilage with some of its physiological implications. J Bone Joint Surg 1970;52-B:554-563.

Muir H. The chondrocyte, architecture of cartilage: Biomechanics, structure, function, and molecular biology of cartilage matrix macromolecules. BioEssays 1995;17:1039-1048.

Myers SL et al. Experimental assessment by high frequency ultrasound of articular cartilage thickness and osteoarthritic changes. J Rheumatol 1995;22(1):109-116.

Neurath M, Stofft E. New aspects of the functional anatomy of the menisci. Unfallchirurg (Abstract) 1992;95(1):17-20.

Nerlich AG et al. Localization of collagen X in human foetal and juvenile articular cartilage and bone. Histochemistry 1992;98:275-281.

Newton G et al. Characterization of human and mouse cartilage oligomeric matrix protein. Genomics 1994;24:435-439.

Nuki G. Osteoarthritis: a problem of joint failure. J Rheumatol 1999;58(3):142-147.

O'Connor WJ et al. The use of growth factors in cartilage repair. Orthop Clin N Am 2000;31(3):399-410.

O'Driscoll S, Salter R. The induction of neochondrogenesis in continuous passive motion. J Bone Joint Surg 1984;66A:1248.

O'Driscoll SW et al. The chondrogenic potential of free autogenous periosteal grafts for biological resurfacing of major full-thickness defects in joint surfaces under the influence of continuous passive motion. An experimental investigation in the rabbit. J Bone Joint Surg Am 1986;68(7):1017-1035

Oegema TR et al. The interaction of the zone of calcified cartilage and subchondral bone in osteoarthritis. Microsc Res Techniq 1997;37:324-332.

Ogata K, Whiteside LA. Barrier to material transfer at the bone-cartilage interface: measurement with hydrogen gas in vivo. Clin Orthop 1979;145:273-276.

Ogilvie-Harris DJ, Fitsialos DP. Arthroscopic management of the degenerative knee. Arthroscopy 1991;7:151-157.

Oka M. Biomechanics and repair of articular cartilage. J Orthop Sci 2001;6(5):448-456.

Oka M et al. Development of an artificial articular cartilage. Clin Mater 1990;6(4):361-381.

Olsen BR. Collagen IX. Int J Biochem Cell Biol 1997;29:555-558.

Pal S et al. Structural changes during development in bovine fetal epiphyseal cartilage. Collagen Relat Res 1981;1(2):151-176.

Panula HE et al. Elevated levels of synovial fluid PLA2, stromelysin (MMP-3) and TIMP in early osteoarthrosis after tibial valgus osteotomy in young beagle dogs. Acta Orthop Scand 1998;69:152-158.

Paulsson M, Heinegard D. Noncollagenous cartilage proteins—current status of an emerging research field. Collagen Relat Res 1984;4:219-229.

Peretti GM et al. Biomechanical analysis of a chondrocyte-based repair model of articular cartilage. Tissue Eng 1999;5(4):317-326.

Petersen W, Tillmann B. Collagenous fibril texture of the human knee joint menisci. Anat Embryol (Berl) 1998;197(4):317-324.

Petersen W, Tillmann B. Structure and vascularization of the knee joint menisci. Z Orthop Ihre Grenzgeb (Abstract) 1999;137(1):31-37.

Pfander D et al. Presence and distribution of collagen II, collagen I, fibronectin, and tenascin in rabbit normal and osteoarthritic cartilage. J Rheumatol 1999;26:386-394.

Piperno M et al. Osteoarthritic cartilage fibrillation is associated with decrease in chondrocyte adhesion to fibronectin. Osteoarthr Cartilage 1998;6:393-399.

Pokharna HK, Pottenger LA. Nonenzymatic glycation of cartilage proteoglycans: an in vivo and in vitro study. Glycoconjugate J 1997;4:917-923.

Pokharna HK et al. Lysyl oxidase and Maillard reaction mediated crosslinks in ageing and osteoarthritic rabbit cartilage. J Orthop Res 1995;13:13-21.

Poole AR. Cartilage in Health and Disease. In D McCarty, W Koopman (eds): Arthritis and Allied Conditions: A Textbook of Rheumatology (12th ed). Philadelphia: Lea and Febiger, 1993;279-333.

Poole AR et al. Osteoarthritis in the Human Knee: A Dynamic Process of Cartilage Matrix Degradation, Synthesis and Reorganization. In WB van den Berg et al. (eds): Joint Destruction in Arthritis and Osteoarthritis

(Agents and Actions Supplements, Vol 39). Basel: Birkhäuser, 1993:3-13.

Poole CA. Articular cartilage chondrons: form, function and failure. J Anat 1998;191:1-13.

Poole CA et al. Morphological and functional interrelationships of articular cartilage matrices. J Anat 1984;138(1):113-138.

Poole CA et al. Morphology of the pericellular capsule in articular cartilage revealed by hyaluronidase digestion. J Ultra Struct Res 1985;91:13-23.

Poole CA et al. Immunolocalization of type IX collagen in normal and spontaneously osteoarthritic canine tibial cartilage and isolated chondrons. Osteoarthr Cartilage 1997;5:191-204.

Praemer A et al. Musculoskeletal conditions in the United States. Illinois: Park Ridge, Am Acad Orthop Surg 1992.

Pritzker KP. Animal models for osteoarthritis: processes, problems and prospects. Ann Rheum Dis 1994;53: 406-420.

Pritzker KP et al. Rhesus macaques as an experimental model for degenerative arthritis. P R Health Sci J 1989;8(1):99-102.

Prockop DJ et al. The biosynthesis of collagen and its disorders (first of two parts). N Engl J Med 1979;301(1): 13-23.

Pullig O et al. Expression of type VI collagen in normal and osteoarthritic human cartilage. Osteoarthr Cartilage 1999;7:191-202.

Radin EL et al. Effects of mechanical loading on the tissues of the rabbit knee. J Orthop Res 1984;2(3):221-234.

Radin EL et al. Role of the menisci in the distribution of stress in the knee. Clin Orthop 1984;185:290-294.

Radin EL, Rose RM. Role of subchondral bone in the initiation and progression of cartilage damage. Clin Orthop 1986;213:34-40.

Ragan PM et al. Chondrocyte extracellular matrix synthesis and turnover are influenced by static compression in a new alginate disc culture system. Arch Biochem Biophys 2000;383:256-264.

Rand JA. Role of arthroscopy in osteoarthritis of the knee. Arthroscopy 1991;7:358-363.

Ratcliffe A et al. Differential levels of synovial fluid aggrecan aggregate components in experimental osteoarthritis and joint disuse. J Orthop Res 1994;12:464-473.

Ratcliffe A et al. Synovial Fluid Analyses Detect and Differentiate Proteoglycan Metabolism in Canine Experimental Models of Osteoarthritis and Disuse Atrophy. In WB van den Berg et al. (eds): Joint Destruction in Arthritis and Osteoarthritis (Agents and Actions Supplements, Vol 39). Basel: Birkhäuser, 1993;63-67.

Ratcliffe A, Mow VC. Articular Cartilage. In WD Comper (ed): Extracellular Matrix I. Tissue Function. Amsterdam: Harwood academic publishers. 1996;234-302.

Redler I et al. The ultrastructure and biomechanical significance of the tidemark of articular cartilage. Clin Orthop 1975;112:357-362.

Rodrigo JJ et al. Improvement of full-thickness chondral defect healing in the human knee after debridement and microfracture using continuous passive motion. Am J Knee Surg 1994;7:109-116.

Rodkey WG. Basic biology of the meniscus and response to injury. Instr Course Lect 2000;49:189-193.

Roeddecker K et al. Meniscal healing: a histological study in rabbits. Knee Surg Sport Traum Arthrosc 1993;1(1):28-33.

Roth V, Mow VC. The intrinsic tensile behaviour of the matrix of bovine articular cartilage and its variation with age. J Bone Joint Surg 1980;62A(7):1102-1117.

Roughley PJ et al. The presence of a cartilage-like proteoglycan in the adult human meniscus. Biochem J 1981;197(1):77-83.

Roughley PJ et al. Proteolytic Degradation in Human Articular Cartilage: its Relationship to Stromelysin. In WB van den Berg et al. (eds): Joint Destruction in Arthritis and Osteoarthritis (Agents and Actions Supplements, Vol 39). Basel: Birkhäuser, 1993: 149-159.

Ryan LM, McCarty DJ. Calcium Pyrophosphate Crystal Deposition Disease: Pseudogout, Articular Chondrocalcinosis. In DJ McCarty, WJ Koopman (eds): Arthritis and Allied Conditions: A Textbook of Rheumatology, (12th ed). Philadelphia: Lea & Febiger, 1993:1835-1855.

Sah RL et al. Biosynthetic response of cartilage explants to dynamic compression. J Orthop Res 1989;7(5):619-636.

Saied A et al. Assessment of articular cartilage and subchondral bone: subtle and progressive changes in experimental osteoarthritis using 50 MHz echography in vitro. J Bone Miner Res 1997;12(9):1378-1386.

Salter DM. Tenascin is increased in cartilage and synovium from arthritic knees. Br J Rheumatol 1993;32:780-786.

Salter RB. History of rest and motion and the scientific basis for early continuous passive motion. Hand Clin 1996;12(1):1-11.

Salter RB. The physiologic basis of continuous passive motion for articular cartilage healing and regeneration. Hand Clin 1994;10(2):211-219.

Salter RB. The biologic concept of continuous passive motion of synovial joints. The first 18 years of basic research and its clinical application. Clin Orthop 1989;242:12-25.

Schinagl RM et al. Depth-dependent confined compression modulus of full-thickness bovine articular cartilage. J Orthop Res 1997;15(4):499-506.

Scott JE. Proteoglycan-fibrillar Collagen Interactions in Tissues: Dermatan Sulphate Proteoglycan as a Tissue Organiser. In JE Scott (ed): Dermatan Sulphate Proteoglycans: Chemistry, Biology, Chemical Pathology. London: Portland Press, 1993:165-192.

Seedhom BB, Hargreaves DJ. Transmission of the load in the knee joint with special reference to the role of the menisci: Part II. Experimental results, discussion and conclusions. Eng Med 1979;8:220-228.

Setton LA et al. Altered Structure-function Relationships for Articular Cartilage in Human Osteoarthritis and an Experimental Canine Model. In WB van den Berg et al. (eds): Joint Destruction in Arthritis and Osteoarthritis (Agents and Actions Supplements, Vol 39). Basel: Birkhäuser, 1993:27-48.

Setton LA et al. Altered mechanics of cartilage with osteoarthritis: human osteoarthritis and an experimental model of joint degeneration. Osteoarthr Cartilage 1999;7(1):2-14.

Sell DR, Monnier VM. Structure elucidation of a senescence cross link from human extracellular matrix. J Biol Chem 1989;264:21597-21602.

Shepherd DE, Seedhom BB. Thickness of human articular cartilage in joints of the lower limb. Ann Rheum Dis 1999;58(1):27-34.

Skaggs DL et al. Radial tie fibers influence the tensile properties of the bovine medial meniscus. J Orthop Res 1994;12(2):176-185.

Smith JW et al. Observations on the distribution of the protein polysaccharide complex and collagen in bovine articular cartilage. J Cell Sci 1967;2:129-136.

Smith RL et al. Rabbit knee immobilization: bone remodeling precedes cartilage degradation. J Orthop Res 1992;10(1):88-95.

Solursh M. Ectoderm as a determinant of early tissue pattern in the limb bud. Cell Differ 1984;15(1):17-24.

Solursh M. Cartilage stem cells: regulation of differentiation. Connec Tiss Res 1989;20(1-4):81-89.

Solursh M. Extracellular matrix and cell surface determinants of connective tissue differentiation. Am J Med Genet 1989;34(1):30-34.

Sokoloff L. The Biology of Degenerative Joint Disease. University of Chicago Press, Chicago 1969.

Sommerlath KG. Results of meniscal repair and partial meniscectomy in stable knees. Int Orthop 1991;15(4):347-350.

Spilker RL et al. A transversely isotropic biphasic finite element model of the meniscus. J Biomech 1992;25:1027-1045.

Steadman JR et al. The microfracture technic in the management of complete cartilage defects in the knee joint. Orthopade 1999;28(1):26-32.

Steinmeyer J, Knue S. The proteoglycan metabolism of mature bovine articular cartilage explants superimposed to continuously applied cyclic mechanical loading. Biochem Biophys Res Commun 1997;240(1):216-221.

Steinmeyer J et al. Effects of intermittently applied cyclic loading on proteoglycan metabolism and swelling behaviour of articular cartilage explants. Osteoarthr Cartilage 1999;7(2):155-164.

Stevens SS et al. Computer model of endochondral growth and ossification in long bones: biological and mechanobiological influences. J Orthop Res 1999;17(5):646-653.

Stockwell RA. Chondrocyte Metabolism. In RJ Harrison, RMH McMinn (eds): Biology of Cartilage Cells. Cambridge: Cambridge University Press, 1979:81-123.

Studer D et al. Evidence for a distinct water-rich layer surrounding collagen fibrils in articular cartilage extracellular matrix. J Struct Biol 1996;117:81-85.

Takada N et al. A possible barrier function of the articular surface. Kaibogaku Zasshi (Abstract) 1999;74(6):631-637.

Takahashi M et al. Quantitative analysis of crosslinks pyridinoline and pentosidine in articular cartilage of patients with bone and joint disorders. Arthritis Rheum 1994;37:724-728.

Takahashi M et al. Relationship between pentosidine levels in serum and urine and activity in rheumatoid arthritis. Br J Rheumatol 1997;36:637-642.

Thonar EJ, Sweet MB. Maturation-related changes in proteoglycans of fetal articular cartilage. Arch Biochem Biophys 1981;208(2):535-547.

Tondravi MM et al. Cartilage matrix protein binds to collagen and plays a role in collagen fibrillogenesis. Prog Clin Biol Res 1993;383-B:515-522.

Torzilli PA et al. Characterization of cartilage metabolic response to static and dynamic stress using a mechanical explant test system. J Biomech 1997;30(1):1-9.

Trickey TR et al. Viscoelastic properties of chondrocytes from normal and osteoarthritic human cartilage. J Orthop Res 2000;18(6):891-898.

Tulamo RM et al. Hyaluronate and large molecular weight proteoglycans in synovial fluid from horses with various arthritides. Am J Vet Res 1996;57:932-937.

Uchiyama A et al. Fluorophores from aging human articular cartilage. J Biochem (Tokyo) 1991;110(5):714-718.

Uitto J et al. Conversion of type II procollagen to collagen. Extracellular removal of the amino-terminal and carboxy-terminal extensions without a preferential sequence. Eur J Biochem 1979;99(1):97-103.

Van Tienen T et al. Meniscal lesion repair as a result of porous polymer impants placed in partial thickness defects: a study on dogs (Abstr). 47th Annual Meeting, San Francisco: Orthopaedic Research Society, Feb. 25-28, 2001;46.

Venn MF. Variation of chemical composition with age in human femoral head cartilage. Ann Rheum Dis 1978;37:168-174.

Venn M, Maroudas A. Chemical composition and swelling of normal and osteoarthritic femoral head cartilage. I. Chemical composition. Ann of Rheum Dis 1977;36:121-129.

Visco DM et al. The vascular supply of the chondro-epiphyses of the elbow joint in young swine. J Anat 1989;163:215-229.

Voloshin AS, Wosk J. Shock absorption of meniscectomized and painful knees. A comparative in vivo study. J Biomed Eng 1983;5(2):157-161.

von der Mark K et al. Type X collagen synthesis in human osteoarthritic cartilage. Indication of chondrocyte hypertrophy. Arthritis Rheum 1992;35(7):806-811.

Vunjak-Novakovic et al. Bioreactor cultivation conditions modulate the composition and mechanical properties of tissue engineered cartilage. J Orthop Res 1999;17(1):130-138.

Walker PS, Erkman MJ. The role of the meniscus in force transmission across the knee. Clin Orthop 1975;109:184-192.

Walker JM. Pathomechanics and classification of cartilage lesions, facilitation of repair. J Orthop Sport Phys Ther 1998;28(4):216-231.

Weiss C. Ultrastructural characteristics of osteoarthritis. Fed Proc 1973;32:1459-1466.

Wilkins RJ et al. Chondrocyte regulation by mechanical load. Biorheology 2000;37(1-2):67-74.

Williams JM et al. Increase in levels of serum keratan sulphate following cartilage proteoglycan degradation in the rabbit knee joint. Arthritis Rheum 1988;31:557-560.

Wong M, Carter DR. Mechanical stress and morphogenetic endochondral ossification of the sternum. J Bone Joint Surg Am 1988;70(7):992-1000.

Woo SL et al. Perichondrial autograft for articular cartilage: shear modulus of neocartilage studied in rabbits. Acta Orthop Scand 1987;58(5):510-515.

Wu JJ, Eyre DR. Cartilage type IX collagen is cross-linked by hydroxypyridinium residues. Biochem Biophys Res Commun 1984;123:1033-1039.

Wu JJ, Eyre DR. Covalent interactions of type IX collagen in cartilage. Connect Tissue Res 1989;20:241-246.

Wu JJ, Eyre DR. Structural analysis of cross-linking domains in cartilage type XI collagen. Insight on polymeric assembly. J Biol Chem 1995;270:18865-18870.

Wu JJ et al. Identification of cross-linking sites in bovine cartilage type IX collagen reveals an antiparallel type II-type IX molecular relationship and type IX to type IX bonding. J Biol Chem 1992;267:23007-23014.

Xu Y et al. Characterization of chondrocyte alkaline phosphatase as a potential mediator in the dissolution of calcium pyrophosphate dihydrate crystals. J Rheumatol 1994;21:912-920.

Yang C et al. In vitro fibrillogenesis of collagen II from pig vitreous humour. Biochem J 1995;306(Pt 3):871-875.

Yutani Y et al. Alteration of cartilage specific proteoglycan with non-weight bearing articular cartilage. Osaka City Med J 1994;40(1):19-26.

Zhu W et al. Anisotropic viscoelastic shear properties of bovine meniscus. Clin Orthop 1994;306:34-45.

Chapter 5

The Nature of the Dense Connective Tissues of the Musculoskeletal System: Structure, Function, and Biomechanics of the Intervertebral Disc

Back pain may be broadly attributed to visceral, nonmechanical, and mechanical etiologic factors with the latter regarded as the most common cause of dysfunction (Fairbank and Pynsent 1992; Lawrence et al. 1992) (Table 5-1). In light of this, an understanding of the internal structure of the intervertebral disc (IVD) is clinically important in the management of back pain and dysfunction. Lesions of the IVD, such as disc degradation and tears in its internal structure (annulus fibrosus) (Crock 1986), and extrusion of the IVD (peripheral and central herniations) (Chandraraj et al. 1998) are common pathologies that may contribute to mechanical dysfunction affecting these dense connective tissue-based structures. Human IVDs undergo age-related degenerative changes that contribute to some of the most common causes of impairment and disability for middle-age and older people, including spine stiffness and neck and low back pain (Buckwalter 1995).

The Nonimpaired Intervertebral Disc

The IVD, composed mostly of fibrillar or interstitial collagens, is a component of the tri-joint complex within which are also two facet joints. The IVD across all regions of the vertebral column serves primarily to allow movement between adjacent vertebral bodies, to absorb shock, and to transmit loads through the vertebral column. The morphology and structure of the IVDs reflects their function across the cervical, thoracic, and lumbar regions of the spine. The gross morphology, ultrastructure, and biochemical composition of the IVD at different regions of the spine are elements that must be intact to ensure normal function.

The IVD is the largest avascular structure in the body. Steep gradients in oxygen concentration are evident with the oxygen partial pressure (PO_2) falling to as low as 1% oxygen in the center of the

Table 5-1. Etiology of Back Pain: Visceral, Nonmechanical, and Mechanical

Visceral	Nonmechanical	Mechanical
Gall bladder disease	Tumor	Intervertebral disc herniation
Abdominal aortic aneurysm	Rheumatoid arthritis	Zygoapophyseal joint Osteoarthritis
Pancreatitis		Spondylolithesis
Renal disorders		Pregnancy
Pregnancy		

From Lundon, K Bolton K: Structure and function of the lumbar intervertebral disc in health, aging and pathologic conditions, JOSPT 2001;31(6):291–306.

disc (Ishihara and Urban 1999). The IVD relies on diffusion across the vertebral end-plate as a means of transport for its nutritional supply (Chandraraj et al. 1998). Blood vessels surrounding the periphery of the IVD and within adjacent vertebral bodies provide the route by which nutrients reach the IVD (Ghosh et al. 1977). As the ability of any tissue to undergo repair is related, in part, to its vascularity, the IVD responds to injury with demonstrably prolonged or incomplete repair processes.

Although differences in morphology exist between the IVDs from different regions of the spine (most notably between the cervical and lumbar spine), a basic common structure for the IVD prevails from all sites in the spine (Figure 5-1). All IVDs have three parts: (1) *the nucleus pulposus*, classically described as a central gelatinous mass; (2) *the annulus fibrosus*, a fibrous outer ring; and (3) *the vertebral end-plate*, constituting a cartilaginous layer covering the superior and inferior surfaces of the IVD. A *transitional zone* is evident between the nucleus pulposus and annulus fibrosus (Akeson et al. 1977; Markolf and Morris 1974; Taylor and Akeson 1971). Collagen types I and II distribute radially in opposing concentration gradients in the IVD, with the former predominantly comprising the fiber bundles of the annulus fibrosis and the latter being the principal component of the nucleus pulposus. In addition, minor collagen types, including types III, V, VI, IX , X (Nerlich et al. 1998), XI, XII, and XIV (Duance et al. 1998), may be present within the IVD. Regional differences in structure in the IVDs of the cervical, thoracic, and lumbar spine reflect the functional demands of each area of the spine.

Lumbar intervertebral disc

The IVDs from the lumbar spine are approximately cylindrical, are typically wedge shaped, and taper posteriorly (Figure 5-2). The normal postural lordosis inherent to the lumbar spine may be, in part, attributed to the wedge shape of the lumbar IVD (Figure 5-3).

Thoracic intervertebral disc

At the thoracic spine, the IVDs tend to be less wedge shaped than at the lumbar spine (Figure 5-4). Postural kyphosis typical of this region of the spine is deter-

mined mainly by the shape of the thoracic vertebrae. Regional differences may also be seen in the transverse section of IVDs from the thoracic spine, which assume a more rounded triangular shape (Pooni et al. 1986), as opposed to those from the lumbar spine regions, which assume a more elliptical shape and are able to resist bending movements (Adams and Hutton 1988). The roughly circular cross-section of the thoracic IVD allows the force of torsion to be evenly distributed around its circumference, making it able to withstand forces of this nature. Although facet joint orientation in the lumbar spine acts to limit torsional forces, the IVDs of the lumbar spine are prone to

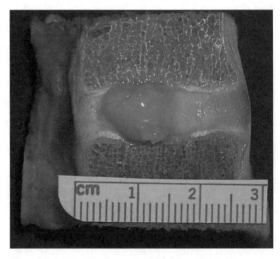

Figure 5-1. Sagital view of an IVD from the lumbar spine in a 30-year-old adult male. Note that when the disc is cut sagitally, the pressure in the nucleus pulposus is released, and it bulges out. (Courtesy Dr. Elisa Bass, PhD, UCSF Orthopaedic Bioengineering Laboratory, San Francisco.)

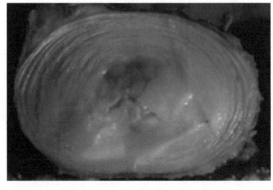

Figure 5-2. Cross-section through a lumbar spine IVD (L4-L5).

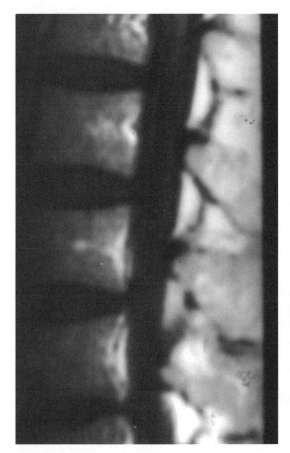

Figure 5-3. IVDs in the L1-L5 region of a 36-year-old non-impaired individual (T1 weighted image, MRI). (From Lundon K, Bolton K. Structure and Function of the Lumbar Intervertebral Disc in Health, Aging and Pathologic Conditions. JOSPT 2001;31[6]:291-306.)

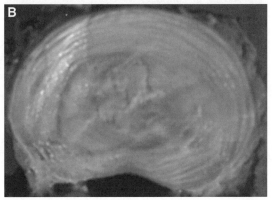

Figure 5-4. A, Cross section through an upper thoracic spine IVD (T2-T3). **B,** Cross-section through a lower thoracic spine IVD (T11-T12).

damage as a result of extremes in these movements (Adams and Hutton, 1983).

Cervical intervertebral disc

The morphology of the cervical IVD differs from the lumbar IVD in that the annulus fibrosus does not consist of concentric lamellae of collagen fibers. The cervical annulus fibrosus instead forms a crescentic mass of collagen that is thick anteriorally, tapers laterally toward the uncinate processes, and is deficient posterolaterally (Mercer and Bogduk 1999). The cross-sectional area of the IVD increases from the cervical (Figure 5-5) to the lumbosacral area that reflects the increased load requiring support by the spinal column in a cephalocaudal direction.

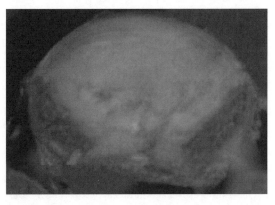

Figure 5-5. Cross section through a cervical spine IVD (C5-C6).

General Morphology of the Intervertebral Disc

Nucleus Pulposus

The nucleus pulposus of a healthy young adult (age 20 to 30 years) is oval shaped and is composed of a highly hydrated gelatinous material (Bogduk and Twomey 1987; Markolf and Morris 1974; Pearce 1992). The inner lamellae of the surrounding annulus fibrosus surround the nucleus pulposus with the transitional zone interspersed between the two regions (Coventry 1945; Inoue 1981). The nucleus pulposus contains predominantly type II collagen as well as some type I collagen as opposed to the annulus fibrosus, which contains more type I than type II collagen (Ghosh et al. 1977). Type I collagen, however, assumes a more remarkable presence in the degeneratively altered nucleus pulposus. The primary function of the nucleus pulposus is to redistribute vertical loads across the IVD (Bogduk and Twomey 1987) with its fluid nature, allowing it to redirect an applied force in multiple directions to be resisted ultimately by the neighboring strong fibrous annulus fibrosus and vertebral end-plate (Adams and Hutton 1988). The nucleus pulposus also contains chondrocytes, and its matrix consists of proteogly-cans (PGs) that behave as a water trap (Bogduk and Twomey 1987); collagen fibers (Eyre, 1988); and other noncollagenous proteins and elastin (Ayad and Weiss 1987; Buckwalter 1982; Coventry 1969; Ghosh et al. 1977). As with all dense regular connective tissues, the biomechanical and functional properties of the nucleus pulposus are derived based on the relative concentration and arrangement of the constituents of its matrix.

Annulus Fibrosus

The components of the annulus fibrosus include matrix collagenous proteins, among which collagen types I, II, and VI represent the major components (Yang et al. 1994). These collagens form ordinary fibrils (collagen type I or II) or microfibrils (collagen VI), either of which can further interact with PGs, elastin, and cells (fibroblasts and chondrocytes) and water to deposit a fiber-reinforced matrix (Eyre and Muir, 1977). At least the outer one third of the annulus fibrosus is innervated (Ashton et al. 1994). A comparison of the constituents of the nucleus pulposus and annulus fibrosus is presented in Table 5-2. The annulus fibrosus is the primary load-bearing com-

---

Clinical Note

Effects of Loading on the IVD

The viscoelastic properties of the IVD can be witnessed clinically and/or vocationally in those individuals positioned in sustained postures such as lumbar flexion in the case of the office worker seated for long periods. Under these conditions the lumbar IVD and zygoapophyseal joints creep, resulting in disc deformation (thinning) and narrowing of the intervertebral space. This physical deformation of the IVD may, in part, be reversed with changes in posture (supine lying at night). In a study of disc height as determined by magnetic resonance imaging (MRI), actual disc height showed an increasing trend from office workers (sedentary) to blue-collar workers (more physical work) at all disc levels except L5-S1 (Luoma et al. 2001). Heavy physical work was shown to hasten the degenerative process in the lumbar spine (Riihimaki et al 1990). Videman et al. (1990) identified that the most benign IVD pathology was related to moderate or mixed physical work loading, whereas back pain and the more serious IVD pathologies were related to the highest and lowest degrees of physical loading. If a load is sustained for a prolonged period or an excessive load is applied, disruption of the IVD may occur by either stretching the collagen fibers, disrupting chemical bonds between adjacent collagen fibers, or affecting the production of proteoglycans (PGs) and collagen by the IVD cells (Adams and Hutton 1988; Bogduk and Twomey 1987; Hutton et al. 1998), resulting in a permanently altered structure. Furthermore, Urban et al. (2001) determined that a loss of cells from the IVDs at the curve apex studied from individuals with neuromuscular scoliosis likely arose because the disc experiences greater mechanical stress due to the deformity.

ponent of the IVD, as it accepts the redistributed forces encountered by the nucleus pulposus. In the thoracic and lumbar spine, the annulus fibrosus is composed of collagen fibers tightly arranged in multiple sheets referred to as *lamellae*, which are arranged in concentric rings around the central nucleus pulposus and bound together by PG gel (Burgeson 1992; Urban and Maroudas 1980). Within each lamellae, the collagen fibers lie parallel to one another, angling between adjacent vertebrae at approximately 65 to 70 degrees vertically (Horton 1958) and lying perpendicular to each other between successive lamellae (Markolf and Morris 1974). In the lumbar spine, the alignment of fibers in successive layers imparts great strength to the annulus fibrosus and contributes to its ability to withstand forces applied to it in any direction (Bogduk and Twomey 1987). The posterior portion of the annulus fibrosus of the lumbar IVD is thinnest and is commonly a site of injury resulting from torsional forces (Bogduk and Twomey 1987). In the cervical IVD, the anterior longitudinal ligament covers the front of the disc, and the posterior longitudinal ligament reinforces the deficient posterior annulus fibrosus with longitudinal and alar fibers (Mercer and Bogduk 1999).

Vertebral End-Plate

The vertebral end-plate is a thin and incomplete layer of cartilage covering the area of the vertebral body that consists of an outer articular area facing the nucleus pulposus and the annulus fibrosus and an inner growth zone on the vertebral body (Bernick and Cailliet 1982). The vertebral end-plate contains interstitial collagens types II and IX but never type I, regardless of degenerative changes (Nerlich et al. 1998). The vertebral end-plate ranges from 0.1 to 1.6 mm in thickness and is strongly attached to the IVD through the annulus fibrosus but is rather weakly attached to the vertebral bodies. The thinnest region of the vertebral end-plate is over the nucleus pulposus (Roberts et al. 1989) and consists of fibrocartilage, as opposed to hyaline cartilage, which is found close to the vertebral body. The vertebral end-plate appears to be important in the metabolism of the avascular IVD in adults (Grignon et al. 2000; Moore 2000).

Biomechanics of the Intervertebral Disc

Response to loading

The IVD, as a dense regular connective tissue structure, displays viscoelastic properties of creep (deformation of a structure subjected to constant load over time) and hysteresis (response to repetitive loading and unloading).

The IVD is vulnerable to four main loading forces: compression (symmetrical and asymmetrical); tension; torsion; and bending. In particular, the IVD is subjected to high compressive forces. Compression of the IVD occurs as a result of the spinal column supporting the weight of the head, thorax, and upper limbs and the contraction of surrounding muscles during movement and physical activities. For instance, standing erect places approximately 500 Newtons (N) of compressive force on the lumbar spine, whereas bending forward to lift 10 kg (30 lbs) puts approximately 2000N on the lumbar spine (Nachemson 1981). Heavy physical work is regarded to increase the compressive forces acting on the disc with a threefold effect: (1) the hydrostatic pressure in the disc rises; (2) the mechanical stress on the disc fibers, end-plate, and subchondral bone increases; and (3) an egress of fluid ultimately raises the osmotic pressure and affects disc cell nutrition (Hutton et al. 1998). Iatridis et al. (1999) also identified that chronically applied compressive forces in the absence of disease process caused changes in the mechanical properties of the IVD. In health, the annulus fibrosus, nucleus pulposus, and vertebral end-plate work as a functional unit to resist compressive forces. The nucleus pulposus redistributes compressive forces that are constrained radially by the fibers of the annulus fibrosus (Hukins and Meakin 2000). Results of Hutton et al. (1998) indicate that the nucleus pulposus is at the forefront of changes brought about by compressive loading. Asymmetrical compressive forces are most likely to occur during the normal activities of daily living (ADLs) (Adams and Hutton 1988). The response of the IVD is nonlinear when subjected to a compressive force in that its response varies depending on the load applied. In this way, the disc offers very little resistance to and is flexible with the application of small loads, but as the load increases, the disc responds by offering greater resistance and thus stability (Osti et al. 1990; Panjabi et al. 1992).

Table 5-2. Ultrastructure of the Normal Intervertebral Disc from the Lumbar Spine

Structure/Component	Water	Proteoglycans (PGs)	Collagen	Elastin	Cells
Nucleus Pulposus (NP)	70%–90%	65% dry weight of NP (Ayad and Weiss, 1987; Fairbank and Pynsent 1992) PGs are key to the inherent mechanical properties of the NP PGs present in the NP include hyaluronic acid, chondroitin sulfate, and keratan sulfate (Buckwalter 1982; Crock 1986; Johnson et al. 1985; Osti et al. 1990)	15%–25% dry weight (Adams and Muir, 1976; Ayad and Weiss 1987) Exists as an irregular mesh network that binds PGs Types II (85%) and small amounts of Types III, V, I and XI collagens are found in the NP (Crock 1986; Beard et al. 1981, Ashton et al. 1994; Buckwalter et al. 1994)	Small quantity of fibers with no specific orientation (Boos et al. 1997)	Chondrocytes responsible for production of matrix including PGs and collagen components Concentration of chondrocytes in the NP is less than that of the surrounding AF and they are found mainly in the vertebral end-plate area (Bushell et al. 1977)
Annulus Fibrosus (AF)	60%–70%	15%–20% of dry weight of AF (Ayad and Weiss 1987; Bogduk and Twomey 1987) PG gel, together with cells and elastin, occupies the spaces between the collagen fibres of the lamellae of the AF; this acts to bind the lamellae together and contributes to the stiffness of the AF (Pokharna and Phillips 1998)	50%–60% of the dry weight of the AF (Ayad and Weiss 1987; Bogduk and Twomey 1987) Types I (predominant collagen of the AF providing resistance to tension), and types II, III, V, VI, IX are found in the AF (Bogduk and Twomey 1987; Boos et al. 1997; Crock 1986)	10% of the dry weight of the AF (Horton 1958) Fibers are arranged in a circular, oblique, and vertical manner within the lamellae (Horton 1958)	Chondrocytes and fibroblasts are dispersed among the collagen fibres of the individual lamellae and between the lamellae themselves (Boden et al. 1990) Fibroblasts are found predominantly in the periphery of the AF; chondrocytes towards the NP (Buckwalter et al. 1976)

Concentration of type II collagen progressively increases toward the center of the annulus as type I collagen concentration decreases (Bogduk and Twomey 1987; Coventry et al. 1945; Crock 1986; Grignon et al. 2000)	Elastin fibers are closely related to the densely packed collagen fibres; they are oriented parallel to these fibres (Boos et al. 1997)	Elastin confers resilience/elasticity to the AF (Grignon et al. 2000; Kazarian 1975)

From Lundon K and Bolton K: Structure and function of the lumbar intervertebral disc in health, aging and pathologic conditions JOSPT 2001;31(6):291–306.

Axial rotation (torsion) occurs around the central axis of the spine, the location that appears to lie in either the posterior aspect of the IVD or the spinal canal (Adams and Hutton, 1983). Excessive rotational strain is restricted largely by the zygoapophyseal (facet) joints. Bending (flexion and extension movements) encompasses the movements of flexion, extension, and lateral flexion. Although the zygoapophyseal joints provide the principle resistance to flexion and extension at the lumbar spine (Bogduk and Twomey 1987), the fibers of the annulus fibrosus also severely stretched, and the tension developed in the annulus fibrosus refers increasing pressure to the nucleus pulposus (Nachemson 1960).

Effect of Age Changes in the Intervertebral Disc and Vertebral Body

Effect of growth, development and aging on function of the intervertebral disc

During processes of skeletal growth and maturation, the clear gelatinous nucleus pulposus becomes a firm fibrous plate. In early adulthood, fissures and cracks appear in the disc with extensions into the central regions of the IVD from the periphery (Buckwalter et al. 1994). PG aggregates from the human newborn and infant IVD annulus fibrosus resemble those from hyaline cartilage with a central hyaluronan filament and multiple attached monomers (Buckwalter et al. 1994). In contrast, aggregates with this presentation were observed to be rare in the infant nucleus pulposus and disappeared with increasing age (Buckwalter

et al. 1994). In comparison with PGs from newborn human articular cartilage, PGs from newborn human nucleus pulposus formed smaller aggregates and had shorter, more variable aggrecan molecules. In the first 6 to 8 months of life, the proportion of aggregated monomers was shown to decline by 40% in the human nucleus pulposus, whereas the nucleus pulposus from adolescent and older humans demonstrated monomer clusters but no large aggregates similar to those found in articular cartilage or in the infant nucleus pulposus (Buckwalter et al. 1994). Therefore within the first year of human life, the populations of aggregates and large aggrecan molecules analogous to those found in articular cartilage decline until few, if any, of these molecules remain in the central disc tissues of skeletally mature individuals (Buckwalter et al, 1994). In infants, clusters of notochordal cells and syncytial cords occupy the inner regions of the nucleus pulposus with chondrocyte-like cells assuming the places made available by the loss in the former by the time adolescence is reached. The decline in viable cells in the central region of the IVD in particular occurs after skeletal maturity (Trout et al. 1982). A loss of viable cells occurs within the nucleus pulposus with advancing age, and research shows that approximately 2% of cells from an infant nucleus pulposus were observed to be undergoing necrosis at any one time, compared with more than 50% of cells that were in this state in an adolescent and young adult (Buckwalter 1995). A general decrease in PG and water concentration in the IVD, particularly in the central regions of the disc, can be seen by the time early adult life is reached (Gower and Pedrini 1969), in addition to increased levels of noncollagenous

---

Clinical Note

Nature of Loading on the IVD

At higher rates of loading, the capacity of the disc to dissipate energy and therefore absorb shock loads is lower (Race et al. 2000). The pressure within the nucleus pulposus rises when the IVD is subject to vertical compression forcing it to bulge radially, exerting pressure on the vertebral end-plate and causing the inner and outer boundaries of the annulus fibrosus to move outward (Hukins and Meakin 2000). If the compression force is asymmetrical, then a radial bulging of the IVD becomes pronounced in the area where the force is concentrated (Adams and Hutton, 1988). This can be witnessed during lumbar spine flexion, where compression forces are exerted greatest in the anterior and least in the posterior IVD regions.

Clinical Note

Intradiscal Pressure

The measurement of intradiscal pressure in response to the site and rate of loading as it relates to changes in disc integrity has been of clinical interest within the field of physical rehabilitation. Regional overload has been considered responsible for progressive structural weakness of the posterolateral annular fibers of the lumbar disc. *In vivo* pressure changes of the L3-L4 disc have been measured in several static postures and during performance of common exercises and movements (Nachemson and Morris 1964). The greater the distance between the load and the body (i.e., the greater the lever arm), the greater is the rise in intradiscal pressure as measured at the third lumbar IVD. In addition, it was determined that the greatest intradiscal pressure at the L3-L4 segment was created by sitting bent forward at a 20-degree angle while holding a weight (Nachemson 1966). Finally, the combination of a high loading rate applied in compression and sagittal flexion to the L2-L3 motion segment was observed to significantly increase peak intradiscal pressure (Wang 2000).

---

proteins (Dickson et al. 1967). By adolescence the PG population of the nucleus pulposus consists of clusters of short aggrecan molecules and nonaggregated PGs that may in part be explained by a decline in the concentration of link proteins at this time in life (Donahue et al. 1988). Most of the water loss occurs during childhood and adolescence with only a small loss occurring during adult life (Twomey and Taylor 1985). Declining nutrition for the support of the center of the disc and matrices may be caused by a progressive age-related decrease in the number of arteries from the periphery of the annulus fibrosus that supplies the region of the IVD from the periphery. Recall that the disc cells rely on diffusion of nutrients from blood vessels on the periphery of the annulus fibrosus and from vessels within the vertebral bodies (Hassler 1969). In addition the decrease in water content may further interfere with diffusion of nutrients and cell nutrition.

The gross structure and ultrastructure of the IVD changes dramatically with age (Buckwalter 1995), and the distinction between pure age-related and other pathologic changes is not always clear (Vernon-Roberts 1992). General changes in ultrastructure with age of the IVD include a diminished water content; decreased pyridinoline (a collagen maturation cross-link); and increased pentosidine (nonenzymatically initiated age-related cross-link) (Pokharna and Philips 1998). A progressive, age-related accumulation of collagen, both in the annulus fibrosus and the nucleus pulposus (Adams and Muir 1976; Olczyk 1992), and an increase in collagen fiber diameter (Trout et al. 1982) are believed

to account for the increasing stiffness of the IVD (Bogduk and Twomey 1987). Splits and clefts with a horizontal orientation develop approximately halfway between the vertebral end-plate and the center of the disc, usually in the posterior zone close to the junction of the nucleus pulposus and annulus fibrosus (transitional zone). As these clefts enlarge the central portion of the disc becomes progressively separated from the adjacent disc tissue (Twomey and Taylor 1985), and the extension of these clefts through the annular fibers in a posterior or posterolateral direction may eventually extend through the annulus fibrosus to become continuous with the epidural space of the spinal canal (Vernon-Roberts 1988).

Nucleus pulposus aging

The most extensive change with age occurs in the central nucleus pulposus and inner fibers of the annulus fibrosus of the IVD (Buckwalter 1995). Histological studies have identified that the nucleus pulposus becomes progressively more fibrotic and less distinct from the annular region with aging (Coventry et al. 1945), and by the age of 40 the nucleus pulposus has essentially become a fibrous pad (Miller et al. 1988), which is related to a loss of water (Eyre and Muir 1977; Gower and Pedrini 1969). Because of this gradual degeneration of the nucleus pulposus into a more "solid and dry" mass, the nucleus pulposus is less able to redistribute pressure as it did as a fluid body and is conducive to a weakened IVD (Bogduk and Twomey 1987). This results in poor pressure transmission and reduced ability to exert radial pressure on the annulus fibrosus, thereby causing unequal loading of different portions of the annulus fibrosus. Similar to articular cartilage, the nucleus pulposus of the IVD contains a high concentration of PGs that act to impart an important biomechanical role to the tissue. PG concentration of the IVD, particularly in the central region decreases, and a decrease in the proportion of PGs that form aggregates also occurs. The mechanism of IVD dehydration is not clearly understood but possibly relates to a change in chemical composition of the nucleus pulposus and, in turn, its hydrophilic capacity (Adams et al. 1977; Buckwalter et al. 1994).

Annulus fibrosus aging

The biochemical changes with age seen in the annulus fibrosus are similar but less extreme than those of the nucleus pulposus with processes such as dehydration and an increase in the collagen content of the annulus fibrosus taking place (Gower and Pedrini 1969; Olczyk 1992). The boundary between the annulus fibrosus and nucleus pulposus ultimately becomes almost indistinguishable (Gower and Pedrini 1969; Pearce, 1992). This is achieved as the inner annulus expands at the expense of the nucleus pulposus, while the size of the outer annulus remains approximately unchanged (Buckwalter 1995). Lesions identified as rim or peripheral (Osti 1992); circumferential (Pearce 1992); and radial (Osti 1992) of the annulus fibrosus are associated with age changes and may predispose the individual to disc protrusions.

Vertebral end-plate aging

With age, fissure formation, fractures, and horizontal cleft formation become common. Overall, the vertebral end-plate becomes progressively thinner, and focal areas of degeneration may progress to become full-thickness defects (Vernon-Roberts 1988), progressing to calcification (Bernick and Cailliet 1982). At approximately age 20, the vertebral end-plate has become sealed off from the vertebral body with progressive dehydration of the vertebral end-plate observed with aging when compared with those from adolescents and young adults (Bishop and Pearce 1993).

In association with aging of the vertebral bodies, irregular osteophytes may develop on the anterior or posterior rim of the vertebral bodies that have decreased bone density. This may increase the pressure on the vertebral end-plate, leading to microfracture and a degenerative condition referred to as *disc osteophyte complex*. Eventually, the superior and inferior surfaces of the vertebral body may become concave as a result of the degeneration of the vertebral end-plate (Hansson and Roos 1981).

In summary, the IVD assumes a more fibrous nature with advancing age attributable to dehydration, an increase in collagen, reduction in PGs, and reduction in elastin content (Bogduk and Twomey 1987; Johnson et al. 1985). Lumbar disc degeneration first appears in males during the teen years and in females, during the third decade (Miller et al. 1988). In general, age changes occur earlier and progress more rapidly in the L5-S1 region. Furthermore, a history of specific activity involve-

Clinical Note

Aging and the IVD

Among the most common complaints of middle-age and older individuals are problems of stiffness and pain in the neck and back (Jette 1990). The IVD displays extensive change that manifests with age (Vernon-Roberts and Pirie 1977) most clearly seen in the central regions incorporating the nucleus pulposus and the transitional zone between the nucleus pulposus and the annulus fibrosus. Age-related changes in the ultrastructural composition of the IVD have been associated with an increased probability of herniation of the IVD (Armstrong and Mow 1982). Gross changes in volume and shape of the IVD have been related to impaired mobility of the spine because of altered alignment and loading patterns that ultimately become applied to the facet joints, spinal ligaments, and paraspinous muscles (Buckwalter et al. 1995).

ment in power sports across the life span appear to be associated with greater disc degeneration in the lower thoracic spine but not the lumbar spine (Videman et al. 1997).

The IVD's viscoelastic behavior and response to experimental axial loading also changes significantly with age. Therefore the effect of aging on the function of the IVD has been of considerable research interest (Kazarian 1975; Panjabi et al. 1984; Twomey and Taylor 1982). These biomechanical changes appear to be a direct result of the described alteration with age of the structural components of the IVD. For instance, the decrease in pyridinoline cross links with disc aging may have detrimental effects on matrix resilience and increased pentosidine levels have been implicated in age-related deterioration of connective tissues and loss of disc integrity (Pokharna and Phillips 1998). Other factors that may be superimposed on or coincident with age-related changes occurring in the IVD include increased spinal deformity, smoking, vascular disease, and diabetes (Holm and Nachemson 1988), all factors that may directly or indirectly compromise the vascular supply and consequently, the nutrition to the region surrounding the IVD.

Loading the aging spine

The effect of age on the IVD's ability to resist axial loads is controversial. Creep occurs more rapidly in aged discs when compared with nondegenerate discs (Kazarian 1975). Koeller et al. (1986) were able to demonstrate a twofold increase in creep of the IVD under compression from the age of 30 onward. The nucleus pulposus becomes increasingly dehydrated with age and is less able to exert radial pressure and bear weight when subjected to a vertical force. The annulus fibrosus, which may be additionally weakened by radial transverse tears, is then forced to share a greater proportion of the load (Bogduk and Twomey 1987).

Intervertebral Disc: Common Pathologies

The normal processes of aging can often be difficult to distinguish from other pathologies that affect the IVD. In addition, pathology of the IVD affecting the cervical spine differs from that affecting other regions, namely the IVD from the lumbar spine. The motion and integrity of the IVD is interdependent with other supporting spinal structures, including the zygoapophyseal joints, associated ligaments, neural structures, and muscles. In the lumbar spine, prolapse of the IVD is common. Low back pain has been shown to be associated specifically with signs of lumbar disc degeneration and with posterior disc bulges (Luoma et al. 2000); however, degenerative changes in the IVD evaluated by magnetic resonance imaging (MRI) may also be witnessed in individuals who are asymptomatic (Boden et al. 1990). In the cervical spine, frank prolapse is uncommon, and degenerative changes include end-plate sclerosis, disintegration and collapse of the disc, bulging annulus fibrosus, development of osteophytes from margins of the vertebral body, uncovertebral or zygoapophyseal joints, and narrowing of the intervertebral foramina by chondro-osseous spurs (Brooker and Barter 1965; Goodman 1988; Gore et al. 1987; Lestini and Wiesel 1989; McNab 1975; Scoville 1966).

Intervertebral Disc Herniation

IVD herniation can present as either peripheral or central lesions that manifest from adolescence onward into old age and, in the lumbar spine, may cause back pain and sciatica (Figures 5-6 and 5-7). However, a significant number of disc herniations can be witnessed on MRI that are asymptomatic, depending on the position of the disc herniation, its relationship to the nerve root, and the type of herniation (McCall 2000). Because of such a widespread age group that is vulnerable to this condition, these changes are not only a consequence of age-related dehydration of the IVD (Bogduk and Twomey 1987). The risk of IVD herniation is, however, known to increase when the disc is loaded in a flexed position. Simunic et al. (2001) identified that the combined degree of flexion and the level of hydration of the IVD play important roles in influencing the tendency of the nucleus pulposus to break loose and extrude through a preexisting annular division. Central herniation of the IVD refers to *intrabody nuclear herniation* as opposed to *peripheral herniation*, the most common form encountered in clinical symptomatology and the form in which extruded nuclear material encroaches on the spinal cord and the intervertebral foramen

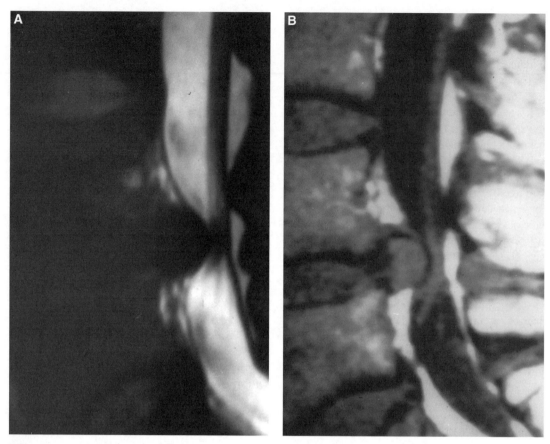

Figure 5-6. A, Disc extrusion (herniation) at the L4-L5 region in a 45-year-old male. A full-thickness tear of the annulus fibrosus gives the "toothpaste" sign. (T2 weighted image, MRI). **B,** Disc extrusion (herniation) at the L4-L5 region in a 45-year-old male: the "toothpaste" sign (T1 weighted image, MRI). (From Lundon K, Bolton K. Structure and Function of the Lumbar Intervertebral Disc in Health, Aging and Pathologic Conditions. JOSPT 2001;31[6]:291-306.)

(Chandraraj et al. 1998). Intradural disc herniations comprise 26% to 30% of all herniated discs, with 5% found in the thoracic, 3% in the cervical; and 92% in the lumbar regions (Negovetic et al. 2001). The factors involved in the evolution of a disc herniation include degradation of the nucleus pulposus and a lesion in the annulus fibrosus or vertebral end-plate (Bogduk 1992 ; Vernon-Roberts 1988). The nuclei pulposi of prolapsed discs in older individuals have been noted to contain more collagen, with its solubility distinctly higher compared with normal tissues of the same age (Olczyk, 1992). Other factors such as congenital defects at the vertebral end-plate (Vernon-Roberts 1988) and trauma may accelerate degradation of the IVD, which then can lead to disc herniation. Although herniation of the IVD is not known to be exclusively age-related, Harada and Nakahara (1989) identified that the

nature of herniated disc material is age-related. The study of older and young individuals determined that herniated disc samples were typically composed of a combination of tissues, including avulsed vertebral end-plate, annulus fibrosus, and nucleus pulposus (Harada and Nakahara 1989).

Disc Degeneration

Degradation of the nucleus pulposus of the lumbar spine IVD may occur after an inflammatory repair response that results from fracturing the vertebral end-plate for which a significant association has been demonstrated (Kerttula et al. 2000). Furthermore, exposure of the matrix of the nucleus pulposus to circulation also may permit the body to mount an immune response against components of

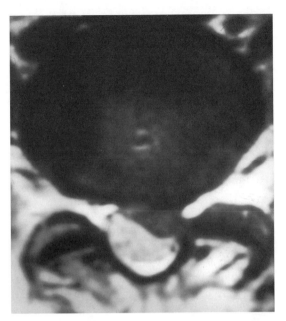

Figure 5-7. Axial view of IVD extrusion (herniation) at the L4-L5 region in a 45-year-old male seen in Figure 5-6 with impingement on the thecal sac. (From Lundon K, Bolton K. Structure and Function of the Lumbar Intervertebral Disc in Health, Aging and Pathologic Conditions. JOSPT 2001;31[6]:291-306.)

the nucleus pulposus leading to disc degeneration. Disc degradation (Adams and Hutton 1983) results from dehydration and deterioration of the nucleus pulposus function (Bogduk and Twomey 1987) after inflammation, proteolysis and depolymerisation of the nucleus pulposus matrix. Disc degeneration is regarded as universal as age advances; however, the individual may be asymptomatic. Potential triggering events include altered mechanical loading of the spine through repeated torsion or compression injuries, leading to annular defects or vertebral end-plate fractures respectively and accelerating disc degeneration. Tears in the IVD occur with age, may demonstrate reduced elastic moduli compared with groups without tears, and are associated with changes in the mechanics of the intervertebral joints in flexion, extension, and torsion (Thompson et al. 2000). Altered metabolism of the IVD resulting from these events is marked by the degradation of PGs, which is reflected by an increase in the blood level of PG components of which keratan sulfate may be an epitope (Kuiper et al. 1998). In addition, evidence shows greater compressive loading across the life span, particularly

in men (Miller et al. 1988), and/or changes in blood flow (avascular nutritional pathways) precede disc degeneration (Chandraraj et al. 1998). Disc degradation may be followed by processes including isolated disc resorption or internal disc disruption. Isolated disc resorption is the consequence of degradation that is limited to the nucleus pulposus, and is characterized by narrowing and marked degeneration of a single disc (Crock 1986). Although the nucleus pulposus itself lacks innervation, an insidious deterioration of the nucleus pulposus affects its mechanical function and ultimately will cause abnormal movement patterns and back pain stemming from abnormal stresses on pain sensitive structures such as the outer annulus fibrosus, zygoapophyseal joints, and their surrounding ligaments. Even more extensive damage to the disc can occur if the degradative process related to isolated disc resorption extends peripherally to involve the annulus fibrosus, resulting in internal disc disruption. The destruction of the nucleus pulposus and progressive erosion of the annulus fibrosus are hallmarks of this condition (Bogduk 1992; Crock 1986). Herniation, protrusion, or bulging are events that are part of this degradation process. If the internal disc degradation extends the length of a radial fissure to the outer annulus fibrosus, weakness occurs in this region and disc herniation results (Bogduk 1992) (see Figure 5-6; Figure 5-8).

Lesions of the IVD: Morphological Characteristics

Lesions of the IVD may present in a variety of morphological forms (Table 5-3). Since the IVD is essentially an avascular structure, its response to injury and ability to repair itself is limited. Furthermore, the level of the IVD may contribute to its vulnerability to changes. For instance, PGs of lumbosacral discs demonstrate a catabolic rate exceeding biosynthesis that is different from the upper levels of the lumbar spine discs (Taylor et al. 2000).

Posterior or posterolateral protrusion

IVDs from the lumbar and low thoracic regions are vulnerable to posterior protrusions that typically occur in young people when the nucleus pulposus is still gelatinous (Bogduk and Twomey 1987). The size and direction of the protrusion lead to variable clinical sequelae, including pain and neurological symptoms (Vernon-Roberts 1988).

Schmorl's Nodes

The nucleus pulposus, under pathologic conditions such as a deficient vertebral end-plate, may protrude into the adjacent vertebral body either from above or below. At these sites that are vascular weak spots, the early formation of central intrabody nuclear herniations may occur (Chandraraj et al. 1998). Acquired lesions, including fracture of the trabeculae in the vertebral body and necrosis of marrow tissues, congenital lesions

or Scheuermann's disease may be conducive to the development of Schmorl's nodes, most of which are balloon or mushroom shaped, less than 5 mm in diameter, and found posterior to the central axis of the vertebra (Vernon-Roberts 1988). If causative forces persist, the herniation progresses, influenced by the degree of reactive inflammation associated with such a herniation. Formation of a cartilaginous cap or calcification of the protrusion may act to arrest its expansion; however, the lesion may also fibrose and calcify (Vernon-Roberts 1988).

Anterior and Lateral Protrusions

Anterolateral bulging of the disc without rupturing the annulus fibrosus, although an infrequent occurrence, may happen after extrusion of the nucleus

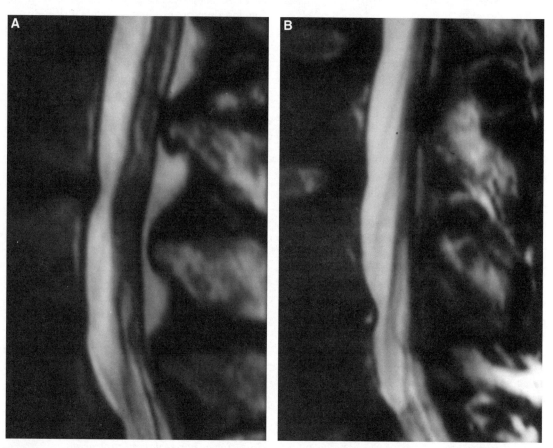

Figure 5-8. A, Bulging IVD (L4-L5) in a 42-year-old female demonstrating a lax but otherwise intact annulus fibrosus (T2 weighted image, MRI). **B,** Disc protrusion (L5-S1) with a partial defect in the annulus fibrosus in a 45-year-old female with nuclear material contained by the outer annular fibers (T2 weighted image, MRI). (From Lundon K, Bolton K. Structure and Function of the Lumbar Intervertebral Disc in Health, Aging and Pathologic Conditions. JOSPT 2001;31[6]:291-306.)

Table 5-3. Basic Clinical Presentation of Intervertebral Disc Lesions

Type of IVD Lesion	Nature of Lesion (Definition)
1. Disc herniation	A process by which part of the nucleus pulposus is expelled through the annulus fibrosus and enters the vertebral canal. Compression of surrounding structures, including spinal nerve roots, is typical.
2. Disc protrusion	Nuclear material does not completely penetrate the annulus fibrosus, but stretches the peripheral lamellae of the annulus fibrosus beyond the normal perimeter of the disc.
3. Disc prolapse/herniation	Frank rupture of nuclear material into the vertebral canal.

From Lundon K, Bolton K: Structure and function of the lumbar intervertebral disk in health, aging and pathologic conditions. JOSPT 2001;31(6):291–306.

pulposus in a posterior or vertical direction (Vernon-Roberts 1988).

Summary

The IVD allows bending and torsion of the spine while simultaneously resisting compression from gravity and muscular activity. The IVD from the different regions (cervical, thoracic, and lumbar spine) differ in their morphology and three-dimensional architecture, although a common basic structure is evident. In the lumbar spine, the IVD is a composite structure of the nucleus pulposus, a central gel-like region surrounded by peripherally located concentric rings of highly ordered, dense collagen fibers known as the annulus fibrosus. The nucleus pulposus is a highly hydrated gel of collagen fibers enveloping PGs and is similar to that found in hyaline (articular) cartilage. The cartilaginous vertebral end-plate of the IVD has a composition similar in part to that of hyaline cartilage. The nucleus

Clinical Note

Sources of Pain Associated with Intervertebral Disc Pathology

Mechanical compression or distension of the nerve root at the lumbar spine, dorsal root ganglion, or smaller nerves surrounding the disc have been attributed to disc herniation or bulge leading to neural compromise and consequent sciatic pain (Luoma et al. 2000). The presence of disc extrusion and/or ipsilateral severe nerve compression at one or multiple sites and visualized by lumbar MRI was shown to be strongly associated with distal leg pain (Beattie et al. 2000). Disc degeneration or bulging was not significantly associated with specific pain patterns in the presence of mild to moderate nerve compression. Pain may also stem from intradiscal pathology that may be a result of pain sensitive nerve endings in the fibers of annulus fibrosus, even in the inner parts of a degenerated disc (Coppes et al. 1997). Mechanical stimulation of the posterior annulus fibrosus has been shown to reproduce symptoms of severe and chronic back pain (Schwarzer et al. 1995) identifying the lumbar IVD as an intrinsic source of pain without nerve root involvement (Jaffray and O'Brien, 1986). This pain has been attributed to inflammation or chemical disturbances and mechanical deformation of damaged disc tissue resulting from internal disc disruption (Adams et al. 2000). Application of in vivo loading to the posterolateral annulus fibrosus and depressurization of the nucleus pulposus has been associated with discogenic pain (McNally and Adams 1996) lending support to the use of extension exercises that aim to cause an anterior migration of nuclear tissue. CT scans and MRI techniques are often used to visualize general morphological change at the IVD. In one study, MRI demonstrated that both symptomatic and asymptomatic disc herniation can be accompanied by structural abnormalities of the IVD (Boos et al. 1997). A significant number of disc herniations that can be witnessed on MRI are asymptomatic, depending on the position of the disc herniation, its relationship to the nerve root, and the type of herniation (McCall 2000) (see Figure 5-8, A and B). Other studies have shown that some herniated IVD fragments reduce in size over time in symptomatic subjects (Komori et al. 1996; Maigne et al. 1992). However, only a mild correlation could be made between symptoms and morphological changes observed by MRI.

pulposus and annulus fibrosus represent a mixed connective tissue matrix of at least two collagen types. The principal collagen type found in the nucleus pulposus is type II collagen. This collagen type represents more than 85% of the total collagen present in the nucleus pulposus with the remainder being type I collagen. The annulus fibrosus contains mostly type I collagen. In addition, types III, V, VI, IX , X , XI, XII, and XIV collagen have been found in the IVD. The complex morphology and ultra-structure of the IVD across different regions of the spine in the human provide the critical elements that permit normal mobility and transmission of force through the vertebral column. Alterations in IVD structure are manifested in a variety of clinical conditions routinely encountered in orthopaedic physical therapy practice. These structural and biomechanical changes are typically related to degenerative changes that occur in association with aging and trauma. The IVD assumes a more fibrous nature with advancing age attributable to dehydration, an increase in collagen, and reduction in PGs and elastin content. Identifying the relationships between the condition of the IVD and spinal pain is clinically important to improve and deliver appropriate clinical management of IVD pathologies.

References

Adams MA, Hutton WC. The mechanical function of the lumbar apophyseal joints. Spine 1983;8(3):327.

Adams MA, Hutton WC. Mechanics of the Intervertebral Disc. In P Ghosh P (ed), The Biology of the Intervertebral Disc, Volume II. Boca Raton, Fla: CRC Press, 1988;39-71.

Adams MA et al. Effects of backward bending on lumbar intervertebral discs. Spine 2000;25(4):431-437.

Adams P, Muir H. Qualitative changes with age of proteoglycans in human lumbar discs. Ann Rheum Dis 1976; 35(4):289-296.

Adams P et al. Biochemical aspects of development and ageing of human lumbar intervertebral discs. Rheumatol Rehabil 1977;16(1): 22-29.

Akeson WH et al. Biomechanics and biochemistry of the intervertebral disks: the need for correlation studies. Clin Orthop 1977;129:133-140.

Armstrong, CG, Mow VC. Variations in the intrinsic mechanical properties of human articular cartilage with age, degeneration, and water content. J Bone and Joint Surg 1982;64A:88-94.

Ashton IK et al. Neuropeptides in the human intervertebral disc. J Orthop Res 1994;12:186-192.

Ayad S, Weiss JB. Biochemistry of the Intervertebral Disc. In MIV Jayson (ed), The Lumbar Spine and Back Pain (3rd ed), New York: Churchill Livingstone, 1987.

Beard HK, Stevens RL. Biochemical Changes in the Intervertebral Disc. In MIV Jayson (ed), The Lumbar Spine and Back Pain (2nd ed), London: Pitman Medical, 1980;407-436.

Beard HK et al. Immunofluorescent staining for collagen and proteoglycans in normal and scoliotic intervertebral discs. J Bone Joint Surg Br 1981;638(4):529-534.

Beattie PF et al. Associations between patient report of symptoms and anatomic impairment visible on lumbar magnetic resonance imaging. Spine 2000;25(7): 819-828.

Bernick S, Cailliet R. Vertebral end-plate changes with aging of human vertebrae. Spine 1982;7(2):97-102.

Bishop PB, Pearce RH. The proteoglycans of the cartilaginous end-plate of the human intervertebral disc change after maturity. J Orthop Res 1993;11(3):324-331.

Boden SD et al. Abnormal magnetic resonance scans of the lumbar spine in asymptomatic subjects. A prospective investigation. J Bone Jt Surg 1990;72A:403-408.

Bogduk N. The Sources of Low Back Pain. In MIV Jayson (ed), The Lumbar Spine and Back Pain (4th ed). New York: Churchill Livingstone, 1992;61-88.

Bogduk N, Twomey LT. Clinical Anatomy of the Lumbar Spine, New York: Churchill Livingstone, 1987.

Boos N et al. Tissue characterization of symptomatic and asymptomatic disc herniations by quantitative magnetic resonance imaging. J Orthop Res 1997;15: 141-149.

Brooker A, Barter R. Cervical spondylosis: a clinical study with comparative radiology. Brain 1965;88: 925-936.

Buckwalter JA et al. Elastic fibres in human intervertebral discs. J Bone Joint Surg 1976; 58A(1):73-76.

Buckwalter JA. Fine Structural Studies of the Human Intervertebral Disc. In AA White, SL Gordon (eds), Idiopathic Low Back Pain. St. Louis: Mosby, 1982.

Buckwalter JA et al. Age-related changes in cartilage proteoglycans: quantitative electron microscopic studies. Microsc Res Tech 1994;28(5):398-408.

Buckwalter JA. Spine update aging and degeneration of the human intervertebral disc. Spine 1995;20(1):1307-1314.

Burgeson RE, Nimni NE. Collagen types. Molecular structure and tissue distribution. Clin Orthop 1992;282: 250-272.

Bushell GR et al. Proteoglycan chemistry of the intervertebral disks. Clin Orthop 1977;129:115-123.

Chandraraj S et al. Disc herniations in the young and end-plate vascularity. Clin Anat 1998;11:171-176.

Chelberg MK et al. Identification of heterogeneous cell populations in the normal human intervertebral disc. J Anat 1995;186(I):43-53.

Coppes MH et al. Innervation of "painful" lumbar discs. Spine 1997;22:2342-2350.

Coventry MB. Anatomy of the intervertebral disc. Clin Orthop 1969;67:9-15.

Coventry MB et al. The intervertebral disc: its microscopic anatomy and pathology. Part I: anatomy, development and physiology. J Bone Joint Surg Br 1945;27(1): 105-112.

Crock HV. Internal disc disruption: a challenge to disc prolapse 50 years on. Spine 1986;11(6):650-653.

Crock HV. Repraisal of intervertebral disc lesions. Austral Med J 1970;1:983-989.

Dickson IR et al. Variations in the protein components of human intervertebral disk with age. Nature 1967;215: 52-53.

Donahue PJ et al. Characterization of link protein(s) from human intervertebral-disc tissues. Biochem J 1988;251:739-747.

Duance V et al. Changes in collagen cross-linking in degenerative disc disease and scoliosis. Spine 1998;23(23):2545-2551.

Eyre DR, Muir H. Quantitative analysis of types I and II collagen in human intervertebral discs at various ages. Biochemica et Biophysica Acta 1977;492:29-43.

Eyre DR. Collagens of the Disc. In P Ghosh (ed), The Biology of the Intervertebral Disc, Volume I. Boca Raton, Fla: CRC Press, 1988;171-188.

Fairbank JCT, Pynsent PB. Syndromes of Back Pain and Their Classification. In MIV Jayson (ed), The Lumbar Spine and Back Pain (4th ed), New York: Churchill Livingstone, 1992.

Farfan HF et al. The effects of torsion on the lumbar intervertebral joints: the role of torsion in the production of disc degeneration. J Bone Joint Surg Am 1970;52A(3):468-497.

Ghosh P et al. Collagens, elastin and noncollagenous protein of the intervertebral disc. Clin Orthop 1977;129: 124-132.

Goodman BW. Neck pain. Prim Care 1988;925-936.

Gore D et al. Neck pain: a long-term follow-up of 205 patients. Spine 1987;12:1-5.

Gower WE, Pedrini V. Age-related variations in protein-polysaccharides from human nucleus pulposus, annulus fibrosus, and costal cartilage. J Bone Joint Surg Am 1969;51A(6):1154-1162.

Grignon B et al. The structure of the cartilaginous end plates in elderly people. Surgic Radiol Anat 2000;22(1):13-19.

Hansson T, Roos B. Microcalluses of the trabeculae in lumbar vertebrae and their relation to their bone mineral content. Spine 1981;6(4):375-380.

Harada Y, Nakahara S. A pathological study of lumbar disc herniation in the elderly. Spine 1989;14(9):1020-1024.

Hassler O. The human intervertebral disc. A micro-angiographical study on its vascular supply at various ages. Acta Orthop Scandinavica 1969;40:765-772.

Haughton VM et al. Flexibility of lumbar spine motion segments correlated to type of tears in the annulus fibrosus. J Neurosurg 2000;92:81-86.

Holm S, Nachemson A. Nutrition of the intervertebral disc: acute effects of cigarette smoking. An experimental animal study. Uppsala J Med Sci 1988;93:91-99.

Horton GW. Further observations on the elastic mechanism of the intervertebral disc. J Bone Joint Surg Br 1958;40B:552-557.

Hukins DWL. Disc Structure and Function. In P Ghosh (ed), The Biology of the Intervertebral Disc, Volume I. Boca Raton, Fla: CRC Press, 1988;1-37.

Hukins DWL, Meakin JR. Relationship between structure and mechanical function of the tissues of the intervertebral joint. Amer Zoologist 2000;40(1):42-52.

Hutton W et al. The effect of compressive force applied to the intervertebral disc in vivo. Spine 1998;23(23): 2524-2537.

Iatridis J et al. Compression induced changes in intervertebral disc properties in a rat tail model. Spine 1999;24(10):996-1002.

Inoue H. Three-dimensional architecture of lumbar intervertebral discs. Spine 1981;6(2):139-145.

Inoue H, Takeda T. Three-dimensional observation of collagen framework of lumbar intervertebral discs. Acta Orthop Scand 1975;46(6):949-956.

Ishihara H, Urban JP. Effects of low oxygen concentration and metabolic inhibitors on proteoglycan and protein synthesis rates in the intervertebral disc. J Orthop Res 1999;17(6):829-835.

Jaffray D, O'Brien JP. Isolated intervertebral disc resorption. Spine 1986;11:397-401.

Jensen GM. Biomechanics of the lumbar intervertebral disk: a review. Phys Ther 1980;60(6):765-773.

Jette AM et al. Musculoskeletal impairments and physical disablement among the aged. J Gerontol 1990;45(6):M203-M208.

Johnson E et al. Elastic fibres in the annulus fibrosus of the adult human lumbar intervertebral disc. A preliminary report. J Anat 1985;143:57-63.

Kazarian L. Creep characteristics of the human spinal column. Orthop Clin North Am 1975;6(1):3-18.

Kerttula LI et al. Posttraumatic findings of the spine after earlier vertebral fracture in young patients: clinical and MRI study. Spine 2000;25(9):1104-1108.

Koeller W et al. Biomechanical properties of human intervertebral discs subjected to axial dynamic compression: influence of age and degeneration. J Biomech 1986;19:807-816.

Komori H et al. The natural history of herniated nucleus pulposus with radiculopathy. Spine 1996;21(2):225-229.

Kuiper JI et al. Keratan sulfate as a potential biomarker of loading of the intervertebral disc. Spine 1998;23(6): 657-663.

Lawrence VA et al. Acute low back pain and economics of therapy: the iterative loop approach. J Clin Epidemiol 1992;45(3):301-311.

Lestini W, Wiesel S. The pathogenesis of cervical spondylosis. Clin Orthop 1989;239:69-93.

Lundon K, Bolton K. Structure and function of the lumbar intervertebral disc in health, age and pathologic conditions. JOSPT 2001;31(6):291-306.

Luoma K et al. Low back pain in relation to lumbar disc degeneration. Spine 2000;25(4):487-492.

Luoma K et al. Disc height and signal intensity of the nucleus pulposus on magnetic resonance imaging as indicators of lumbar disc degeneration. Spine 2001;26(6):680-686.

Maigne J et al. Computed tomographic follow-up study of forty-eight cases of nonoperatively treated lumbar intervertebral disc herniation. Spine 1992;17(9):1071-1074.

Markolf KL, Morris MD. The structural components of the intervertebral disc. J Bone Joint Surg Am 1974;56A(4):675-687.

McCall I. Lumbar herniated disks. Radiol Clin North Am 2000;38(6):1293-1309.

McDevitt C. Proteoglycans of the Intervertebral Disc. In P Ghosh (ed), The Biology of the Intervertebral Disc, Volume II. Boca Raton, Fla: CRC Press, 1988.

McNab I. Cervical spondylosis. Clin Orthop 1975;109:69-77.

McNally DS, Adams MA. In vivo stress measurement can predict pain on discography. Spine 1996;21:2580-2587.

Mercer S, Bogduk, N. The ligaments and annulus fibrosus of human cervical intervertebral discs. Spine 1999;24(7):619-628.

Miller JA et al. Lumbar disc degeneration: correlation with age, sex, and spine level in 600 autopsy specimens. Spine 1988;13(2):173-178.

Moore RJ. The vertebral end-plate: what do we know? Europ Spine J 2000;9(2):92-96.

Nachemson A. Lumbar intradiscal pressure: experimental studies on post-mortem material. Acta Orthop Scand Suppl 1960;43:1-104.

Nachemson A, Morris JM. In vivo measurements of intradiscal pressure. J Bone Joint Surg 1964;46A(5):1077-1092.

Nachemson A. The load on lumbar discs in different positions of the body. Clin Orthop 1966;45:107-122.

Nachemson, A. Disc pressure measurements. Spine 1981;6:93-97.

Negovetic L et al. Intradural disc herniation at the T1, T2 level. Croat Med J 2001;42(2):193-195.

Nerlich A et al. Immunolocalization of major interstitial collagen types in human lumbar intervertebral discs of various ages. Virchows Arch 1998;432:67-76.

Olczyk K. Age related changes in collagen of human intervertebral discs. Gerontology 1992;38(4):196-204.

Osti OL et al. Annulus tears and intervertebral disc degeneration: An experimental study using an animal model. Spine 1990;15(8):762-767.

Osti OL et al. Annular tears and disc degeneration in the lumbar spine. J Bone Joint Surg Br 1992;74B(5):678-682.

Panjabi M et al. Biomechanical Studies in Cadaveric Spines. In MIV Jayson (ed), The Lumbar Spine and Back Pain (4th ed). New York: Churchill Livingstone, 1992;133-135.

Panjabi MM et al. Effects of disc injury on mechanical behaviour of the human spine. Spine 1984;9(7):707-713.

Panjabi M et al. Intrinsic disc pressure as a measure of integrity of the lumbar spine. Spine 1988;13(8):913-917.

Panjabi M et al. Effects of disc degeneration on the stability of a motion segment. Transact Annual ORS 1992;29(8):212.

Pearce RH. Morphologic and Chemical Aspects of Aging. In JA Buckwalter et al. (eds), Musculoskeletal Soft-Tissue Aging: Impact on Mobility. Rosemont, Ill: American Academy of Orthopaedic Surgeons, 1992;363-379.

Pokharna HK, Phillips FM. Collagen cross-links in human lumbar intervertebral disc aging. Spine 1998;23(15):1645-1648.

Pooni JS et al. Comparison of the structure of human intervertebral discs in the cervical, thoracic and lumbar regions of the spine. Surg Radiol Anat 1986;8(3):175-182.

Race A et al. Effect of loading rate and hydration on the mechanical properties of the disc. Spine 2000;25(6):662-669.

Riihimaki H et al. Radiographically detectable degenerative changes of the lumbar spine among concrete reinforcement workers and house painters. Spine 1990;15:114-119.

Roberts S et al. Biochemical and structural properties of the cartilage end-plate and its relation to the intervertebral disc. Spine 1989;14(2):166-174.

Schwarzer AC et al. The prevalence and clinical features of internal disc disruption in patients with chronic low back pain. Spine 1995;20:1878-1883.

Scoville W. Types of cervical disk lesions and their surgical approaches. JAMA 1966;196:479-481.

Simunic DI et al. Biomechanical factors influencing nuclear disruption of the intervertebral disc. Spine 2001;26(11):1223-1230.

Steffen T et al. Lumbar intradiscal pressure measured in the anterior and posterolateral annular regions during asymmetrical loading. Clin Biomech 1998;13(7):495-505.

Taylor TKF, Akeson WH. Intervertebral disc prolapse: a review of morphologic and biochemical knowledge concerning the nature of prolapse. Clin Orthop 1971;76:54-75.

Taylor TKF et al. Spinal biomechanics and aging are major determinants of the proteoglycan metabolism of intervertebral disc cells. Spine 2000;25(23):3014-3020.

Thompson R et al. Disc lesions and the mechanics of the intervertebral joint complex. Spine 2000;25(23):3026-3035.

Trout JJ et al. Ultrastructure of the human intervertebral disc: II. Cells of the nucleus pulposus. Anat Rec 1982;204:307-314.

Twomey L, Taylor J. Flexion creep deformation and hysteresis in the lumbar vertebral column. Spine 1982;7(2):116-122.

Twomey L, Taylor J. Age changes in lumbar intervertebral discs. Acta Orthop Scand 1985;56(6):496-499.

Twomey L et al. Age changes in the bone density and structure of the lumbar vertebral column. J Anat 1983;136(I):15-25.

Urban J, Maroudas A. The chemistry of the intervertebral disc in relation to its physiological function. Clin Rheum Dis 1980;6:51-76.

Urban M et al. Intervertebral disc composition in neuromuscular scoliosis: changes in cell density and glycosaminoglycan concentration at the curve apex. Spine 2001;26(6):610-617.

Vernon-Roberts B. Disc Pathology and Disease States. In P Ghosh (ed), The Biology of the Intervertebral Disc, Volume II. Boca Raton, Fla: CRC Press, 1988.

Vernon-Roberts B. Age-related and Degenerative Pathology of the Intervertebral Discs and Apophyseal Joints. In MIV Jayson (ed), The Lumbar Spine and Back Pain (4th ed). New York: Churchill Livingstone, 1992.

Vernon-Roberts B, Pirie CJ. Degenerative changes in the intervertebral discs of the lumbar spine and their sequelae. Rheumatol Rehabil 1977;16(1):13-21.

Videman T et al. Lumbar spinal pathology in cadaveric material in relation to history of back pain, occupation, and physical loading. Spine 1990;15:728-740.

Videman T et al. Lifetime exercise and disk degeneration: an MRI study of monozygotic twins. Med Sci Sports Exercise 1997;29(10):1350-1356.

Wang JL et al. Viscoelastic finite-element analysis of a lumbar motion segment in combined compression and sagittal flexion. Spine 2000;25(3):310-318.

Yang C et al. Structural and functional implications of age-related abnormal modifications in collagen II from intervertebral disc. Matrix Biol 1994;14:643-651.

Chapter 6

Dynamics of the Nonmineralized Connective Tissues of the Musculoskeletal System

Connective Tissue Biomechanics

The material to be discussed in this chapter deals with the physical behavior of the dense, nonmineralized connective tissues. The rationale for addressing the general principles underlying the biological and biomechanical nature of the dense connective tissues (tendons, ligaments, capsules, articular cartilage, intervertebral disc) is that this information is important for both prevention and management of injury to these tissues, the knowledge of which is the cornerstone of orthopaedic physical therapy practice.

Relation of Architecture to Function

The property of *extensibility* is a hallmark of the connective tissues, and the ability of networks of fibrous collagen within these tissues to reorient themselves to imposed forces contributes to the nonlinear stress-strain curves (Figure 6-1) that are typical of these tissues (Wainwright et al. 1976). One property common to the extensible connective tissues of the musculoskeletal system is that they become progressively stiffer as they become extended and the collagen fibers become aligned with the direction of stretching. Collagen fibers can form cross-helical, cross-ply or quasirandom networks in the extensible connective tissues with strain-induced reorientation of these networks, giving rise to the nonlinear mechanical properties of connective tissue at finite strains (Purslow et al. 1998). In connective tissues that have as diverse a presentation ranging from the perimysial connective tissue that separates muscle fascicles (Purslow

1989) to the annulus fibrosus of the intervertebral disc (Klein and Hukins 1982), a cross-ply or cross-helical arrangement of collagen fibers is evident, with respect to the long axis of the muscle fiber or cranio-caudal axis of the body respectively.

The dense regular connective tissues display both viscous and elastic rheological properties and thus are considered *viscoelastic* in nature, displaying both time and frequency dependent properties (Dorrington 1980; Wainwright et al. 1976). These properties can be demonstrated by the application of a fixed extension to the tissue, with the result that the initial stress generated decreases with time or by the application of a fixed stress whereupon the initial extension in the tissue increases with time, a phenomenon referred to as *creep*. Therefore stress-relaxation and load deformation represent two kinds of mechanical events characteristic of a viscoelastic tissue. *Mechanical creep*, defined as the elongation of tissue with a constant load over time beyond intrinsic extensibility is regarded to play a role in conventional tissue expansion during the application of a chronic stretching force (Wilhelmi et al. 1998). In creep, the continued extension of the material under constant load means that tissue reorientation caused by increasing overall strain in the specimen can occur, driven by the strain energy imparted to the specimen which increases with time (Purslow et al. 1998).

Mechanisms Underlying Connective Tissue Extensibility

Reorientation of collagen fibers caused by finite extension of connective tissues is a well-documented phenomenon (Aspden 1986); the

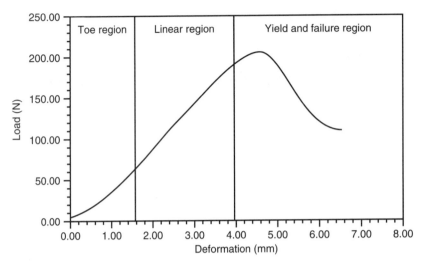

Figure 6-1. Basic stress-strain or load-deformation curve for tendon. (From Woo SL-Y et al. Anatomy, Biology and Biomechanics of Tendon, Ligament, and Meniscus. In SR Simon. Orthopaedic Basic Science. Rosemont, Ill: American Academy of Orthopaedic Surgeons, 1994;51.)

time-dependent aspect of the properties of extensible connective tissues is what becomes more difficult to explain. In one study a lack of obvious reorientation was observed during the time course of either a strong stress-relaxation or creep transient indicating that long-range reorientation of collagen fibers is not the only principal structural event associated with the viscoelastic behavior of these tissues (Purslow et al. 1998). Collagen fiber reorientation following loading has thus been identified as not the exclusive source of the viscoelastic properties of extensible connective tissues. The nonlinear (strain-dependent) nature of the stress-relaxation response in these tissues suggests that relaxation processes both *within* the collagen fibers themselves and/or at the *fiber-matrix (molecular relaxations within the PG matrix surrounding the collagen fibers) interface* may be responsible for their viscoelastic nature (Purslow et al. 1998). Therefore viscoelastic properties of extensible connective tissues may reside both within the collagen fibers and at the interface between fiber and matrix.

Role of the Collagen Fiber

The mechanical (supportive and connective) behavior of regular dense connective tissue (RDCT) is governed largely by fibers, of which the majority are collagen. As mentioned above, the characteristics of these fibers and their interaction with other components of the matrix determine tissue strength. Ligaments and tendons present with a multimodal collagen fibril diameter distribution that endows them with optimal functional properties (see Chapter 3). In general, a fiber bundle can either fail by *tear*, where collagen fibrils break as their tensile strength is exceeded, or by creep, which occurs when fibrils slide past each other and the tissue they form disaggregates (Ottani et al. 2001). In addition to the physical properties of collagen and architectural arrangement of fibers (cross-helical, cross-ply, or quasirandom network), mechanical properties of connective tissues, in terms of their measured tensile strength, are well correlated with the average diameter of their collagen fibrils (Parry and Craig 1984). The proportion of collagen fibrils of different sizes, often reflecting collagen fiber maturity, contributes to connective tissue mechanics. The benefit of tissues having a higher fraction of small diameter fibrils (that would ultimately ensure a better interfibrillar binding by virtue of their higher surface/volume ratio) would be that they could accommodate for both tensile strength if also associated with large diameter fibrils and creep resistance (Ottani et al. 2001). In contrast, fibrils that have more spatial layout (as are found in nerve sheaths, blood vessels and interstitial connective tissues) have smaller, uniform fibrils ranging approximately from 25 to 1000 nm and presenting with distinctive, unimodal distribution. These fibrils typically run in small, wavy bundles and often form three-dimensional isotropic networks that, as a result of soft highly compliant matrices, are able to resist multidirectional stresses with high, cyclical deformations without permanent effects (Ottani et al. 2001). Although gliding freedom of individual collagen fibers in collagen-based tissues varies with their configuration, it is critical to the maintenance of normal connective tissue mobility (Akeson et al. 1980). In addition, the proportion of collagen and other fibers plays a role in connective tissue biomechanics. For instance, although collagenous fibers in particular assist in the production of force in structures such as the ligament and tendon, elastic fibers also contribute to the ability of tissues and organs to regain their original form after mechanical deformation.

Response of Connective Tissue to Physical Stress and Activity

Mechanical Stress as Physical Stimulus

The formation and maintenance of collagen in dense connective tissue is highly dependent on stress as a physical stimulus. In fact, mechanical stresses are important environmental cues for both normal cellular functions and pathophysiological changes in numerous conditions in connective tissue–based structures (e.g., atherosclerosis). The effects of immobilization and conditions of stress deprivation, particularly in association with trauma to the dense connective tissues, is of equal clinical significance. Even in the absence of trauma, the effects of immobilization and deprivation of stress on connective tissue integrity can be of serious clinical consequence.

Increasing evidence exists that mechanotransduction processes in response to mechanical stresses share many common features with processes of cell adhesion, such as an increase in tyrosine phosphorylation of proteins in the focal adhesion sites. Integrins may function as mechanotransducers in cells (Shyy and Chien 1997) and other cell components such as intermediate filaments are directly implicated in providing cell resilience and the maintenance of tissue integrity, each of which has direct implications for the connective tissues. By maintaining the shape and plasticity of the cell, the intermediate filament network acts as an integrator within the cell space. In this way, the state of mechanical force imposed on the tissue or a cell can alter the shape of certain elements of the cytoskeleton and thus participate in the control of cell functions (Galou et al. 1997).

The response of collagen to mechanical elongation often is demonstrated using the tendon or ligament as a representative dense connective tissue. The mechanical behavior of tendon or ligament is studied by elongating the structure to the point of rupture, while measuring increases in length and tension during stretch. To make comparisons between the mechanical properties of a structure, force and elongation are presented as *stress* and *strain* respectively (Box 6-1). One achieves a *stress-strain* curve that depicts values of change in *length* and *tension* of a structure (Figure 6-2). Five distinct regions fall within either an elastic or plastic range that are ascribed to a stress-strain curve (see Figure 6-2).

Box 6-1.

Stress is defined as the amount of tension or load per unit cross-sectional area that is placed on a specimen. The role of stress as a physical stimulus affecting intact connective tissues can be summarized by two simple observations:

i) increasing stress levels causes increased collagen formation and content in tendon and ligaments (Woo et al., 1975).
ii) deprivation of stress causes weakening (disorganization of collagen fibers in tendon) of connective tissues (Enwemeka, 1992).

Strain is the elongation of a structure or material that occurs in response to stress.

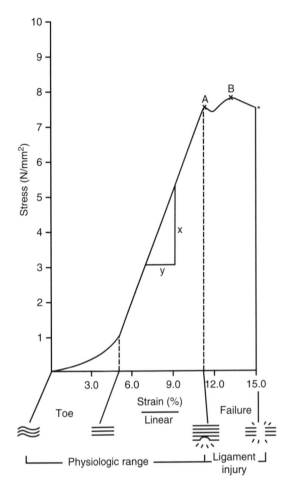

Figure 6-2. Normal stress-strain curve for ligament illustrating toe, elastic, and plastic regions. (From Binkley J. Overview of ligament and tendon structure and mechanics. Implications for the clinical practice. Physiother Canada 1989;41[1]:24-30.)

The Elastic Range: Toe and Linear Regions

Toe Region

Relatively low force is required to elongate the tissue (resulting in approximately 1.2% to 1.5% strain) within this physiological range and is characterized by the straightening of the fibril crimp at the level of the collagen fascicle (see Chapter 3) in the ligament or tendon (Chazal et al. 1985; Diament et al. 1972). The toe-linear region of the stress-strain curve is also the region within which physiologic limits of elongation in tendon are defined. Restoration of the initial length of the connective-tissue-based structure (e.g., ligament or

tendon) takes place, as does the internal fibril crimp on release of stress in the toe region. As can be seen in the curve, the relationship between force and elongation in the toe region is nonlinear. The elastic properties of the structure are fully demonstrated. Normal functional range for ligament and capsules is hypothesized to be within the toe region (Binkley 1989).

Linear Region

The linear region of the curve represents the behavior of the collagen fibrils (parallel) after the crimp has been removed via the applicaton of increased stress to the structure (Chazal et al. 1985; Diament et al. 1972). The stiffness of tendon/ligament is essentially consistent with stress experienced, rapidly increasing with elongation. Full recovery from elongation in the linear region is expected, meaning that the lengthening of ligament or tendon in this region is still within its physiologic limits. Once the linear region of the tendon's stress-strain curve is reached, however, the collagen can be permanently lengthened by internal microfailure (denaturing and weakening the fibers), which occurs when the tissue is subjected to excessive strain and/or temperature. The crimp form is permanently lost when strain exceeds 3% or 4%, where denaturation of collagen fibers having lost their crimp can be visualized ultrastructurally. Any strain occurring in this region can be attributed to stretching of the denatured fibers, based on observations made on discrete collagen fibers taken from tendon and subjected to stress. Since deformation to the end of the linear range is completely reversible, elongation of connective tissue into this range does not cause gross injury nor does it result in any residual length increase *at a macroscopic level* (Binkley 1989).

The Plastic Range: Progressive, Major, and Complete Failure Regions

A distinct increase occurs in the slope of the curve in the progressive failure region. Extensive internal microfailure within the structure occurs in this region; however, the appearance of the tendon/ligament at the gross level remains initially intact. Irreversible lengthening and failure of ligament or tendon occurs here and is represented by a decrease in slope of the curve as portions of the tissue collagen begin to fail, leading to the *yield point* (Butler et al. 1978). As further stress is applied, a maximal load point is reached whereupon complete failure of the structure occurs rapidly. Elongation into the plastic range results in permanent tissue lengthening or complete failure (macrofailure) where one sustains a rupture of the tissue material.

In summary, mechanical forces can bring forth structural changes equivalent to those produced by heat of chemical changes. Recovery has been proposed to result from strain occurring between collagen molecules (if less than 3%), and minimal displacement of these collagen molecules takes place, which permits associated bonds to re-organize during recovery. These events would not occur at higher strain levels. Permanent denaturation can be seen between 4% and 10% strain.

Connective Tissue: Evidence for the Biological Response to Mobilization and Physical Activity

The repair and maintenance of connective tissues is the responsibility of the mesenchymally derived fibroblast whose activity is regulated, in part, by the mechanical environment in which it dwells. Dynamic strain is integral to fibroblast stimulation and in the organization of the overall extracellular matrix (ECM) of connective tissues (Figures 6-3 and 6-4). The purpose of appropriate mobilization at any age therefore is to impact synthesis of proteoglycans (PGs) and collagen by fibroblasts, improve the motion of collagen fibers, and prevent the development of anomalous cross-links between

fibers and other macromolecular elements of the ECM that are associated with periods of extended immobilization. Recall that the role of PGs is to attract and hold water molecules and in turn lubricate the connective tissue fibers, ultimately limiting the number of cross-links formed by creating increased distance between fibers and other elements of the ECM.

The positive effects of physical strain on tendon and other connective tissue–based structures are recognized; however little knowledge exists on how mechanical strain specifically affects tendon cells (Zeichen et al. 2000). Although little is known about the mechanisms that occur between mechanical stimulation and cellular (fibroblastic) responses, studies from flow-mediated endothelial mechanotransduction have showed that effects occur within seconds and include a variety of electrophysiological and biochemical responses in the cells (Davies 1995). Based on the findings of Quinn et al. (1998), cell-matrix interactions in the cell-associated matrix may be an important aspect of the chondrocyte response to mechanical compression that might involve macromolecular transport limitations and morphological changes associated with fluid flow and local compaction of the matrix around cells (Figure 6-5). Furthermore, a biphasic response at 60 minutes and at 15 minutes but not at 30 minutes to cyclic biaxial mechanical strain applied to dishes of cultured tendon cells was observed, indicating that the application of time-dependant mechanical stress to tendon fibroblasts resulted in an alteration of cellular proliferation that was sustained even after 24 hours in the group subject to 60 minutes of cyclic strain (Zeichen et al. 2000).

Clinical Note

Principles of Recovery

If a physical stress is applied to a tissue but the stress is removed before rupture (see *yield phase*), the structure will *recover* its original length with rest or when the load is removed. The structure returns to its original length and is said to have *recovered*.

The term *recovery* refers only to the return of the tendon or ligament to its original length at a gross or macroscopic level, and does *not* rule out the presence of some internal microfailure, which is a clinically desirable effect when the intent of the therapeutic stress is to effect an increase in local mobility.

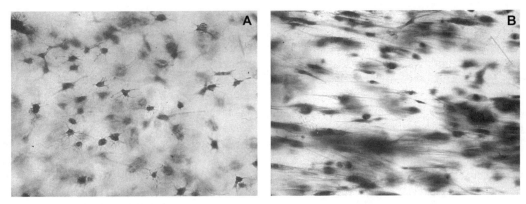

Figure 6-3. A, Effect of low level mechanical loading on cellular (fibroblast) alignment within collagen matrix. **B,** Effect of high level of mechanical loading on fibroblast morphology within collagen matrix. (From Eastwood M et al. Effect of precise mechanical loading on fibroblast populated collagen lattices: morphological changes. Cell Motility and the Cytoskeleton 1998;40:13-21. Copyright John Wiley and Sons.)

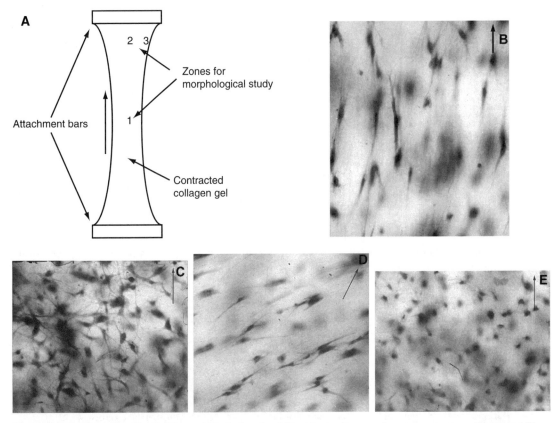

Figure 6-4. A, The zones (1 to 3) for morphological study of fibroblastic alignment in response to stress. **B,** Aligned fibroblasts from zone 1. **C,** Nonaligned fibroblasts from zone 2. **D,** Aligned fibroblasts from zone 3. **E,** Loss of cellular alignment and bipolarity from zone 1 with the removal of the mechanical load. The arrows in **B, C, D,** and **E** indicate the direction of the long axis of the collagen gel. (From Eastwood M et al. Effect of precise mechanical loading on fibroblast populated collagen lattices: morphological changes. Cell Motility and the Cytoskeleton 1998;40:13-21. Copyright John Wiley and Sons.)

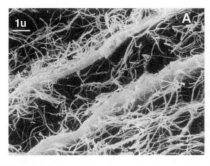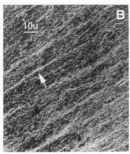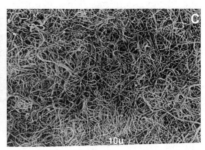

Figure 6-5. Scanning electron micrographs of collagen lattices under mechanical stress: **A,** Random orientation of collagen fibrils in between two aligned bipolar fibroblasts. **B,** Highly aligned fibroblasts, indicated with a small arrow is a cell, whereas the larger arrow indicates the general orientation of the cells and the direction of the major axis. **C,** Cell-free collagen gel, loaded and fixed under tension; note the random orientation of collagen fibrils. (From Eastwood M et al. Effect of precise mechanical loading on fibroblast populated collagen lattices: morphological changes. Cell Motility and the Cytoskeleton 1998;40:13-21. Copyright John Wiley and Sons.)

Biological Concept of Continuous Passive Motion on Synovial Joints

Over the past three and a half decades the concept of continuous passive motion (CPM) of synovial joints stimulating pluripotential mesenchymal cells to differentiate into articular cartilage and accelerating the healing of articular tissues has been explored. In addition to the effects on articular cartilage healing and regeneration, accelerated healing of periarticular tissues such as tendons and ligaments has been demonstrated with the use of CPM of synovial joints after injury and surgical repair. In addition, CPM appears to prevent adhesions and joint stiffness (Salter 1989). In both adolescent and adult animal models, healing of articular cartilage defects with the greatest amount of hyaline cartilage regeneration was observed in a CPM managed group compared with immobilized and intermittent active motion groups (Salter et al. 1980). The application of CPM during the early

postoperative period was shown to be most beneficial when there was a slow rate of motion as opposed to a faster rate; furthermore 1 week of CPM begun immediately after injury achieves the same benefits as 3 weeks of CPM, with reparative tissue remaining intact at one year postoperative (Salter et al. 1978). The use of CPM postoperatively was shown to decrease the atrophic changes associated with immobilization and significantly increase the strength of repair tissue at 6 and 12 weeks relative to controls after a medial collateral ligament replacement using the semitendinosus tenodesis in the rabbit model (Salter and Minster 1982).

Postarthroplasty

The acceptance of the need for early, protected motion after total joint arthroplasty, particularly total knee joint replacement (TKR), has resulted in the use of instruments such as the CPM machine

---

Clinical Note

Continuous Passive Motion

The CPM is ideally instituted immediately postoperative (while the patient is still under general anesthesia) and is continued nonstop for a minimum period of 1 week, after which active exercises of the involved joint are encouraged. The optimal rate of motion of the various CPM devices for humans is one complete cycle every 45 seconds (Salter 1989).

under these conditions. This acceptance of the role of early motion has been shown to result in range of motion (ROM) to be achieved more easily, fewer postoperative manipulations are needed, and patients leave the hospital sooner. However, although patients appear to achieve their motion earlier, the ultimate ROM gained at 6-12 months postoperative TKR is not different between groups who received early CPM intervention and those who did not (Ecker and Lotke 1989).

Effect of Joint Motion and Loading

The work of Houlbrooke et al. (1990) sought to identify whether the loss of PGs in immobilized nonweightbearing joints was caused by a lack of compression, movement, or both. This study showed that movement alone without weightbearing was in fact sufficient to maintain glycosaminoglycan (GAG) content as was weightbearing without movement during a period of immobilization. A significant loss in articular cartilage GAG in nonweightbearing joints occurred under conditions of immobilization (Houlbrooke et al. 1990). This finding is in contrast to the findings of Palmoski et al. (1980) where GAG content decreased in joints that were free to move but not subject to weightbearing. In this study the loading of the joint, which occurred from contraction of the muscles that span the knee and stabilize the limb in stance and not merely joint movement, was determined to be required at least partially to maintain the integrity of the articular cartilage (Palmoski et al. 1980). Movement alone also was shown to be insufficient in maintaining PG levels in articular

cartilage in that when a joint that normally bears weight was subject to a period of nonweightbearing, a loss in matrix PGs in the articular cartilage occurred, which ultimately led to a loss in function of the structure (Kiviranta 1987). The disparity in the findings of these studies may be attributed to differences in experimental design and simulation of the nonweightbearing, mobilized state that was represented by amputation (Palmoski et al. 1980) as opposed to a free but nonweightbearing limb held in sling (Houlbrooke et al. 1990).

Mobilization and Manipulation of Nonmineralized Connective Tissues

The healing of connective tissue and appropriate scar formation was observed to be related to tissue movement in early studies (Stearns 1940). Passive physical mobilization of specific connective tissue structures has been employed in the management of soft tissue conditions such as acute and chronic tendonitis (Chamberlain 1982). Although deep friction massage is used to augment ligament and tendon healing and repair (Cyriax and Russell 1980), the underlying mechanisms are not well understood. Physiological effects of soft tissue friction techniques include local hyperemia, massage analgesia, and reduction of adherent scar tissue (Norris 1993) and facilitating tendon healing by accelerating the inflammatory process to completion, which then encourages subsequent stages of healing to ensue (Prentice 1994). Augmented soft tissue mobilization (ASTM) techniques may facilitate tendon healing via the recruitment and

---

Clinical Note

Mobilization of the Nonweightbearing, Immobilized Joint

The clinical implications of dealing with an individual presenting with restricted ROM after immobilization and no weightbearing become evident when the known biological effects of such conditions on articular cartilage are considered. The study results of Houlbrooke et al. (1990) support maximizing ROM exercise across joints, even in the absence of weight bearing, with the intent to maintain the integrity of the articular cartilage matrix. Furthermore, this study demonstrated that weightbearing alone is equally beneficial in the maintenance of the integrity of articular cartilage matrix under conditions where an immobilized (e.g. cast, splint) joint exists.

activation of fibroblasts that ultimately promote healing and early recovery of limb function (Davidson et al. 1997). Fibroblast proliferation and activation are key events in the tendon healing process and are responsible for the production of cellular mediators of healing and synthesis of collagen (Leadbetter 1992). In one study where augmented soft tissue mobilization techniques were applied to inflamed tendons, stimulation of fibroblast proliferation was dependent on the magnitude of the applied pressure (Gehlsen et al. 1999). Therapeutic pressure may provide the initial stimulus for the healing cascade and the application of heavy pressure appears to best promote fibroblast proliferation that may be of particular significance for patients experiencing cumulative trauma disorders such as Achilles tendonitis, rotator cuff tendonitis, and golfer's or tennis elbow (Gehlsen et al. 1999). Furthermore, application of physical force through both stress and motion has been shown to modulate the synthesis of PGs and collagen by the fibroblasts (Woo et al. 1975). Mechanical stretching of fibroblasts therefore stimulates their proliferation (Jain et al. 1990) and biochemically modifies their resident environment (Eastwood et al. 1998) by affecting their synthesis of ECM proteins (Thie et al. 1989). Mechanical stimulation can alter cellular function including ion transport (Schwartz et al. 1991); release of second messengers (Letsou et al. 1990); protein synthesis (Thie et al. 1989); and gene expression (Komuro et al. 1991). Furthermore, the tensegrity model holds that the cytoskeleton may function to transmit forces or messages of these forces from cell surface structures to the nucleus of the cell (Ingber 1993). In this way mechanotransduction processes, in response to mechanical stresses share many common features with processes in cell adhesion, such as an increase in tyrosine phosphorylation of proteins, in focal adhesion sites (Shyy and Chien 1997). Intermediate filaments have been shown to be directly involved in cell resilience and maintenance of tissue integrity (Galou et al. 1997). By maintaining the shape and plasticity of the cell, the intermediate filament network acts as an integrator within the cell space. The state of mechanical force imposed on a tissue or a cell can alter the shape of certain elements of the cytoskeleton and thus participate in the control of cell function (Galou et al. 1997).

Friction Massage

Massage has been defined by Beard and Wood (1974) as "certain manipulations of the soft tissues of the body, which are most effective when performed with the hands and administered for the purpose of producing effects on the nervous and muscular systems, as well as the local and general circulation of the blood and lymph." A more specific application of massage movements referred to as *friction* has been advocated for conditions of inflammation and other connective tissue pathology such as ligament injuries (Mennell 1947). *Deep friction massage* has been used in clinical practice to impact select musculoskeletal structures such as ligaments and tendons in an effort to encourage therapeutic movement over a defined region (Cyriax and Russell 1980). The intent of friction massage is to obtain or restore mobility within specific sites of connective tissue–based structures and prevent the formation of adhesions after injury to these structures (Chamberlain 1982). The technique requires the transverse application of deep localized massage to specific structures that varies in length and force depending on the acuteness of the injury and phases of healing (Cyriax and Russell 1980). The impact of friction massage ranges from modulation of synthesis of matrix components of connective tissues (inflammatory to repair phase) to alteration of scar formation by influencing the laying down of new collagen fibers and intermolecular cross-linking processes and encouragement of connective tissue lubrication (repair to remodeling phases).

Manual Therapy: Effect on Connective Tissues

The use of manual therapy techniques by physical therapists, including mobilization and manipulation, on connective tissues is employed largely to relieve pain and increase mobility of joints (Kaltenborn and Evjenth 1989; Maitland 1986). Although therapeutic exercise aims in part to increase the length of muscle, graded manual therapeutic techniques are often directed toward restoring the subtle motions between joint surfaces, including the arthrokinematic motions of spin, glide, and roll (Threlkeld 1992). A main goal of manual therapy is to physically stress and elongate specific nonmineralized connective tissues around a joint or joint complex that may be responsible for restricting joint mobility (Figure 6-6).

In general, the viscoelastic material properties of connective tissue contribute to its behavior in that when loaded more rapidly, it behaves more stiffly (the material deforms less) than tissue that is loaded at a slower rate (Noyes et al. 1974). Sustained stress is known to produce a higher strain compared with cyclic stress in tendon tissue, with both recovering if the strain is below 4% (Rigby et al. 1959). However, the above finding can be altered when a conditioning stretch occurs before loading, resulting in a length increase of 0.4% to 0.8%, which does not recover on removal of the load (Rigby et al. 1959).

Joint Mobilization

Graded mobilizations are small amplitude passive movements that aim to accomplish a gliding or traction at or within a joint (Maitland 1986). The effect of graded mobilizations applied at the end of the available arthrokinematic ROM is to elongate connective tissues (Figure 6-7) as opposed to those applied at the beginning of the available range that intend to treat pain through activation of neural structures (Threlkeld 1992). The structures that tend to shorten and in turn limit joint excursion include ligaments, joint capsules, and periarticular fasciae. The impact of repetitive, low stress, small amplitude movements that are components of mobilization is that synovial fluid may be distributed across articular cartilage and the intervertebral disc (IVD), allowing joint lubrication. Additionally, the cell's experience of movement within the periarticular joint structures such as ligaments and capsule is also affected (Frank et al. 1984; Salter 1989).

The graded mobilizations applied in the range of Maitland grades I and II are applied with the intent to relieve pain but not to permanently elongate connective tissues (Maitland 1986). Mobilization of joints within this range are considered to work within the toe region of the structure's stress-strain curve and clinically may be referred to as "taking out the slack" (Kaltenborn and Evjenth 1989), as temporary relief of the crimp within the structure itself occurs. At higher ranges of graded mobilizations (Maitland grades III and IV), loading affects length of connective tissues through the process of internal *microfailure* mechanisms that result in a change in the resting length of connective tissue through plastic deformation. Microfailure implies that physical disconnection of some of the individual collagen fibers and bundles

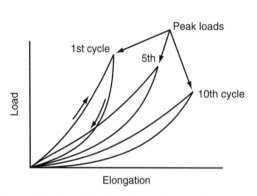

Figure 6-6. Typical loading (*top*) and unloading (*bottom*) curve from cyclic tensile testing of knee ligaments. The two nonlinear curves form any one cycle for a hysteresis loop. The area between the curves is referred to as the area of hysteresis, and represents the energy losses within the tissue. (From Woo SL-Y et al. Anatomy, Biology and Biomechanics of Tendon, Ligament, and Meniscus. In SR Simon. Orthopaedic Basic Science. Rosemont, Ill: American Academy of Orthopaedic Surgeons, 1994;62.)

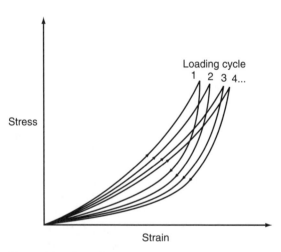

Figure 6-7. Effect of cyclic loading of tendon. Note that the stress-strain curve gradually shifts to the right. Typically, after 10 cycles, the curves become quite repeatable and steady. (From Woo SL-Y et al. Anatomy, Biology and Biomechanics of Tendon, Ligament, and Meniscus. In SR Simon. Orthopaedic Basic Science. Rosemont, Ill: American Academy of Orthopaedic Surgeons, 1994;52.)

occur as a result of progressive loading and ultimate tissue deformation that results in permanent lengthening of tissue. This corresponds to the mid-linear to end-linear phase of the structure's stress-strain curve. This microfailure is considered a form of *therapeutic damage* to the connective tissue that is necessary to accomplish *permanent* lengthening (as opposed to that temporarily accomplished with creep) of a previously restricted tissue. Therapeutic damage affects relationships between collagen, associated macromolecules and ground substance of the ECM and subsequently results in a known cycle of tissue inflammation, repair, remodeling and consolidation. This may be considered a healthy response to therapeutically induced internal tissue failure that must be managed with vigilance to preserve the "new" length of the tissue. Macrofailure, or actual failure of the gross connective tissue structure, in the case of tendon occurs at approximately 8% elongation, whereas microfailure may begin at approximately 3% elongation (Noyes et al. 1983), depicting a narrow range within which appropriate physical stresses should be applied.

Joint Manipulation

The health of joints depends on repeated low stress movements. In the case of the IVD and the zygoapophysial (facet) joints of the spine, these movements ensure the proper flow of fluid and nutrients across and through joint surfaces (Twomey and Taylor 1995). In cases of acute back pain, mobilization and manipulation of the spine has demonstrated some utility in accelerating the process of recovery and return to activity (Twomey and Taylor 1994). Both manipulation and mobilization of joints involves passive joint movements, during which the joint or joint complex is taken through a specific ROM. Although mobilization encompasses low velocity movements within or up to the limit of ROM of a joint, manipulation involves a low amplitude, high velocity thrust at the limit of joint range with the intent to briefly move the joint beyond the point of restriction. Where spinal manipulation has become one of the most widely used techniques for treating vertebral column pain, the impact remains unclear as to specific tissue effects on vertebral malposition or subluxation, reduction of disc bulge/herniation, the freeing of adhesions around a disc or facet joints, repositioning of *meniscoid*

structures or torn articular cartilage within facet joints, and the mechanical stimulation of nociceptive joint fibers (Twomey and Taylor 1995). A Maitland grade V single thrust manipulation would presumably create extensive microfailure (late linear region of the stress-strain curve) within the targeted connective tissue structure.

Connective Tissue Response to Immobilization

Immobilization, in the form of prolonged and uninterrupted rest, has historically been the most common form of therapy for musculoskeletal disorders (Bick 1968). It may be considered one of the most important advances in the understanding of healing of musculoskeletal tissues that prolonged immobilization may, in fact, act to delay recovery. Prolonged immobilization adversely affects the health of normal tissues, and it is known that appropriate and early resumption of activity promotes optimal repair and function of injured tissues. Although the adverse functional effects of prescribing immobilization for musculoskeletal ailments were noted as early as the nineteenth century (Keith 1919), joint immobilization continues to be employed in the care of many musculoskeletal conditions but is restricted to limited periods and with greater consideration of the biology of the healing tissue and the whole body effects. The biologic basis for the link between application of load and the cellular and metabolic response continues to remain open to investigation (Zeichen et al. 2000). Motion inflicted too early after injury or during repair of connective tissues can have detrimental effects by increasing the inflammatory reaction and may even damage repair tissue, leading to failure of the healing process. The ramifications after excessive joint mobilization has been called *fracture disease* and features chronic edema, muscle atrophy, joint stiffness, and in extreme cases, joint fusion and disuse osteoporosis (Kamps et al. 1994). The corollary of this situation is that when connective tissue–based structures are deprived of stress, significant morphologic, biochemical, and biomechanical changes occur. Recall that periarticular connective tissues encompass a wide variety of structures, including tendons, ligaments, fascia, capsules, and synovial structures, all of which share the common ultrastructural composition of collagen fibers in addition to other ECM components such as PGs and water. Circumstances that make immobilization of joints and associated connective tissue structures impossible to avoid may include casting and splinting of injured sites, with the natural intent and consequence being restricted joint motion. Even in cases of short periods of immobilization, as might be indicated after a simple elbow dislocation, splinting of the reduced elbow for 2 weeks was noted to enhance patient comfort and did not adversely affect the eventual outcome, whereas splinting for more than 3 weeks resulted in worse function at 61-month follow-up (Schippinger et al. 1999). In extreme cases, alterations associated with prolonged immobilization of a joint may lead to full restriction of joint motion and subsequent intraarticular ankylosis, typically occurring within a period in excess of 1 year (Enneking 1972). Of further note is that immobilization of extremities in the elderly is apt to result in contractures more often, after less trauma, and after shorter periods than in younger individuals (Akeson et al. 1968).

Clinical Note

Effects of Long-Term Immobilization on Mechanical Properties of Ligaments

Clinical management of ligaments after periods of immobility and disuse should incorporate protective measures in the early rehabilitation period and careful design of long-term goals for the appropriate time when strenuous activities should be resumed. Significant alterations occur in the mechanical properties and projected functional capacity of a ligament unit after short-term (8 weeks) immobilization with changes related to the severity of immobility imposed (Figure 6-8). These changes can persist with incomplete recovery noted 5 months after resumed activity, requiring up to 12 months (in the nonhuman primate model) until ultimate strength properties return to normal (Noyes 1977). From this report, a period that may extend beyond a year may therefore be required for the maturation of the healing process and the full recovery of strength of ligamentous tissue after even short-term immobilization. Furthermore, the ultimate failure of the ligament unit from immobilized limbs occurred largely through the underlying cortical bone beneath the ligament-bone junction, through the body of the ligament, or by both modes, but not in a major mode through the ligament-bone junction (Noyes 1977). In this study, a change in the relationship between load and ligament elongation after immobilization was shown in terms of a decrease in ligament stiffness (slope of the load-deformation curve) or as an increase in ligament extensibility (compliance or elongation per unit load) that was related to the degree of immobility imposed. In fact, reduced load-to-failure to about one third of that of normal controls is evident at the bone-ligament-bone complex after periods of immobilization (Akeson et al. 1987). An extended period is therefore required after relative or complete states of immobility before the functional capacity of a ligament unit at any site returns to normal. Disuse-induced changes after fracture, ligament repair or other disorders may extend well beyond the period in which normal activity is undertaken and beyond the return of muscle function that may appear sufficient for the reengagement of ambulation and other activities. Although engagement in physical activity and appropriate mechanical forces is observed as having a favorable influence on the healing and repair processes of injured connective tissues, specific parameters of exact timing, magnitude and mode of application remain difficult to qualify. A critical period in the healing phase and return of ligament integrity may be experienced when plaster immobilization is discontinued and joints and supporting ligament structures are subject to large forces. Detrimental effects may be sustained with too early and strenuous ambulation before the regaining of muscle strength and coordination to control the joint and protect the ligament structures (Noyes and Sonstegard 1973). Therefore sufficient time for the healing of soft tissues must be permitted, and undue forces must be avoided in the early phases of healing, particularly following removal of casts. Additionally, appropriate strengthening of supporting muscles after injury acts to improve joint stability and allows the optimal healing and repair of injured ligaments.

In summary, the concept that connective tissue healing occurs as rapidly as a few weeks to months after injury refers more to the early deposition of collagen and the reconnection of tissue in terms of its histology. However, remodeling of this connective tissue continues to extend beyond that period and is essential to achieve or regain the ultimate strength and mechanical integrity inherent to connective tissue–based structures.

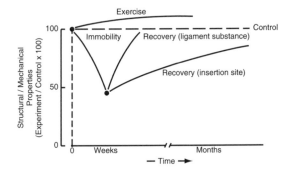

Figure 6-8. Summary of the homeostatic responses of the components of the bone-ligament-bone complex when subjected to different levels of physical activity. (From Woo SL-Y et al. Ligament, Tendon, and Joint Capsule Insertions to Bone. In SL-Y Woo, JA Buckwalter. Injury and Repair of the Musculoskeletal Soft Tissues. Rosemount, Ill: American Academy of Orthopaedic Surgeons, 1988;156.)

Periarticular Tissues: Biological Response to Immobilization

Significant biochemical changes occur in periarticular connective tissues after periods of enforced joint immobilization, including a significant loss of water, hyaluronic acid, chondroitin-4 and chondroitin-6 sulfate, and dermatan sulfate (Akeson et al. 1967; Akeson et al. 1973). An increase in joint stiffness and decrease in water and total hexosamine content in periarticular connective tissues were observed as the time of immobilization increased in the rabbit knee joint (Akeson et al. 1974). Immobilization of the knee joint for 9 weeks resulted in a reduction of the mechanical properties of the lateral collateral ligament with specific reductions in ligament stiffness (Amiel et al. 1982). Furthermore, an increase in collagen turnover (synthesis and degradation) was found in the immobilized medial collateral ligament and patellar tendon with the findings of reduced stiffness attributed to a change in ligament substance itself rather than a result of tissue atrophy (Amiel et al. 1982).

These findings are relatively uniform across connective tissue–based structures such as tendon, capsule, ligament, and fascia (Akeson et al. 1968), and it has been demonstrated that while collagen mass may decline by 10%, collagen turnover may increase with accelerated processes of degradation and synthesis under conditions of immobilization

(Akeson et al. 1987). Therefore contracture of connective tissue after immobilization of joints alone is not the result of fibroplasia and scar formation. Instead, significant increases in the quantity of reducible intermolecular collagen cross-links in the immobilized rabbit knee periarticular connective tissues have been demonstrated (Akeson et al. 1977). Forced motion of contractures causes physical disruption of either the adhesions between gross structures, the intermolecular cross-linking, or both between fibers in periarticular connective tissue (Woo et al. 1975). The excessive intermolecular cross-links interfere with joint extensibility and do not allow free gliding between fibers or between the fibers and other components of the ECM. Therefore to stretch contracted connective tissue to a specified length requires higher stress than in the noncontracted state because of the decreased extensibility of the tissue, resulting from excessive or greater than normal cross-linking in the connective tissue matrix.

In tissues such as ligaments that are recognized for their relatively high order of fibril arrays in health any new fibrils formed under conditions of immobilization display a disordered arrangement which results in a change in overall physical properties including a reduced ultimate load to failure of the tissue (Akeson et al. 1987). In tissues such as synovium and capsule, which are inherently more extensible, the disordered deposition of fibrils appears to impede flexibility by producing fiber-fiber gliding impediments at specific points along the structure (Figure 6-9) (Akeson et al. 1987). This haphazard laying down of newly synthesized collagen fibers in immobilized ligaments is thought to occur because of the absence of the usual controls on orientation of matrix imposed by physical forces. The relatively rapid changes in connective tissue of ligament after immobilization can be seen in Figure 6-10. Although the loss in mechanical properties of this tissue after immobilization is rapid, the recovery period is significantly longer.

A significant decrease in the linear stress, maximum stress, and stiffness of immobilized but weight-bearing ligaments in rat model experiments was observed compared with contralateral control ligaments after a 40-day period of immobilization (Binkley and Peat 1986). In addition, a significant decrease in the proportion of smaller, cross-sectional area fibrils and a significant increase in the

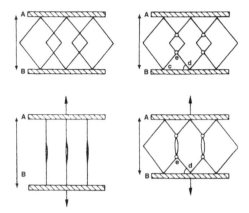

Figure 6-9. A diagram showing the idealized weave pattern of collagen fibers. It can be demonstrated that fixed contact at strategic sites (e.g., points d and e) can severely restrict the extension of this collagen weave. (From Akeson WH. Immobility effects on synovial joints. The pathomechanics of joint contracture. Biorheology 1980;17:95-110. Copyright IOS Press.)

proportion of larger-diameter fibrils was seen after a period of immobilization, findings attributed to decreased synthesis and degradation of collagen during immobilization (Binkley and Peat 1986). Collagen fibril size and density has been shown to be altered with increased levels of mechanical stress, demonstrating the link between ultrastructure and mechanical properties of connective tissues (Figure 6-11).

Synovial Joints: Biological Response to Immobilization

Fibroblasts and chondrocytes of connective tissues rely on physical forces to influence their rate of synthesis and degradation of matrix components. In this way synovial joints require physical stress to maintain the biochemical matrix composition and biomechanical characteristics of tissues associated with normal joints. Although the effects of

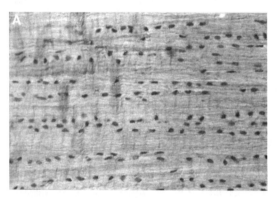
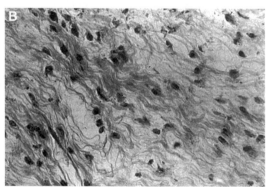

Figure 6-10. A, Anterior cruciate ligaments from contralateral control, nonimmobilized rabbit knee (magnification X1000). **B,** Anterior cruciate ligaments from 9-week immobilized rabbit knee (magnification X1000). (From Akeson WH. Immobility effects on synovial joints. The pathomechanics of joint contracture. Biorheology 1980;17:95-110. Copyright IOS Press.)

Clinical Note

Effect of Immobilization on Mechanical Properties of Knee Ligaments

After immobilization, ligaments reach their linear regions and maximum stress at lower than normal levels of applied forces, indicating that ligament laxity and complete ligament failure may occur with comparatively low levels of force (Binkley and Peat 1986). Ligaments become more compliant after several weeks of stress deprivation (Amiel et al. 1982). Clinical implications for physical rehabilitation of injured or repaired ligaments after a period of immobilization are such that cautious return to activity is indicated during efforts aimed at reducing joint stiffness because of the inferior mechanical properties of ligaments.

immobilization on muscle and bone are well recognized, changes in nonmineralized connective tissue–based structures associated with synovial joints has received less attention. If joints are immobilized for any length of time, then the extensibility of connective tissue is lost and abnormal cross-links develop between connective tissue fibers. When synovial joints are subject to extended periods of immobilization, many changes occur, including proliferation of fibrofatty connective tissue within the joint space, adhesions between synovial folds, adherence of fibrofatty connective tissue to cartilage surfaces, atrophy of cartilage, ulceration at points of cartilage-cartilage contact, disorganization of cellular and fibrillar ligament alignment, weakening of ligament insertion sites owing to osteoclastic resorption of bone and Sharpey's fibers, regional osteoporosis of the involved extremity, increased force requirement for joint cycling and increased ligament compliance (Akeson et al. 1987). Immobilization of the rabbit knee in extension induced changes in GAG metabolism in weight-bearing cartilage of the knee joint similar to those reported to occur in human osteoarthritis (Eronen et al. 1978). Although the reasons for this pathology are unknown, immobilization of the knee joint in extension causes a continuous compression of the weight-bearing cartilages in the joint; distraction of a joint has been shown to enable diminished osteoarthritic changes in rabbit knees from developing during periods of

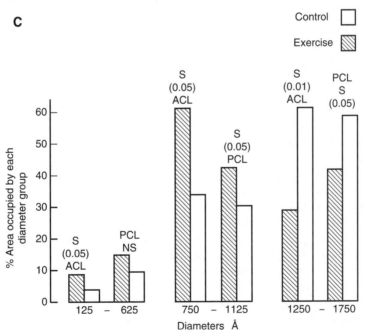

Figure 6-11. **A** and **B,** Transverse sections through exercised ACL (*left*) and nonexercised control ACL (*right*) (magnification X21,600). *Insets:* Histogram profiles of mean data for number of fibers and percentage area occupied for each diameter group. **C,** Comparison of percentage area occupied by three diameter groupings used for statistical analysis in exercised and control ACL and PCL. (From Frank C et al. Normal Ligament: Structure, Function and Composition. In SL-Y Woo and JA Buckwalter. Injury and Repair of the Musculoskeletal Soft Tissues. Rosemount, Ill: American Academy of Orthopaedic Surgeons, 1988;75, 77.)

immobilization (Videman and Michelsson 1977). A gradual increase in joint stiffness and a corresponding gradual reduction in tissue water and GAG content seen after joint immobilization identify the stress and motion dependence of ground substance in connective tissue homeostasis (Akeson et al. 1974; Akeson et al. 1977).

Joint Hypomobility

The Etiologic Factors and Pathogenesis of Joint Contractures

A number of structures are implicated when a joint is described as having a contracture, including the joint capsule, ligaments, and the muscles and their tendons, which adapt to a deformed joint position. Connective tissue homeostasis is disrupted, resulting in changes in fibrous structures when diarthrodial joints are subjected to prolonged periods of immobilization. Of great clinical relevance is that immobilization across joints after musculoskeletal trauma causing inflammation triggers contracture formation more rapidly and to a greater extent than by immobilization without superimposed trauma (Cummings et al. 1983). In contrast to conditions of immobilization alone, when trauma to connective tissue–based structures occurs, fibroplasia and excessive scar formation contribute to early contracture formation. Several mechanisms may underlie the development of a contracture and ultimate restriction in ROM of an affected joint. Damage incurred at the synovium, capsule, cartilage, and bone appear to greatly contribute to joint stiffness after long-term immobilization. Potential contributors to joint contracture include proliferation of intraarticular connective tissue (pannus) and the associated adhesions formed in its association with cartilage (Langenskiold et al. 1979; Schollmeier et al. 1994); an increase in cross-linking between collagen fibrils, the extracellular matrix or lack of hydration between collagen fibers (Akeson 1961; Akeson et al. 1977; Amiel et al. 1980); and adaptive shortening of the joint capsule (Cummings et al. 1983). With prolonged immobilization of a physically traumatized joint, fibro-fatty connective tissue proliferates and encroaches the joint space, and these changes are first seen at 2 weeks. As immobilization continues,

fibrous adhesions occur and further affect the mobility of the joint (Farmer and James 2001).

The development of joint contractures is commonly observed after immobilization with splints or casts; however, other mechanisms include neuromuscular disorders with associated muscle imbalances, disorders causing joint pain such as trauma, sepsis, inflammatory disorders, degenerative processes, congenital disorders, prolonged bed rest, and a variety of disturbances that result in mechanical incongruity of joint surfaces (Akeson et al. 1987). In fact, in neuromuscular conditions, immobilization, muscle weakness or paralysis and spasticity are the three main factors leading to the development of contractures variously affecting the joint itself, contractile tissue, and/or connective tissue (Farmer and James 2001). A general loss in lubricating and buffering volume of water and GAGs in concert with increased inter- and intramolecular cross-links of collagen contribute to joint stiffness (Akeson et al. 1980). In an experimental model of joint stiffness in the dog, the water concentration was reduced in tendon, synovial membrane, capsule, skin, and fascia by 2% to 3% after 4 to 12 weeks of immobilization (Akeson 1961). Recall that water and PGs impart important viscoelastic properties to connective tissues, acting as lubricants and spacing buffer systems between collagen fibers. Therefore both qualitative and quantitative changes in the periarticular collagenous structures around a joint occur. The deposition of collagen at focal points in relation to the capsule and ligament structures may restrict joint motion by not being properly aligned and may ultimately produce an effective shortening of the connective tissue–based structures.

Management of Contractures: Elongation of Shortened Connective Tissues

When joints are immobilized for any length of time, the connective tissue of joint structures loses its extensibility, allowing the development of abnormal cross-linking between connective tissue fibers. The development of a soft tissue contracture can significantly impede the rehabilitation process, making requisite efforts to lengthen the shortened connective tissue to regain lost ROM around the joint. The viscoelastic characteristics inherent to connective tissue of tendon make it the most responsive to the combined application of low load and high temperature to achieve an increase in length of the tissue (Warren et al. 1971). Although it has been shown that elevating the temperature of collagenous tissue renders it more extensible (Lehmann et al. 1970; Rigby 1964), the combined application of a sustained load and elevated temperatures of up to 45° C (113° F) was proven to produce residual length increases in collagenous tissue greater than that incurred by comparable levels of loading alone (Lehmann et al. 1970). The effect of different forms of heat on collagen-based tissues is discussed extensively in Chapter 7 of this text.

The two main factors contributing to the development of contractures are the myogenic restriction caused by the muscle, tendon and fascia and the arthrogenic restriction caused by bone, cartilage, synovium, capsule, and ligaments (Trudel and Uhthoff 2000). When a muscle is immobilized to a shortened position, an increased resistance to passive stretch may be detected clinically that may be attributed to connective tissue accumulation. CPM appears to effect a reduced joint infiltration while reducing prospects of abnormal cross-bridging within collagen. In a controlled study the contribution of arthrogenic versus myogenic impediments to ROM at different times after joint immobilization pointed to an increased role of arthrogenic changes contributing to the limitations after immobilization, especially as the period of immobility extended beyond 2 weeks (Trudel and Uhthoff, 2000). The clinical relevance of such findings indicate that attention should be directed to treating the articular structures in the prevention or management of uncomplicated joint contractures that do not involve nerve or skin damage. Furthermore, during immobilization, connective tissue is lost at a slower rate than contractile tissue; therefore a relative increase in the proportion of connective tissue within a muscle after a period of immobilization occurs (Goldspink and Williams 1990). When immobilization is used in conjunction with electrical stimulation, then no connective tissue accumulation occurs, implying that contractile activity is a key factor in the maintenance of a normal proportion of connective tissue with muscle (Farmer and James 2001). In cases of progressive neuromuscular disease such as Duchenne muscular dystrophy, muscle is replaced with collagen and fatty tissue located within the endomysium, perimysium, and epimysium, which ultimately restricts joint motion (McDonald 1998).

Treatment Techniques

Connective tissue accumulates with immobility, but this effect is positively affected by active muscle contraction. However, passive stretching of muscles, unless held in a lengthened position for

---

Clinical Note

Conservative Treatment of the Clinical Contracture

Respect for the negative impact that extended periods of immobilization have on joint complexes provides strong theoretical rationale for early intervention in contracture prevention and management. Despite this knowledge and preventive efforts, the physical therapist continues to be confronted with joint contractures in daily practice. Functional limitations associated with the development of contractures include loss of independence and extremity function, as well as impairment of gross motor tasks such as ambulation, seating, and the ability to transfer. The following key principles guide the conservative treatment of the joint contracture:

1. The stretch of soft tissue contracture affects the viscoelastic nature of the material.
2. When performing stretches on connective tissue structures, the magnitude of loads should be considered in terms of that which permits the slow, steady elongation of connective tissue.

The lengthening of contracted connective tissue may be best accomplished with combined loading and elevation of tissue temperature to within the therapeutic range (up to 45° C/113° F) (Warren et al. 1971).

more than 6 hours per day, cannot easily overcome contracture development in cases where spasticity exists (Farmer and James 2001). Techniques that reduce muscle stiffness but retain muscle function prove most successful in the treatment of a contracture (Farmer and James, 2001). However, where muscle function is not possible, serial plastering, and static/dynamic splinting (orthoses) are circumstantially used based on the underlying conditions to hold a joint at the limit of range. These treatment approaches offer the advantage of being applied for longer periods of time than other methods of passive stretching.

The first line of management of contractures typically includes manual therapies and physical modalities and may also include pharmacologic intervention and surgery. Collagen synthesis inhibitors such as cortisone that act as collagen crosslink inhibitors have negative effects if used extensively to prevent contracture formation. Steroids such as cortisone also can act to inhibit useful collagen synthesis that may defeat the healing of wounds in an indiscriminate manner from the undesirable collagen synthesis associated with contracture formation. Finally, surgical lengthening of shortened connective tissue–based structures may give relief to muscle shortening and provide a therapeutic opportunity for reeducation of movement.

Adaptation of Connective Tissue During Distraction Osteogenesis

The development of contractures and associated decreased ROM is a common clinical complication of distraction osteogenesis that leads to significant functional deficits (Herzenberg et al. 1994). In one investigation aiming to determine the cause of this condition, perimysial fibrosis was observed to be responsible for the ultimate decrease in ROM observed during distraction osteogenesis rather than the muscle fibers themselves (De Deyne et al. 2000).

Joint Hypermobility

Hypermobility Syndrome

Hypermobility syndrome (HMS) refers to the manifestations of joint hyperlaxity, joint hypermobility, or articular hypermobility (Russek 1999). According to one study, HMS was shown to be as

---

Clinical Note

Establishing the Diagnosis of Hypermobility Syndrome

Individuals in whom HMS presents may have complaints of diffuse, largely chronic nature that may have lasted anywhere from between 15 days to 45 years (average time = 6.5 years) (el-Shahaly and el-Sherif 1991). These patients typically lack the positive laboratory findings found in association with rheumatological disorders and in the absence of acute trauma, lack the radiological changes, inflammation, swelling, and decreased mobility typical of orthopaedic pathology (Russek 1999).

The diagnosis of HMS is based on criteria that rates degrees of hypermobility syndrome, the most widely used scale being that of Beighton et al. (1973). The Beighton scale assigns a patient one point for each characteristic including passive extension of the first metacarpophalangeal (MCP) joint past 90 degrees, passive apposition of the thumb to the forearm, hyperextension of the elbow past 10 degrees, hyperextension of the knee past 10 degrees, and trunk flexion that allows the palms to be placed flat on the floor. Each limb is scored separately for the first four items, producing a possible score of 9.

Sprains, subluxations, and dislocations are more common in individuals with HMS (Finsterbush and Pogrund 1982). However the tissue damage that typically accompanies these injuries may not be as severe because of the increased laxity of joint structures (Russek 1999). Individuals with HMS are regarded as more prone to develop osteoarthritis, which affects up to 60% of individuals with this condition (el-Shahaly and el-Sherif 1991).

much as six times more prevalent among women than men (Beighton et al. 1973).

Pathophysiology of Hypermobility Syndrome

HMS may be inherited as a gender-influenced dominant trait with the pathology manifesting in type I collagen metabolism and an increase in the ratio of type III collagen to type I collagen relative to normals (Child 1986).

Management of Hypermobility Syndrome

Education including modification of activities or use of protective splints, braces and taping for vulnerable joints is important in the overall management of individuals with this condition (Biro et al. 1983). Exercise prescription to encourage muscle strengthening and proprioceptive training is also recommended for musculature surrounding affected joints (Biro et al. 1983; Finsterbush and Pogrund 1982). Excessive stretching around vulnerable joints has been observed to be detrimental to this condition, particularly in association with excessive spinal mobility (Howell 1984). No proven role for nonsteroidal antiinflammatory drugs (NSAIDS) exists, with the use of these drugs observed as neither practical nor effective (Child 1986).

Pharmacological Management of Soft Tissue Injuries

The use of medication to manage injury via suppression of the intensity and duration of inflammation and pain to the musculoskeletal soft tissues is commonplace but is not without potential adverse effects on healing and repair processes inherent to these tissues. The use of NSAIDS, corticosteroids, anabolic steroids, and dimethyl sulfoxide are the most common treatment medications for injuries of musculoskeletal soft tissues (Buckwalter 1995).

Nonsteroidal Antiinflammatory Drugs

NSAIDS (e.g., aspirin, ibuprofen) are recommended primarily for the treatment of chronic musculoskeletal disorders; however, they are commonly used for the treatment of acute soft tissue injuries (Abramson 1990). These chemically heterogeneous drugs have analgesic, antipyretic, and antiinflammatory activity (Buckwalter 1995). The reduction of soft tissue inflammation with use of these drugs is believed to occur through a variety of mechanisms including altering the production of cytokines and superoxide radicals, the aggregation and adhesion of neutrophils, and many cell-membrane activities (Abramson 1990). Specifically, NSAIDS appear to decrease the synthesis of prostaglandins by inhibiting cyclooxygenase, the enzyme that catalyzes the conversion of arachidonic acid to a prostaglandin intermediate (Buckwalter 1995).

Corticosteroids

Corticosteroids play a role in the management of chronic inflammatory diseases of the musculoskeletal system. The local injection of corticosteroids and topical application of these drugs for management of musculoskeletal soft tissue injuries is also employed. Although the extreme antiinflammatory potency of these drugs is evident, their use raises the potential for severe complications that exceed that of NSAIDs, including an actual acceleration of the deterioration of connective tissue–based structures.

Summary

Connective tissue has time- and rate-dependent mechanical properties. The property of extensibility is characteristic of the connective tissues, with the ability of internal networks of fibrous collagen within these structures to reorient themselves to imposed forces. Stress relaxation occurs when connective tissue is held under tension at a constant length. When a constant force is applied, lengthening of connective tissue occurs through the effect of creep. Connective tissue when immobilized, forms excessive cross-bridges, reducing its extensibility. Connective tissue is maximally weakened via the application of high forces (e.g., manipulation), as opposed to the minimal structural weakening that occurs when a low force is applied at higher temperatures. The development of connective tissue contractures may require treatment including passive stretching, manipulation, static/dynamic splinting, electrical stimulation, or even surgery, with management techniques dependent on the underlying conditions. Connective tissue healing that is evident within a few weeks to months refers more to the early deposition of collagen and the basic reconnection of tissue identified in terms of its histology; however, remodeling of this connective tissue continues to extend beyond that period and is essential to achieve or regain the ultimate strength and mechanical integrity inherent to connective tissue–based structures.

References

Abramson SB. Nonsteroidal Anti-inflammatory Drugs: Mechanisms of Action and Therapeutic Considerations. In WB Leadbetter et al (eds), Sports Induced Inflammation. Clinical and Basic Science Concepts. Park Ridge, Illinois: American Academy of Orthopaedic Surgeons, 1990;421-430.

Akeson WH. An experimental study of joint stiffness. J Bone Joint Surg 1961;43-A(7):1022-1034.

Akeson WH et al. The connective tissue response to immobility: a study of chondroitin-4 and -6 sulfate and dermatin sulfate changes in periarticular connective tissue in control and immobilized knees of dogs. Clin Orthop 1967;51:183-197.

Akeson WH. The connective tissue response to immobility: an accelerated aging response? Exp Gerontol 1968;3: 289-301.

Akeson WH. The connective tissue response to immobility: biochemical changes in periarticular connective tissue of the immobilized rabbit knee. Clin Orthop 1973;93: 356-362.

Akeson WH et al. Biomechanical and biochemical changes in the periarticular connective tissue during contracture development in the immobilized rabbit knee. Connect Tissue Res 1974;2(4):315-323.

Akeson WH et al. Collagen cross-linking alterations in joint contractures: changes in the reducible cross-links in periarticular connective tissue collagen after nine weeks of immobilization. Connect Tissue Res 1977;5:15.

Akeson WH. Immobility effects on synovial joints: the pathomechanics of joint contracture. Third International Congress of Biorheology: Symposium on Soft Tissues around a Diarthrodial Joint. Biorheology 1980;17:95-110.

Akeson WH et al. Effects of immobilization on joints. Clin Orthopaed Rel Res 1987;219:28-37.

Amiel D. The effect of immobilization on the types of collagen synthesized in periarticular connective tissue. Connect Tissue Res 1980;8:27-32.

Amiel D. The effect of immobilization on collagen turnover in connective tissue: a biochemical-biomechanical correlation. Acta Orthop Scand 1982;53:325-332.

Amiel D. Stress deprivation effect on metabolic turnover of the medial collateral ligament collagen. Clin Orthopaed Rel Res 1983;172:265-270.

Aspden RM. Relation between structure and mechanical behaviour of fibre-reinforced composite materials at large strains. Proc R Soc B 1986;212:299-304.

Beard G, Wood EC. Massage, Principles and Techniques. Philadelphia: WB Saunders, 1974.

Beighton P et al. Articular mobility in an African population. Ann Rheum Dis 1973;32:413-418.

Bick EM. Source Book of Orthopaedics. New York: Hafner, 1968.

Binkley JM. Overview of ligament and tendon structure and mechanics: Implications for clinical practice. Physiother Canada 1989;41(1):24-30.

Binkley JM. Peat M. The effects of immobilization on the ultrastructure and mechanical properties of the medial collateral ligament of rats. Clin Orthopaed Rel Res 203:301-308; 1986.

Biro F et al. The hypermobility syndrome. Pediatrics 1983;72:701-706.

Buckwalter JA. Pharmacological treatment of soft-tissue injuries. J Bone Joint Surg 1995;77-A(12):1902-1914.

Butler D et al. Biomechanics of ligaments and tendons. Exer Sport Sci Rev 1978;6:125-181.

Chazal J et al. Biomechanical properties of spinal ligaments and a histological study of the supraspinal ligament in traction. J Biomechan 1985;18:167-176.

Chamberlain GJ. Cyriax's friction massage: a review. J Orthop Sports Phys Ther 1982;4:16-21.

Child AH. Joint hypermobility syndrome: inherited disorder of collagen synthesis. J Rheumatol 1986;13:239-243.

Cummings GS et al. Soft Tissue Changes in Contractures. Orthopedic Physical Therapy Series. Atlanta: Stokesville, 1983.

Cyriax J, Russell G. Textbook of Orthopedic Medicine, Volume 2 (10th ed). Baltimore: Williams and Wilkins, 1980;15-21.

Davidson CJ et al. Rat tendon morphologic and functional changes resulting from soft tissue mobilization. Med Sci Sports Exer 1997;29(3):313-319.

Davies PF. Flow-mediated endothelial mechanotransduction. Physiol Rev 1995;75:519-560.

De Deyne PG et al. The adaptation of perimuscular connective tissue during distraction osteogenesis. Clin Orthopaed Rel Res 2000;379:259-269.

Diament J et al. Collagen: ultrastructure and its relation to mechanical properties as a function of aging. Proceed Royal Society London, 1972;180:293-315.

Dorrington K. The Theory of Viscoelasticity in Biomaterials. In JFV Vincent, JD Currey (eds), The Mechanical Properties of Biological Materials. Cambridge, England: Cambridge University Press, 1980;289-314.

Eastwood M et al. Fibroblast responses to mechanical forces. Proc Instn Mech Engrs 1998;212(H):85-92.

Ecker ML, Lotke PA. Postoperative care of the total knee patient. Orthop Clin North Amer 1989;20(1):55-62.

El-Shahaly HA, el-Sherif AK. Is the benign joint hypermobility syndrome benign? Clin Rheumatol 1991;10: 302-307.

Enneking WF. The intraarticular effects of immobilization on the human knee. J Bone Joint Surg 1972;54-A(5):973-985.

Enwemeka CS. Functional loading augments the initial tensile strength and energy absorption capacity of regenerating rabbit Achilles tendon. Am J Phys Med Rehabil 1992;71(1):31-38.

Eronen I et al. Glycosaminoglycan metabolism in experimental osteoarthrosis caused by immobilization. Acta Orthop Scand 1978;49:329-334.

Farmer SE, James M. Contractures in orthopaedic and neurological conditions: a review of causes and treatment. Disabil Rehabil 2001;23(13):549-558.

Finsterbush A, Pogrund H. The hypermobility syndrome: musculoskeletal complaints in 100 consecutive cases of generalized joint hypermobility. Clin Orthop 1982;168:124-127.

Frank C et al. Physiology and therapeutic value of passive joint motion. Clin Orthop 1984;185:113-125.

Galou M et al. The importance of intermediate filaments in the adaptation of tissues to mechanical stress: evidence from gene knockout studies. Biol Cell 8 1997;9(2):85-97.

Gehlsen GM et al. Fibroblast responses to variation in soft tissue mobilization pressure. Med Sci Sports Exer 1999;31(4):531-535.

Goldspink G, Williams P. Muscle Fibre and Connective Tissue Changes Associated with Use and Disuse. In L Ada, C Canning (eds), Key Issues in Neurological Physiotherapy. Oxford: Butterworth Heinemann, 1990;197-218.

Herzenberg JE et al. Knee range of motion in isolated femoral lengthening. Clin Orthop 1994;301:49-54.

Houlbrooke K et al. Effects of movement and weightbearing on the glycosaminoglycan content of sheep articular cartilage. Austral Physiother 1990;36(2):88-91.

Howell DW. Musculoskeletal profile and incidence of musculoskeletal injuries in lightweight women rowers. Am J Sports Med 1984; 12:278-282.

Ingber D. Cellular tensegrity: defining new rules of biological design that govern the cytoskeleton. J Cell Biol 1993;104:613-627.

Jain MK et al. Mechanical stress and cellular metabolism in living soft tissue composites. Biomaterials 1990;11: 465-472.

Kaltenborn FM, Evjenth O. Manual Mobilization of the Extremity Joints: Basic Examination and Treatment Techniques (4th ed). Oslo: Olaf Norlis Bokhandel Universitatsgaten, 1989;45-48.

Kamps BS et al. The influence of immobilization versus exercise on scar formation in the rabbit patellar tendon after excision of the central third. Am J Sports Med 1994;22:803-811.

Keith A. Menders of the Maimed. London: H Frowde and Hodder and Stoughton, 1919.

Kiviranta I et al. Weight-bearing controls glycosaminoglycan concentration and articular cartilage thickness in the knee joints of young beagle dogs. Arthritis Rheum 1987;30(7):801-809.

Klein JA, Hukins DWL. Collagen fiber orientation in the annulus fibrosus of intervertebral disc during bending and torsion measured by x-ray diffraction. Biochim Biophys Acta 1982;719:98-101.

Komuro IY et al. Mechanical loading stimulates cell hypertrophy and specific gene expression in cultured rat cardiac myocytes. J Biol Chem 1991;266:1268-1275.

Langenskiold A et al. Osteoarthritis of the knee in the rabbit produced by immobilization. Acta Orthop Scand 1979;50:1-14.

Leadbetter W. Cell matrix response in tendon injury. Clin Sports Med 1992;11:533-577.

Lehmann JF et al. Effect of therapeutic temperatures on tendon extensibility. Arch Phys Med 1970;51:481-487.

Letsou GV et al. Stimulation of adenylate cyclase activity in cultured endothelial cells subjected to cyclic stretch. J Cardiovasc Surg 1990;31:634-639.

Maitland GD. Vertebral Manipulation (5th ed). London: Butterworth-Heinemann, 1986;3-102.

McDonald CM. Limb contractures in progressive neuromuscular disease and the role of stretching, orthotics and surgery. Phys Med Rehabil Clin North Amer 1998;9: 187-211.

Mennell JB. Physical Treatment by Movement, Manipulation and Massage (5th ed). Philadelphia: Blakiston, 1947.

Merriless MJ, Flint MH. Ultrastructure study of tension and pressure zones in a rabbit flexor tendon. Am J Anat 1980;157:396.

Norris CM. Sports Injuries. New York: Butterworth-Heinemann, 1993;109-111.

Noyes FR, Sonstegard DA. Biomechanical function of the pes anserinus at the knee and the effect of its transplantation. J Bone Joint Surg 1973;55-A:1225.

Noyes FR et al. Biomechanics of anterior cruciate ligament failure: an analysis of strain-rate sensitivity and mechanisms of failure in primates. J Bone Joint Surg (Am) 1974;56:236-253.

Noyes FR. Functional properties of knee ligaments and alterations induced by immobilization: A correlative biomechanical and histological study in primates. Clin Orthop 1977;123:210-242.

Noyes FR et al. Intraarticular cruciate reconstruction I. Perspectives on graft strength, vascularization and immediate motion after replacement. Clin Orthop 1983;172:71-77.

Ottani V et al. Collagen structure and functional implications. Micron 2001;323:251-260.

Palmoski MJ et al. Joint motion in the absence of normal loading does not maintain normal articular cartilage. Arthr Rheumat 1980;23(3):325-333.

Parry DAD, Craig AS. Growth and Development of Collagen Fibrils in Connective Tissue. In A Ruggeri, P Motta (eds), Ultrastructure of the Connective Tissue Matrix. The Hague:Martinus Nijhoff, 1984;34-64.

Prentice W. Therapeutic Modalities in Sports Medicine (3rd ed). St Louis: Mosby, 1994;336-349.

Purslow PP. Strain induced reorientation of an intramuscular connective tissue network: implications for passive muscle elasticity. J Biomech 1989;22:21-31.

Purslow PP et al. Collagen orientation and molecular spacing during creep and stress-relaxation in soft connective tissues. J Experiment Biol 1998;201:135-142.

Quinn TM et al. Mechanical compression alters PG deposition and matrix deformation around individual cells in cartilage explants. J Cell Sci 1998;111:573-583.

Rigby BJ et al.. The mechanical behaviour of rat tail tendon. J Gen Physiology 1959;43:265-283.

Rigby BJ. The effect of mechanical extension upon the thermal stability of collagen. Biochim Biophys Acta 1964;79:634-636.

Russek LN. Hypermobility syndrome. Phys Ther 1999;79(6):591-599.

Salter RB et al. Further studies in continuous passive motion [abstract]. Orthop Trans 1978;2:292.

Salter RB et al. The biological effect of continiuous passive motion on the healing of full-thickness defects in articular cartilage. J Bone Joint Surg 1980;62A:1232.

Salter RB, Minster RR. The effect of continuous passive motion on a semitendinosus tenodesis in the rabbit knee [abstract]. Orthop Trans 1982;6:292.

Salter RB. The biologic concept of continuous passive motion of synovial joints. Clin Orthopaed Rel Res 1989;242:12-25.

Schippinger G et al. Management of simple elbow dislocations: does the period of immobilization affect the eventual results? Langenbecks Arch Surg 1999;384(3):294-297.

Schollmeier G et al. Effects of immobilization on the capsule of the canine glenohumeral joint. A structural functional study. Clin Orthop 1994;304:37-42.

Schwartz MA et al. Fibronectin activates the Na/H antiported by inducing clustering and immobilization of its receptor, independent of cell shape. Proc Natl Acad Sci 1991;88:121-122.

Shyy JYJ, Chien S. Role of integrins in cellular responses to mechanical stress and adhesion. Curr Op Cell Biol 1997;9(5):707-713.

Stearns ML. Studies of the development of connective tissue transparent chambers in the rabbit ear II. Am J Anat 1940;67:55-97.

Thie MW et al. Mechanical confinement inhibits collagen synthesis in gel-cultured fibroblasts. Eur J Cell Biol 1989;48:294-301.

Threlkeld AJ. The effects of manual therapy on connective tissue. Phys Ther 1992;72(12):893-902.

Trudel G, Uhthoff HK. Contractures secondary to immobility: is the restriction articular or muscular? An experimental longitudinal study in the rat knee. Arch Phys Med Rehabil 2000;81:6-13.

Twomey L, Taylor JR. Physical Therapy of the Low Back (2nd ed). New York: Churchill Livingstone, 1994.

Twomey L, Taylor J. Exercise and spinal manipulation in the treatment of low back pain. Spine 1995;20(5): 615-619.

Videman T, Michelsson JE. Inhibition of development of experimental osteoarthrosis by distraction during immobilization. IRCS Med Sci 1977;5:139.

Wainwright SA et al. Mechanical Design in Organisms. London: Edward Arnold, Princeton University Press, 1976.

Warren CG et al. Elongation of rat tail tendon: effect of load and temperature. Arch Phys Med Rehabil, October 1971;(52)465-474.

Wilhelmi et al. Creep vs. stretch: a review of the viscoelastic properties of skin. Ann Plastic Surg 1998;41(2): 215-219.

Woo SL-Y et al. Connective tissue response to immobility. Correlative study of biomechanical and biochemical measurements of normal and immobilized rabbit knees. Arthr Rheumat 1975;18(3):257-264.

Zeichen J et al. The proliferative response of isolated human tendon fibroblasts to cyclic biaxial mechanical strain. Am J Sports Med 2000;28(6):888-892.

Chapter 7

Therapeutic Modalities for the Treatment of Orthopaedic Conditions

Pamela Houghton, BSc (PT), PhD

Therapeutic modalities such as ultrasound, laser, electrical current, and superficial hot and cold agents have all been used extensively for many musculoskeletal conditions. This chapter outlines the issues to be considered when a health care professional is challenged with making a choice of the best modality to be used for a particular musculoskeletal condition. It provides the background information necessary to make the best choice of therapeutic modalities. This chapter begins with a review of the experimental research that provides a description of the physiologic effects of each modality on the neuromuscular and vascular systems, on connective tissue mechanics, and on the cellular processes of inflammation and tissue repair. For certain common musculoskeletal conditions, including ankle sprains, shoulder and epicondylar tendonitis, and acute and chronic low back and neck pain, a brief review of pathophysiology of the musculoskeletal condition is provided. This allows an appreciation of the underlying mechanisms responsible for the clinical signs and symptoms commonly associated with these conditions. Lastly, a review and critical analysis of the clinical research evidence that is available to determine the effectiveness of these therapeutic modalities when applied to human subjects with these musculoskeletal conditions is provided.

Superficial Hot and Cold

Superficial heating agents include modalities such as hot packs, paraffin wax, hydrotherapy baths, infrared lamps, and fluidotherapy, all of which are warmed to a temperature greater than that of the body. When any of these physical agents are applied to the surface of the skin, the temperature of tissues located relatively near the skin surface is elevated because of heat transference mechanisms including conduction, convection, and radiation. Thermal energy supplied by superficial heating agents reaches tissues located within 3 cm of the skin surface and produces negligible direct heating of deeper muscle tissues (Rennie and Michlovitz, 1996). Therefore these superficial heating agents are best used on anatomical locations of the body, such as the hands and feet, with minimal subcutaneous adipose tissue.

Cryotherapy involves the application of ice or cold water to the skin surface. Some forms of cryotherapy include ice packs, which are crushed ice placed into towels and wrapped around the affected body part; ice massage, in which a frozen ice cube is massaged for a short period of time over a relatively small area; ice bath, by which the affected extremity is placed in a water bath that has been cooled using ice to temperatures as low as 5°C (approx. 41° F). In addition to these relatively simple forms of cryotherapy, more sophisticated methods of delivering cold therapy have been developed, such as cold cuffs with chambers through which hypothermic solutions are circulated. Most cryogenic agents exert their physiologic effects by reducing the temperature of skin and subcutaneous structures. Experiments have shown that cryotherapy agents are capable of producing clinically significant hypothermic responses in both joint structures and muscle up to 5 cm below the skin surface (Bierman and Friedlander, 1940; Waylonis 1967).

Both superficial hot and cold therapies are commonly used to treat musculoskeletal conditions. They are relatively inexpensive and easy to use so that patients can be instructed to continue to apply the treatments at home. The general physiologic effects of these superficial thermal agents have been summarized in Table 7-1. The physiologic effects of hot and cold therapies are often opposite. For example, local blood flow, cell metabolism, connective tissue stretch/extensibility, and tissue healing are increased by heating agents and decreased by cryotherapy. However, the effects of these agents on the neuromuscular system, such as alteration in nerve conduction velocity, muscle spasm, pain threshold and pain perception, are changed similarly by hypothermia and hyperthermia.

Effects of Hot and Cold Agents on Blood Flow

When cold is applied to the skin, vasoconstriction of cutaneous arterioles is stimulated immediately. Reduction in blood vessel lumen diameter causes a significant restriction of local blood flow to the skin and subcutaneous tissue. This vascular response to cold therapy is largely under the control of a neural mechanism that is an important part of heat-retention mechanisms of the body. When skin temperature is lowered, peripheral cold thermoreceptors located in subcutaneous tissues cause a reflex stimulation of sympathetic nerves to increase tonic contraction of smooth muscle surrounding cutaneous blood vessels in the local area being cooled. Return of cooled blood into the general circulation reduces core temperature, which in turn stimulates the preoptic area of the hypothalamus to reflexively produce cutaneous vasoconstriction over a greater body surface area, including the contralateral limb. If a large enough area of the body is cooled to produce significant reduction in body temperature, shivering can be stimulated to reelevate body temperature. Also contributing to cold-induced reduction in local blood flow is an increase in blood viscosity that occurs in the presence of lower blood temperatures, which acts to increase the resistance to blood flow.

Continued application of topical cryotherapy for 10 to 15 minutes or longer that reduces skin temperature below 10° C (50° F) reverses the initial vasoconstriction caused when the cold agent was first applied and induces vasodilation and hyperemia. This oscillation between vasodilation and vasoconstriction induced by continued cold application has been termed the *Hunting response* and proposed to be mediated by the axon reflex. Persistent vasoconstriction produces noxious stimuli, which in turn causes nerve impulses to be transmitted antidromically (in a reverse direction along axons) toward skin arterioles to inhibit vasomotor tone and cause reperfusion of the area with warm blood and restoration of the normal skin temperature. Other explanations of mechanisms that underlie vasodilation observed after cold therapy have been proposed. The reduced temperatures produced in the smooth muscle surrounding the cutaneous blood vessels located in the skin beneath the cold agent could interfere directly with the contractile ability of the vessels and thereby release vasoconstrictive tone normally present in cutaneous vasculature. Additionally, vasodilation observed after exposure to cold agents may occur in response to metabolic demand. This reactive hyperemia occurs as waste products accumulate and oxygen and nutrient demands increase.

Elevating skin temperature with a superficial heating agent such as a hot pack or paraffin wax

Table 7-1. Summary of Physiologic Effects of Hot and Cold Thermal Agents

	Hot	Cold
Vascular Response		
Local blood flow	↑	↓
Blood viscosity	↓	↑
Capillary permeability	↑	↓
Metabolism		
Metabolic rate	↑	↓
Enzymatic activity	↑	↓
Oxygen demands	↑	↓
Inflammation	↑	↓
Edema	↑	↓
Neuromuscular response		
Nerve conduction	↓	↓
Cutaneous sensation	↑	↓
Pain threshold	↑	↑
Muscle spindle sensivity	↓	↓
Connective tissue		
Synovial viscosity	↓	↑
Collagen plasticity	↑	↓

produces the opposite effects on the cutaneous vasculature. Local application of heat induces peripheral vasodilation via a thermoregulatory reflex mediated by the sympathetic nervous system that causes relaxation of smooth muscle surrounding cutaneous arterioles. Over a longer period of local heat application, inflammatory mediators are released. These humoral substances with potent vasoactive properties include prostaglandins, histamine, and bradykinin, and are believed responsible for initiating a slower onset but longer-lasting local erythema.

Effects of Hot and Cold Agents on Pain

Cryotherapy has long been recognized for its ability to reduce painful sensations or "numb the area" (Miller and Webers, 1990; Sluka et al. 1999). Analgesia produced by cold therapy is mediated in a large part by a cold-induced block of conduction of noxious stimuli along pain fibers. A reduction in local temperature surrounding peripheral nerves has been shown to produce a reduction in nerve conduction velocity and an inhibition of post synaptic transmission (Lee et al. 1978). Cold application to mixed motor and sensory nerves reduces the speed of action potential propagation to the greatest extent in small myelinated nerves and is least effective on unmyelinated C fibers. This results in a blunting of the pain caused by the loss of sharp, well-localized, noxious sensations that are primarily transmitted in fast-conducting A-delta fibers. Changes in nerve transmission produced by local application of cold therapy is only temporary, with restoration of precooled conduction rates occuring within 15 minutes of cold application. Prolonged or intense cold application to superficial nerves can compromise nerve viability and produce lasting hypoesthesia and paresthesia because of neuropraxia or axonotmesis (McMaster 1982).

Also postulated is how cold therapy reduces pain via lowering the excitability of cutaneous thermoreceptors causing an increase in pain threshold (Miller and Webers 1990). In addition, analgesia also may occur indirectly because of the antiinflammatory effects of cryotherapy, which, together with the cold-induced reduction in metabolic rate, decreases the availability of inflam-

matory mediators. Having fewer inflammatory mediators present in the injured tissue reduces the activation of pain receptors by these chemical irritants that can augment the activation of nociceptors (Kowal 1983).

Application of local heat also has been shown to have analgesic effects. Heat-induced analgesia is thought to be mediated primarily through neuromuscular reflexes. The application of superficial heating agents to the skin has been shown to elevate the pain threshold of free nerve endings acting as cutaneous thermoreceptors and also has been shown to alter sensory afferent nerve conduction velocity (Lee et al. 1978). The relevance of these finding to therapeutic use is not readily apparent since both increases and decreases in conduction have been recorded after heat therapy. Transmission of mild, comfortable thermal stimuli along myelinated sensory afferents may act to gate the pain stimuli at the level of the spinal cord and block further transmission up to higher brain centers, thus reducing pain perception. Vascular changes induced by temperature elevations also can indirectly contribute to pain reduction. Heat induced vasodilation produces an increased local blood flow that would wash out metabolites and other chemical irritants that can activate pain receptors.

Benson and Copp (1974) compared the analgesic effects of cold and hot agents and found that cold was superior to heat in raising the pain threshold of healthy volunteers. They also demonstrated that at 30 minutes after treatments the heat-treated areas actually had more pain sensitivity than control-treated shoulders whereas cold-treated shoulders had a sustained anesthetic effect. They concluded that cryotherapy should be the modality of choice when treating superficical areas and that heat application may even exacerbate pain symptoms in the long term.

Effects of Hot and Cold Agents on Post Traumatic Inflammation and Edema

Local vasoconstriction induced by hypothermia reduces fluid filtration into the interstitium and hence less potential exists for edema to develop. In addition, the reduced metabolism that occurs when tissue temperatures are lowered results in less production of waste metabolites, which reduces the osmotic draw of fluid into the interstitium that contributes to tissue edema. A reduction in metabolic rate also impedes many of the inflammatory processes, resulting in a reduced release of inflammatory mediators and ultimately reduced edema formation after tissue injury. Lower rates of metabolism reduce oxygen demand of tissues, which reduces the chances of further injury of tissues with limited blood perfusion caused by ischemia. Studies of humans (Taber et al. 1992; Hecht et al. 1983) and animals (McMaster and Liddle 1980) have shown that mild tissue cooling is effective in reducing acute inflammation and tissue swelling but that more intense cold application actually produced greater tissue edema than control limbs not exposed to tissue cooling. Thus if cryotherapy application results in excessive tissue cooling, thermal injury can occur and can exacerbate tissue swelling.

Chemical reactions in cells are influenced by temperature. Van Hoff's law states that chemical activity and metabolic rate will increase two to three times for each 10°C rise in tissue temperature (Rennie and Michlovitz 1996). The increased metabolic rate induced by local heating therefore will stimulate the inflammatory response to tissue injury. Increased production of waste products and hyperthermia-induced degranulation of inflammatory cells will result in the accumulation of potent vasoactive substances (prostaglandins and histamine) that stimulate endothelial cell contraction and increase capillary permeability. These hemodynamic changes, coupled with an increase in capillary hydrostatic pressure caused by vasodilation of arterioles perfusing to collectively produce a marked increase in fluid filtration from within the vascular system into the interstitial space. The end result is a marked increase in tissue edema. Swelling of tissue at the site of injury challenges the ability to supply adequate oxygen to the healing tissue, and the tissue stretching produced by the edema stimulates free nerve endings and causes pain. Since these heat-induced effects on pain and swelling can interfere with the repair process, the application of superficial heating agents to a tissue that is in the acute inflammatory phase of tissue repair (generally within the first 24-72 hours after injury) is generally not recommended.

Effects of Hot and Cold Agents on Tissue Repair

While cold application is beneficial during the early phases of healing, continued hypothermia throughout the healing process can impair tissue healing and interfere with the development of optimal tissue strength post injury (Esclamado et al. 1990). Persistent inhibition of the inflammatory process deprives the healing process of key chemical mediators responsible for stimulating new tissue formation. In addition, vasoconstriction produced by cryotherapy reduces local blood flow at the site of injury and interferes with the delivery of oxygen to fuel tissue healing.

Elevation of local tissue temperature at the site of tissue injury in the later stages of the healing process has been purported to accelerate tissue repair. A key mechanism of action by which a thermal agent accelerates the healing process is through heat-induced vasodilation, which provides improved blood supply and optimal tissue oxygenation. Figure 7-1 displays a schematic representation of where superficial heating modalities best influence the healing process. Other beneficial effects of therapeutic heat include alteration of enzymatic activity of chronic wound fluid, stimulation of fibroblast proliferation and metabolism, and improved phagocytic activity of inflammatory cells (Rabkin and Hunt 1987). Recently, improved healing of chronic wounds has been demonstrated by the application of heat using a specially designed noncontact dressing that creates a moist wound environment and delivers sufficient thermal energy to maintain normal tissue temperature (Cherry et al. 1999; Santilli et al. 1999; Kloth et al. 2000).

Effect of Hot and Cold Agents on Tissue Extensibility: Range of Motion

After injury, connective tissue will shorten progressively, and joint contractures can develop if stretching exercises through the full range of motion are not performed. The loss of mobility also can result from the development of adhesions that interfere with the ability of tissue components to physically interrelate with each other (see Chapter 6). Temperature elevation in combination with stretch can alter the viscoelastic properties of connective tissue (Strickler et al. 1990). Alteration of

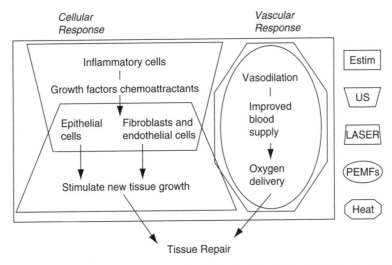

Figure 7-1. Diagram depicts the primary mechanism of action of electrical stimulation (Estim), pulsed ultrasound (US), laser, pulsed electromagnetic fields (PEMFs) and superficial heating agents (heat). PEMFs and heat accelerate tissue healing primarily through vascular response which results in increased local blood supply whereas laser and US stimulate new tissue growth by activating key cells involved in tissue repair. Electrical stimulation can stimulate both vascular and cellular responses.

the viscous properties of connective tissue permits elongation that persists after the external force is removed. Application of moderate heating can denature the immature bonds formed between newly deposited collagen fibers in scar tissue and allow more tissue extensibility. Greater residual length changes with less damage will occur when a stretch is applied during the time the tissue temperature is elevated (Lentell et al. 1992; Hoyrup and Kjorvel 1986).

The effects of cold therapy on contractile and noncontractile tissue components both help and hinder joint flexibility (Kowal 1983). Hypothermia inhibits connective tissue plasticity, which interferes with joint flexibility. Increased joint range of motion may however be facilitated by local application of cold therapy before stretching exercise because of decreased pain perception, which allows more effective stretching forces to be tolerated. In addition, increased joint mobility can be realized secondarily because of the ability of thermal agents to inhibit contractile components of muscles that may limit joint mobility caused by tonic muscle spasm. Vapocoolant sprays deliver a fine stream of fluoromethane or ethylchloride that rapidly cool the skin via evaporation. These sprays are ideal cryotherapy agents used to improve range of motion since they can activate neuromuscular

reflexes that inhibit muscle spasm and reduce pain but do not penetrate through tissue layers sufficiently to reduce tissue temperature and interfere with connective tissue extensibility.

Electrical Stimulation

The application of electrical currents through at least two conductive electrodes placed on the skin to affect a variety of tissues of the integumentary and musculoskeletal system such as ligaments, tendons, nerves, and muscles is known as *transcutaneous electrical nerve stimulation* (TENS). While technically all forms of electrical stimulation applied to the skin surface that do not employ the use of indwelling electrodes should be called "TENS," this term is most often associated when electrical currents are used to treat pain. Numerous waveforms and electrical stimulus parameters have been developed, including interferential current, high voltage galvanic pulsed current, direct current, and asymmetrical biphasic pulsed current. Ultimately, all these devices, regardless of the stimulus parameters used, can deliver electrical energy to various tissues located beneath the skin surface. Most obvious are the effects of electrical stimulation on excitable tissues such as nerves and muscle. These tissues of the neuromuscular system are particularly responsive to externally applied electrical currents producing intense sensory perceptions and strong muscle contractions. Other more subtle effects of electrical energy are those produced on cells of skin and connective tissues that are involved in the healing processes and on vessels of the vascular and lymphatic systems.

Effects of Electrical Stimulation on Blood Flow

Several studies report improved cutaneous blood flow after treatment with some form of electrical stimulation (Mohr et al. 1987; Faghri et al. 1998; Clemente et al. 1991). Treatment with high voltage pulsed current (HVPC) with negative polarity produced greater increases in local blood flow in rats than did positive polarity stimulation (Taylor et al. 1992). Some reports suggest elevations in blood flow can be enhanced by stimulating the muscle pump with the use of relatively high intensity stimulation that is sufficient to produce intermittent neuromuscular contraction (Currier et al. 1986; Faghri et al. 1998; Clemente et al. 1991). However, reports also suggest that low intensity stimulation without muscle contraction can produce significant blood flow changes (Mohr et al. 1987; Hecker et al. 1985; Indergand and Morgan 1994).

The effect of electrical stimulation has been examined on both skin (Indergand and Morgan 1994; Olson et al. 1999; Hecker et al. 1985) and skeletal blood flow (Levine et al. 1990; Tracy et al. 1988; Walker et al. 1988; Liu et al. 1987) of healthy volunteers and these reports have produced equivocal results suggesting that the effect of electrical stimulation has differential effects on blood vessels located in skin and muscle. Different types of electrical waveforms such as Interferential Current (Olson et al. 1999; Nussbaum et al. 1990; Lamb and Mani 1994), HVPC and medium frequency burst current or "Russian current" (Currier et al. 1986) also have been assessed for their ability to improve local blood flow in healthy volunteers. Apart from HVPC, none of these specialized waveforms has been shown to have preferential hemodynamic effects. Thus electrical stimulation either with or without muscular contraction has not been shown conclusively to change blood flow to skin or skeletal muscle of healthy volunteers.

However, Gilcreast et al. (1998) and Faghri et al. (1998) have demonstrated that electrical stimulation can enhance perfusion of ischemic limbs. In addition, Kjartansson et al. (1988) and Im et al. (1990) showed enhanced survival rates of skin flaps pretreated with electrical stimulation, which they attributed to improved blood perfusion. Therefore electrical stimulation appears to have differential effects on blood flow in healthy volunteers compared to those with impaired circulation.

Effect of Electrical Stimulation on Pain

Transcutaneous delivery of electrical currents often is used to reduce the amount of pain perceived. Extensive research has examined the mechanism by which TENS reduces pain; it is a topic too extensive to be covered in this chapter. Briefly, TENS is believed to produce analgesic effects by two mechanisms. One involves activation of sensory nerves that interacts with pain stimuli at the level of the spinal cord and inhibits pain perception. The second involves the electrically induced release of the endogenous opiates, enkephalins and endorphins, which act within the central nervous system to enact potent analgesic effects.

Effects of Electrical Stimulation on Inflammation and Edema

In vitro studies have demonstrated that electrical stimulation can activate several activities of the inflammatory cells involved in the initial phases of tissue repair (Orida and Feldman 1982; Reich et al. 1991; Zhuang et al. 1997). It can induce migration to the site of injury through galvanotaxis as well as stimulate inflammatory cell degranulation and release of important chemical mediators such as growth factors and chemoattractants. Electrical stimulation also can induce inflammatory cell proliferation so that a greater number of these cells are able to respond to the tissue injury (Figure 7-2).

Experiments investigating edema produced by injuries placed experimentally in animal models demonstrated that HVPC using negatively charged electrodes applied locally over the edematous area reduced edema for up to 17 hours post treatment (Bettany et al. 1990a; Bettany et al. 1990b; Mendel

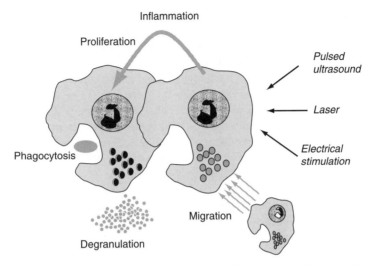

Figure 7-2. A schematic representation of the pro-inflammatory effects of pulsed ultrasound, laser, and electrical stimulation. They include attraction of white blood cells to migrate into the site of injury, stimulation of leucocyte proliferation, degranulation of white blood cells and release of various chemical mediators, and activation of phagocytic activity which assists debridement of necrotic or foreign material.

et al. 1992; Taylor et al. 1992; Karnes et al. 1992; Fish et al. 1991). Edema reduction under the negative pole has been attributed to a phenomenon called cataphoresis – the movement of negatively charged cells and macromolecules such as serum albumin into the capillary lumen because of repulsion by a similarly charged cathode (Cook et al. 1994). Reed (1988), using hamster cheek pouches, also documented that the application of electrical current reduced microvessel leakage and posttraumatic edema formation. Whether electrical stimulation can produce similar effects on swelling present following musculoskeletal injuries in human subjects has not been investigated sufficiently. In one clinical study that examined swelling postacute injury in humans HVPC treatment was found to be as effective as compression therapy at reducing posttraumatic swelling (Griffin et al. 1990).

Effects of Electrical Stimulation on Tissue Repair

Endogenous bioelectrical potentials have been measured across the skin of many animals and humans (Foulds and Barker 1983). These potentials appear to be important in the healing process, as a strong correlation exists between their presence and rapid progression of the wound-healing process. Exogenous application of electrical current to chronic wounds is believed to reproduce the endogenous potential. Numerous studies performed both *in vitro* on cultures of single cell types and on animal models into which artificially produced wounds are created surgically have demonstrated that electrical stimulation can stimulate a number of cellular processes known to be important for wound healing.

In vitro studies on macrophages (Orida and Feldman 1982), epithelial cells (Cooper and Schliwa 1985; Hinsenkamp et al. 1997; Zhao et al. 1997), and fibroblasts (Bourguignon and Bourguignon 1987; Cheng et al. 1982; Falanga et al. 1987; Dunn et al. 1988; Erickson and Nuccitelli 1984; Hinsenkamp et al. 1997; Zhao et al. 1997) collectively suggest that electrical stimulation contributes to accelerated wound repair. Basic science research would suggest that electrical current might activate tissue repair by stimulating cell division (Bourguignon and Bourguignon 1987; Cheng and Goldman 1998; and Zhao et al. 1999a&b), and promoting cell differentiation (Hinsenkamp et al. 1997). Electrical currents also may act by directly stimulating cells important in healing to migrate into the site of injury (Orida and Feldman 1982) where they enhance the release of key chemical mediators, including histamine (Reich et al. 1991) and growth factors (Zhuang et al. 1997).

Cell culture studies have provided insight into possible intracellular mechanisms that underlie physiologic responses to electrical currents. A summary of these intracellular actions of electrical current is provided in Figure 7-3. They include activation of transcription and translation of messenger ribonucleic acid (mRNA) to make available important protein precursors (Zhao et al. 1999b), increased adenosine triphosphate (ATP) production to supply necessary energy demands (Cheng et al. 1982), increased membrane permeability that would allow increased intracellular stores of calcium (Zhuang et al. 1997), and increased production of membrane receptors for important cytokines such as epidermal growth factor (Falanga et al. 1987).

In vivo studies have revealed that local application of electrical current to wounded skin (Alvarez et al. 1983; Bach et al. 1991; Mertz et al. 1993; Chu et al. 1990; Burgess et al. 1998; Smith et al. 1984), or surgically incised ligaments (Fujita et al. 1992; Litke and Dahners 1994; Akai et al. 1988) and tendons (Nessler and Mass 1987; Owoeye et al. 1987) results in improved collagen deposition

(Alvarez et al. 1983; Bach et al. 1991; Fujita et al. 1992; Nessler and Mass 1987), enhanced wound epithelialization (Mertz et al. 1993; Brown et al. 1988; Chu et al. 1990) accelerated collagen maturation and organization (Akai et al. 1988), and greater tensile strength (Litke and Dahners 1994; Owoeye et al. 1987; Burgess et al. 1998; Smith et al. 1984). The application of electrical current has been shown to stimulate several activities of fibroblasts. For a summary of effects of electrical stimulation on fibroblasts see the schematic diagram in Figure 7-3. These fibroblastic effects of electrical stimulation include enhanced collagen synthesis and secretion (Alvarez et al. 1983; Bach et al. 1991; Cheng et al. 1982; Bourguignon and Bourguignon 1987), increased fibroblast proliferation (Bourguignon and Bourguignon 1987), increased number of receptor sites for certain growth factors (Falanga et al. 1987), and alteration of the direction of fibroblast migration (Dunn et al. 1988; Erickson and Nuccitelli 1984).

Epithelial cell activity during repair also seems to be affected by electrical current. In particular, *in vitro* studies have shown that cell proliferation (Zhao et al. 1999a), and cell differentiation (Hinsenkamp et al. 1997) can be activated in epidermal cells by electrical stimulation. In addition, keratinocyte migration can be influenced by the application of an electrical field (Cooper and Schliwa 1985; Zhao et al. 1997) and the synthesis and secretion of growth factors by epithelial cells can be augmented by the application of an electrical current (Zhuang et al. 1997).

In addition to the direct cellular effects of electrical stimulation on the tissue repair process, vasodilation induced by electrical stimulation also assists tissue repair by supporting increased demands for oxygen and nutrients. Enhanced local blood flow also could wash out waste products produced by the injured tissue and remove inflammatory mediators that may contribute to local edema and produce pain. While increased local perfusion can produce many benefits in injured tissue, an increase in arterial perfusion also could exacerbate venous congestion and facilitate edema formation. In particular, where a preexisting impairment in venous return exists because of valvular insufficiency or muscle pump failure. While the majority of experimental research studies report the beneficial effect of electrical stimulation on soft tissue

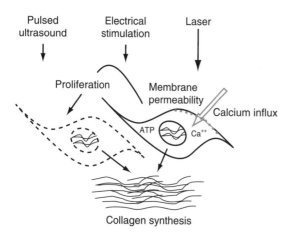

Figure 7-3. A schematic representation of proposed effects of pulsed ultrasound, electrical stimulation, and laser on fibroblastic activity. Diagram represents a summary of results obtained from several in vitro and in vivo research studies. Intracellular mechanisms, including alteration in membrane permeability, increased calcium influx (Ca++), and enhanced oxidative metabolism (ATP), are believed to result in stimulation of fibroblastic activities such as DNA synthesis and cell proliferation and collagen synthesis and secretion.

repair, a few studies have failed to detect a significant improvement in histologic composition of tissues treated with electrical current during the healing process (Steckel et al. 1984; Brown and Goggia 1987). In general, however, experimental research consistently reports that electrical stimulation acts to augment the wound-healing process by directly stimulating cell processes during all the phases of tissue repair (see Figure 7-1).

Electromagnetic Fields

Electromagnetic fields interact with electrically charged molecules present in tissue resulting in the production of electrical currents. These induced ionic currents produced by the movement of charged molecules within tissues in turn also produce significant tissue temperature elevations. Shortwave diathermy (SWD) involves the delivery of high frequency electromagnetic waves at a characteristic frequency (27.12MHz) that produces tissue temperature elevations in structures located at some distance from the skin surface (greater than 3 cm). Pulsed electromagnetic fields (PEMFs) administered in an interrupted mode induce electrical currents in deep structures without producing an accumulation of heat within the tissues. This method of producing electrical currents has a distinct advantage since it does not require placing specialized electrodes in direct contact with the skin; rather, a single large electrode is placed at the site of injury and perpendicular to, but not in contact with, the skin surface.

Effects of Electromagnetic Fields on Tissue Repair

The basic cellular and physiological mechanisms by which electromagnetic fields act on tissue repair are poorly understood. Studies suggest that similar cellular events produced by TENS occur after treatments with PEMFs. *In vitro* studies have shown that PEMFs increase fibroblast and endothelial cell proliferation and induce differentiation of skin fibroblasts in culture (Rodemann et al. 1989). This accelerated activity of fibroblasts and endothelial cells has been shown to result in enhanced inflammatory processes (Detlavs et al.

1996), increased collagen synthesis and angiogenesis (Patino et al. 1996), and accelerated wound closure rate (Ottani et al. 1988). Therefore whether the electrical current is produced by capacitive coupling of two oppositely charged electrodes applied in contact with the skin or by the induction of electrical current produced in body fluids by the indirect application of electromagnetic fields does not seem to matter. The net result is accelerated deposition of new tissue during the proliferative phase of the tissue repair process.

Effects of PEMFs on Blood Circulation

Clinical studies have demonstrated that the application of PEMFs result in alterations in tissue perfusion, elevations in local tissue oxygen pressures, and reduced tissue edema. Changes in local blood flow induced by electromagnetic fields are believed to be a key mechanism by which PEMFs activate the healing process (see Figure 7-1). These circulatory changes have been demonstrated consistently in animal experiments (Mayrovitz and Larsen 1992), healthy human subjects (McMeeken 1992), and in patients with peripheral vascular disease (Santoro et al. 1992). Administration of the PEMFs produces minimal tissue temperature elevations; therefore circulatory changes induced by this modality are believed to occur as a result of induced electrical current as opposed to the thermal or magnetic fields produced concurrently by PEMFs.

Laser

Laser is an acronym for light amplification by stimulated emission of radiation. This modality represents a type of man-made light energy that is characterized by monochromaticity, polarization, and coherency. The type of laser used therapeutically to treat musculoskeletal conditions involves delivery of relatively low-light energy (from a few milliwatts [mW] to 100-200 mW) for short periods of time (seconds) and produces insignificant changes in tissue temperature (measured to be 0.5-0.75°C). Thus biologic effects produced by this type of low-level laser therapy result from the interaction of light energy with tissue and are not caused by tissue heating. As such, this type of laser often is referred to as "cold" or "soft" lasers. Conversely, surgical type lasers such as CO_2 laser use thermal energy as a cutting or vaporizing tool, generating temperatures greater than 300°C at the site of impact of the beam.

Therapeutic lasers utilize wavelengths of light throughout the visible and infrared portion of the electromagnetic spectrum (630 nm to 904 nm) including, but are not limited to, ruby, helium neon (HeNe), argon, krypton, neodymium:yttrium-aluminum garnet (Nd:YAG), galium aluminum arsenide (GalAlAs), and galium arsenide (GalAs), devices. To date the most commonly utilized and investigated types of therapeutic lasers include visible light produced by HeNe gas or the infrared light produced from the semiconductor diodes of GalAs or GalAlAs lasers. HeNe (632.8 nm) is said to have the ability to directly penetrate the skin to a depth of only 0.8 mm. Approximately 96% of light energy emitted by a HeNe laser is absorbed in the epidermal layer of the skin (3.6 mm thick) (Basford 1993). The remaining 4% of available HeNe light energy will penetrate into the dermal layers of the skin and may reach as deep as a few centimeters. Longer wavelength infrared light produced by GalAs (820-905 nm) lasers can penetrate more deeply (2 to 4 mm) (Kolarova et al. 1999). Estimates reveal that as much as 27% of GalAs light energy can penetrate through the outer skin layer and reach subcutaneous structures (Basford 1995). Because of the relatively superficial action of the shorter wavelength light of HeNe lasers, deeper penetrating light produced by GalAs laser is more frequently used clinically to treat musculoskeletal conditions involving structures located deep within the joint and muscle. Lasers are often available in both continuous and pulsed modes. A continuous laser is one that emits a constant relatively low power for a period of at least 0.5 seconds. By contrast, a pulsed source emits a series of extremely high power pulses (Watts) that are very short in duration (nanoseconds) with a relatively long time off between pulses. Studies have postulated that pulsing this high intensity laser allows for a greater amount of light energy to penetrate to deeper tissue structures without an accumulation of heat. Other pulsed lasers simply interrupt the continuous laser beam so that the laser is on for 20% to 50% of the time and effectively reduce the total power of laser delivered. The merits or benefits of this type of pulsed laser have not been demonstrated.

Effect of Laser on Pain

Reduced pain perception and altered peripheral nerve activity have been associated with laser therapy (Zarkovic et al. 1989). Some have found evidence using animal models to suggest that laser-induced analgesia may be mediated by an alteration in nerve conduction velocity (Rochkind et al. 1989), whereas others have not (Ebert and Roberts 1997). The effects of laser on nerve impulse conduction also have been studied in healthy human subjects. Lundeberg et al. (1987), Greathouse et al. (1985), Basford et al. (1990), and Kramer and Sandrin (1993) all failed to detect an effect of either HeNe or infrared laser on nerve conduction velocity. However, Snyder-Mackler et al. (1989) and King et al. (1990) reported a small but significant increase in conduction time with the application of HeNe laser to acupuncture points at relatively low intensities. Further search for evidence to support a humoral mechanism of laser-induced analgesia has produced equivocal results (Zarkovic et al. 1989; Maeda 1988). Therefore an opiate-mediated mechanism for laser-induced analgesia has not been demonstrated conclusively.

Effects of Laser on Tissue Repair

The most consistent research evidence that suggests laser can have important biostimulatory effects on the healing process comes from *in vitro* studies in which the effects of various forms of laser have been examined on cells maintained in culture. These *in vitro* studies have involved many different cell types known to be important in facilitating the healing process of musculoskeletal tissues including several types of inflammatory cells such as macrophages (Bolton et al. 1991; Young et al. 1989), neutrophils (Shiroto et al. 1989), mast cells (Trelles et al. 1989; Bouma et al. 1996), and lymphocytes (Passarella et al. 1985; Ohta et al. 1987) as well as fibroblasts (Noble et al. 1992; Pourreau-Schneider et al. 1990; Webb et al. 1998; Lam et al. 1986; Colver et al. 1989; Skinner et al.

1996), endothelial cells (Bouma et al. 1996; Graham and Alexander 1990) and epithelial cells (Rood et al. 1992; Yu et al. 1996).

Biologic processes observed to be altered by administration of laser to cell cultures include protein synthesis (Skinner et al. 1996; Colver et al. 1989; Lam et al. 1986), cell growth and differentiation (Pourreau-Schneider et al. 1990; Rood et al. 1992), cell proliferation (Ohta et al. 1987; Webb et al. 1998), cell motility (Noble et al. 1992), phagocytosis (Karu et al. 1989; Shiroto et al. 1989), and cell degranulation (Trelles et al. 1989; Bolton et al. 1991; Young et al. 1989; Yu et al. 1996). Intracellular mechanisms of action to produce these cellular changes have also been investigated and proposed. They include activation of DNA synthesis to facilitate cell proliferation (Sroka et al. 1999; Skinner et al. 1996; Ohta et al. 1987), increase in transcription and translation of mRNA to make available important protein precursors (Yu et al. 1996), and change in membrane permeability to stimulate physiologic changes such as nerve depolarization and stimulation of the influx of extracellular stores of calcium (Young and Dyson 1990c). Calcium influx is, in turn, known to be an important intracellular signal for numerous cell processes including cell movement and phagocytosis, secretion of cytoplasmic granules containing potent chemical mediators, alteration in receptor binding affinity to facilitate intercellular communication, and activation of mitochondrial production of ATP via oxidative metabolism to make available energy to fuel increased needs of the photo-activated cell.

The direct actions of laser observed in *in vitro* studies are believed to underlie several cellular processes known to be important during the inflammatory phase of tissue repair. The application of laser to a site of injury has been associated with an accelerated accumulation of mast cells within the tissues at the site of treatment (El Sayed and Dyson 1990, El Sayed and Dyson 1996). This proinflammatory effect of laser has been associated with light-induced proliferation of leukocytes and white blood cell migration to the site of injury in response to the stimulated release of chemoattractive agents. Several reports have documented the ability of laser to stimulate cell degranulation causing the release of potent inflammatory mediators such as prostaglandins, growth factors, and

histamine from various different types of leukocytes involved in the inflammatory phase of tissue repair. Laser irradiation of rat skin stimulated mast cell accumulation at the site of irradiation and a greater percentage of those mast cells present were found to be degranulated in previously traumatized skin (El Sayed and Dyson 1990). Laser applied to macrophages in culture stimulates the release of chemical mediators into the cell culture supernatant that in turn was shown to be capable of activating fibroblast cell function (Bolton et al. 1991; Young et al. 1989). Similarly, cell cultures of T lymphocytes exposed to laser were found to release an angiogenic factor that stimulated endothelial cell proliferation (Agaiby et al. 2000).

Other effects of laser on inflammation include the ability of laser to activate the phagocytic abilities of white blood cells (Karu et al. 1989; Shiroto et al. 1989, Mester et al. 1985). Laser-induced activation of the natural debridement action of leukocytes helps to clean foreign or dead and devitalized tissues within the injury site and promote faster resolution of the inflammatory phase of repair (see Figure 7-2). The ability of laser to reduce experimentally induced inflammation and edema has been investigated, and laser was found to produce a small but significant decrease in edema formation produced by an inflammatory irritant (Honmura et al. 1992). Antiinflammatory effects of laser have also been documented by improvements in the histologic appearance of synovial membrane biopsies obtained from patients undergoing total knee arthroplasty because of rheumatoid arthritis (Amano et al. 1994).

In vivo studies examining the effects of laser on reparative processes occurring in experimental injuries placed surgically into connective tissue of skin (Utsunomiya 1998; Braverman et al. 1989; Kovacs et al. 1974; Bischt et al. 1994; El Sayed and Dyson 1996; Lyons et al. 1987; Longo et al. 1987; Saperia et al. 1986; Hunter et al. 1984; McCaughan et al. 1985; Schultz et al. 1985; Yu et al. 1997; Dyson and Young 1986) tendons (Reddy et al. 1998), joint capsule (Hayashi et al. 1995), and cartilage (Schultz et al. 1985) have been performed in several species including dogs (Utsunomiya 1998), rabbits (Braverman et al. 1989; Kovacs et al. 1974; Reddy et al. 1998; Hayashi et al. 1995), rats (Bischt et al. 1994; El Sayed and Dyson 1996; Kovacs et al. 1974; Lyons et al. 1987; Longo et al. 1987), pigs (Saperia et al. 1986; Hunter et al. 1984), guinea pigs (McCaughan et al. 1985; Schultz et al. 1985) and mice (Yu et al. 1997; Dyson and Young, 1986).

In summary, several reports have demonstrated that laser treatment of injured tissues resulted in increased collagen deposition (Bischt et al. 1994; Saperia et al. 1986; Reddy et al. 1998) and that this augmentation of collagen production was associated with a concomitant improvement in the tensile strength of surgically incised skin (Kovacs et al. 1974; Lyons et al. 1987; Braverman et al. 1989) and tendons (Reddy et al. 1998). For a review of the effects of laser therapy on fibroblast activity and collagen production see Figure 7-3. Several other studies have reported no benefit of laser on wound healing and breaking strength (Hall et al. 1994; Surinchak et al. 1983; Broadley et al. 1995; Allendorf et al. 1997). These negative findings tended to occur more commonly in studies where laser treatment regimes result in the administration of relatively low amounts (less than 1 Joules/cm^2) of light energy to the wound bed (Saperia et al. 1986; Hunter et al. 1984) or where the sham control group to which the effects of laser treatments are compared was located within the same animal (Braverman et al. 1989; Hall et al. 1994; McCaughan et al. 1985).

Although numerous research studies suggest laser therapy can have profound physiologic effects on the body, inconsistent results have generated some skepticism about the effectiveness of this relatively new modality. A number of factors can impact the tissue response to laser irradiation. Some stimulus parameters believed to influence the effects of laser therapy include laser wavelength, intensity, pulse frequency, and treatment schedule. In addition to the laser parameters provided by the equipment, the biologic response to laser also is affected by factors within the host tissue such as tissue type, local blood flow, and basal level of tissue activity. Clearly more research is required to fully appreciate the influence that these and other factors have on the ability of laser therapy to produce the desired response. Once factors influencing the response to laser are understood, a more systematic approach to assessment of laser therapy effectiveness can be used. In this way, perhaps more consistent and meaningful results will become available in future clinical trials.

Ultrasound

Therapeutic ultrasound is produced by a crystal located in a sound head or transducer that vibrates to create high frequency acoustic waves not detected by the human ear. The delivery of high frequency sound waves to tissues through an appropriate coupling medium produces mechanical energy. Therapeutic ultrasound administered as a continuous sound wave, produces kinetic energy and the oscillations of tissue components in turn produces hyperthermia. In addition to the thermal effects of continuous ultrasound, the physical movement produced by the sound waves is responsible for the mechanical effects described as acoustic microstreaming, micromassage, and cavitation. When ultrasound is delivered in the "pulsed mode" using an automated on/off cycle, the heat produced by kinetic energy is allowed to dissipate; therefore no net tissue heating is produced. Physiological effects produced by pulsed ultrasound are attributed primarily to the mechanical properties of ultrasound rather than the thermal effects of this agent.

Therapeutic ultrasound involves the delivery of a spatial average intensity of between 0.1-3 W/cm^2 of sound energy, which is generally greater than intensities used in most diagnostic ultrasound machines (0.04-0.1W/cm^2). The most common frequencies in ultrasound devices used for therapeutic purposes are 1 and 3 MHz; however, lower frequency (30 to 45kHz) or "long wave" ultrasound machines are available. In general, since higher frequency sound waves produced by a 3 MHz sound head would be absorbed more quickly in the superficial structures, these devices should be used only when targeting structures located just beneath the skin surface (2 cm) (ter Haar and Hopewell 1982). Lower frequency sound heads (1 MHz) produce ultrasound waves that have been purported to transmit more readily through subcutaneous structures and have been shown to penetrate to depths of 3 to 5 cm below the skin surface including articular structures and skeletal muscles of healthy, non-obese, human subjects (ter Haar and Hopewell 1982).

Effects of Ultrasound on Blood Flow

While many sources describe changes in local circulation as one of the thermal effects of continuous ultrasound, little scientific evidence exists to support these claims. An examination of research studies that have been performed to assess changes in skeletal blood flow in response to ultrasound treatments has for the most part produced inconclusive results (Robinson and Buono 1995; Hogan et al. 1982; Rubin et al. 1990). In fact, some reports suggest that ultrasound induces vascular changes such as production of blood stasis (Dyson et al. 1971), hemolysis (Williams et al. 1986), increased vascular permeability, transient vasoconstriction (Hogan et al. 1982; Rubin et al. 1990), and production of oxygen free radicals (Maxwell 1992), all of which could interfere with local tissue perfusion. However, most of these potentially deleterious effects of ultrasound were associated with the application of relatively high intensities (2-3 W/cm^2) of ultrasonic energy (Dyson et al. 1971; Williams et al. 1986).

Effects of Ultrasound on Pain

Musculoskeletal Pain

Ultrasound has been shown to increase the pain threshold (Mardiman et al. 1995) and reduce pain perception (Williams et al. 1987) in healthy volunteers. The analgesic effects of ultrasound are proposed to be caused by the ability of ultrasound to change nerve conduction velocity. Kramer (1984) investigated the effects of both pulsed and continuous ultrasound and concluded that changes in nerve conduction velocity was more likely the result of the thermal heating effect of ultrasound. By contrast, Oztas and colleagues (1998) reported lower nerve conduction velocities after administration of continuous ultrasound at either 0.8 W/cm^2 or 1.5 W/cm^2 for 5 minutes 5 days a week for a 2-week period. These authors expressed concern about a tendency for patients with carpal tunnel syndrome treated with either dose of continuous ultrasound to experience a further impairment of motor nerve conduction. An alternative explanation of results from these reports is that changes in nerve conduction velocity are dependent on whether the ultrasound is delivered in a continuous or pulsed mode or whether tissue heating occurs.

Other mechanisms of ultrasound-induced analgesia also have been proposed, such as ultrasound-induced release of endogenous opiates. A more rapid resolution of the inflammatory stage of tissue repair causing less tissue swelling also may contribute to the reduction in pain reported by patients following ultrasound treatment of their musculoskeletal injury.

Effects of Ultrasound on Tissue Repair

Several experimental studies performed in both cell culture and animal models have examined the physiologic effects of ultrasound. Cell culture studies have provided convincing evidence that ultrasound can alter the activity of cells known to be important in the inflammatory phase of healing. Stimulation of phagocytic activity of inflammatory cells such as macrophages and neutrophils has been reported (Crowell et al. 1997). This debridement action of ultrasound would be important in the initial stages of recovery from injury to clear the area of dead or devitalized material. In addition, ultrasound has been shown to stimulate degranulation of inflammatory cells like macrophages (Young and Dyson 1990b) and mast cells (Dyson and Luke 1986). This results in the release of numerous chemical mediators that in turn have been shown to activate other key cells in the healing process such as fibroblasts (Young and Dyson 1990b). Thus the effects of ultrasound during inflammation appear to help to accelerate the healing process by stimulating the natural debridement process and by causing the release of the body's endogenous source of growth factors and other cytokines at the local site of injury (see Figure 7-2).

Examination of the temporal pattern of changes in the histologic composition of tissues obtained from animal models after injury suggests that ultrasound treated tissues remain in the inflammatory phase of repair for a much shorter period of time (Young and Dyson 1990a). In this way, ultrasound treatment has been suggested to promote a more rapid progression through the inflammatory phase of healing allowing the deposition of new tissue to occur at the site of injury sooner and completion of the repair process to occur more rapidly. The effects of ultrasound on this phase of repair may be best described as "proinflammatory" and based on results obtained from both *in vitro* and *in vivo* experimental models, these proinflammatory effects of ultrasound are effective in augmenting both the quantity and quality of the healing process. Some studies have failed to find a significant effect of ultrasound on acute inflammation (Snow and Johnson 1988; Goddard et al. 1983) while other reports describe the effects of ultrasound as "antiinflammatory." El Hag et al. (1985) and Hashish et al. (1986) both reported that swelling and trismus were reduced when ultrasound was applied to the jaw of patients who had undergone minor dental surgery to extract wisdom teeth. Fyfe and Chahl (1985) reported significant reductions in experimentally induced edema on rat abdomens within 30 minutes of treatments using pulsed ultrasound. However, by contrast these same investigators (Fyfe and Chahl 1982) also reported subsequently that application of similar treatment regime to edema produced experimentally in rat ankle joint caused an initial augmentation of swelling at 30 minutes posttreatment and that this swelling was linked with a concurrent histamine release from local mast cells. Also noted in this study was a significant reduction in ankle swelling in ultrasound treated animals compared with control animals that was present 48 hours after ultrasound treatment. This temporal pattern of changes to ankle joint swelling after ultrasound treatment is consistent with the theory that ultrasound initially stimulates the inflammatory phase of repair which in turn results in a more rapid resolution of the edema.

Ultrasound also has been shown to have profound effects on the fibroblast, inducing both fibroblast proliferation and activation of the production of collagen (see Figure 7-3). Cell culture studies clearly show that ultrasound can stimulate fibroblasts to synthesize and secrete collagen (Harvey et al. 1975). Ultrasound also can stimulate fibroblasts to proliferate (De Deyne and Kirsch-Volders 1995), resulting in a greater number of fibroblasts available to produce more collagen. Further study of the mechanisms underlying ultrasound induced fibroblastic activity has revealed that ultrasound can act directly to alter fibroblast function by producing calcium influx (Al-Karmi et al. 1994; Mortimer and Dyson 1988), and altering plasma membrane permeability (Dinno et al. 1989). Ultrasound treatment of experimentally placed skin lesions in animals has been shown in many studies (Byl et al. 1993; Dyson et al. 1968; Young and Dyson 1990a) to be associated with elevated levels of markers of collagen production such as procollagen mRNA expression, and hydroxylproline concentrations (Jackson et al. 1991; Byl et al. 1993). Studies examining the effects of ultrasound on healing tendons has revealed that collagen laid down under the direction of ultrasound is better organized and of greater tensile strength (Enwemeka et al. 1990; Jackson et al. 1991; Gan et al. 1995; Stevenson et al. 1986). Producing scar tissue of greater breaking strength is an important functional advantage when referring to the healing of soft tissues such as ligaments and tendons. However, care needs to be taken when extrapolating to the clinical situation any results obtained using experimentally produced injuries of ligaments and tendons of animals. Many authors have highlighted important differences between collagen organization present in most human tendons versus those in animal models (Enwemeka et al. 1990; Turner et al. 1989; Roberts et al. 1982; Shamberger et al. 1981). Most studies performed using animal models suggest ultrasound stimulates fibroblastic activity and collagen synthesis and secretion (Young and Dyson 1990a&c; Harvey et al. 1975; Jackson et al. 1991; Byl et al. 1993) and this is consistent with results obtained in cell culture studies (Young and Dyson 1990b; Harvey et al. 1975). A few reports have failed to demonstrate a significant effect of ultrasound on healing.

In summary, ultrasound has been purported to alter scar tissue formation through its actions on cellular processes in all phases of tissue repair but during the inflammatory phase of repair in particular. For a schematic representation of the major effects of ultrasound on the healing process see Figure 7-1. Ultrasound promotes the release of chemical mediators from inflammatory cells that in turn attract and activate fibroblasts to the site of injury, it stimulates fibroplasia during the proliferative stage of repair, and finally it alters collagen organization and improves extensibility and functional capacity of scar tissue when heating effects are applied during the remodeling phase of repair. Some investigators have suggested that the timing of ultrasound treatments during the healing process seems to be an important determinant of functional outcome of tissue repair (Jackson et al. 1991; Gan et al. 1995; Enwemeka et al. 1990). Examination of research literature finds that improved healing results more often are associated with ultrasound treatments administered early in the healing process (Roberts et al. 1982; Shamberger et al. 1981; Turner et al. 1989). Furthermore, Jackson et al. (1991), demonstrated that ultrasound administered during the early inflammatory phase of repair improved ultimate tendon breaking strength and that continued ultrasound treatments after day five of injury did not produce further improvements in tensile strength of repaired tendons. Gan et al. (1995), demonstrated that improvements obtained when ultrasound was administered within 7 days of injury were not observed if the commencement of ultrasound treatments was delayed. Therefore the proinflammatory effect of ultrasound occurring early in the healing process causes the body to produce its own mediators of tissue repair and is the critical action of this modality that is sufficient to kick start scar tissue formation and optimize collagen production, organization, and ultimately functional strength.

Effect of Ultrasound on Tissue Extensibility

Wessling et al. (1987) demonstrated that ultrasound applied to the triceps surae muscle at 1.5 w/cm^2 for 7 minutes in continuous mode during static ankle dorsiflexion stretch can optimize improvements in joint range of motion. Presumably these improvements in joint mobility resulted from the thermal effects of ultrasound. Connective tissue extensibility is increased by tissue heating (Lehmann et al. 1970) and temperatures of the connective tissue of skeletal muscle are known to be elevated sufficiently by the cutaneous application of relatively high intensities of continuous ultrasound (ter Haar and Hopewell 1982). However, Ward and colleagues (1994) failed to find an improvement in joint mobility when similar intensity of ultrasound was administered to patients with burn scar contractures. An explanation for the disparity in the results reported in these two studies is differences in the timing of the ultrasound treatments. Improvements in joint range of motion reported by Wessling and colleagues (1987) occurred when ultrasound was applied simultaneously with the static stretch exercise whereas when ultrasound was administered before the passive stretching

exercises by Ward et al. (1994) no differences in ROM were found. To optimize the effects of heat on connective tissue extensibility authorities generally agreed that the thermal agent is best applied at the same time as the tissue stretch.

Ankle Sprains

Ankle-inversion injury usually results in some degree of tearing of the lateral ligaments of the ankle caused by excessive inward motion of the sole of the foot. Ankle injuries are extremely prevalent, affecting approximately 1% of the population with higher prevalence among younger individuals involved in sporting activities. Inversion sprains with injury to lateral ligaments of the ankle account for more than 10% of emergency attendances. Lateral ankle sprains cause significant pain and suffering so that patients often are unable to weight bear on the injured limb, which significantly limits mobility. The average number of days lost from school, work, or leisure after injury to soft tissues of the ankle is 7 days (Losito and O'Neil 1997).

Treatment of an acute ankle injury is initially directed at reducing joint swelling. Edema produces pressure within the joint capsule and therefore is a major cause of pain and may interfere mechanically with normal joint range of motion. Loss of joint mobility at the ankle produces loss of joint strength, and regaining joint motion and strength is difficult. Inadequate treatment and rehabilitation of the inversion ankle sprain may result in ligament laxity, decreased strength of dynamic ankle stabilizers and proprioceptive deficits. The recovery rate for ankle function after inversion sprain may be related to the effectiveness of edema control at the injury site (Basur et al. 1976; Stamford 1996). Therefore therapeutic interventions that prevent edema formation after injury to the soft tissues of the ankle need to be identified and utilized as soon as possible.

Treatment of Ankle Injuries Using Therapeutic Modalities

Modalities suggested to reduce the formation of edema after a lateral ankle sprain are cryotherapy, pulsed ultrasound, laser, and certain forms of electrical stimulation. Table 7-2 presents a summary of

Table 7-2. Clinical Trials that Have Examined the Effectiveness of the Therapeutic Modalities on Acute Ankle Sprains

Article	Modality	Rx Parameters	N	Rx Grps	Random	Control	Blinded	Outcome Measures	Conclusions
Nyanzi 1999	Pulsed ultrasound	USRx: 20% P, 3.0 MHz, 0.25 W/cm², 10 mins, 3 days	51	Sham USRx	Yes	Yes	Double	Pain↓ ROM↑ Edema↓ Weight Bearing↑	N.S. btwn grps
Bradnock 1995	Pulsed and continuous ultrasound	USRx pulsed: 20% P: 3.0 MHz, 2.0W/cm², 5min, 1 day USRx continuous: 100% C: 45 kHz, 0.95W/cm², 5 min, 1 day	47	Sham USRx -continuous -pulsed	Yes	Yes	Single-Patient	Gait Analysis	USRxContinuous> USRxPulsed = Sham
Makuloluwe 1977	Continuous ultrasound	USRx: 0.8-1.0 MHz, 1.5W/cm², 100%, 4 mins, 2 wks	80	US/iceRx Immobilization	Yes	No	No	Pain↓ Edema↓ ROM↑	US&iceRx > immobilization and Eastoplast
De Bie 1998	GaAs laser	LaserRx: 904nm, 25W, 500Hz, 200nsec, with an irradiated area of 1 cm² high-dose (5J/cm²) and low-dose (0.5J/cm²)	217	Sham LaserRx -high -low	Yes	Yes	Double	Pain↓ Function↑	N.S. btwn grps Sham > LaserRx
Laba 1989	Cold and ultrasound	ColdRx: 2L crushed ice pack in 1 layer of toweling for 20mins Both groups: pulsed US, 1.5W/cm², 5mins combined with exercises, and support.	30	Cold and USRx USRx	Yes	No	No	Pain↓ Edema↓ Recovery↑	N.S. btwn grps
Hocutt 1982	Cold and warm	ColdRx: 40-50°F whirlpool, 12-20mins or ice pack for 15-20mins with bandage HeatRx: warm bath or heating pad for 15min, 1-3x/day and Ace bandage	37	ColdRx or WarmHeatRx; both within 1 hr 1-3 hrs, or >36hrs post trauma	NA	No	No	Function↑	ColdRx & Bandage within 1hr > ColdRx within 1-36hrs or 36hrs, WarmRx within 1hr, 1-36hrs or >36hrs

Study	Modality	Treatment	N	Groups				Outcome	Results
Basur 1976	Cold	ColdRx: gel pack first 48hrs. No temperature given NoRx: All subjects: crepe bandage	60	NoRx ColdRx	Yes	Yes	No	Pain↓ Edema↓ ROM↑	ColdRx > NoRx
Michlovitz 1988	HVPC and ice	ColdRx: Ice: 30mins, daily, 3days Cold and HVPCRx: daily, 3 days -28pps, [-] polarity, 30mins -80pps, [-] polarity, 30mins	30	ColdRx Cold and HVPCRx -high -low	Yes	No	No	Pain↓ Edema↓ AROM↑	N.S. btwn grps
McGill 1988	Pulsed SWD	SWDRx: 82Hz, Intensity: 6, 19.6W, 3doses 15min each, for 3days	37	Sham SWDRx	Yes	Yes	Double	Pain↓ Edema↓	N.S. btwn grps
Wilson 1974	SWD and Pulsed electromagnetic field	SWDRx: dosage according to pts rxn to heating of tissues, 2 doses of 15min each in 1hr for 3 days PEMFRx: 975W, 65microsec, continuous for 1hr for 3 days	40	SWDRx PEMFRx	Yes	No	No	Pain↓ Edema↓ Function↑	PEMFRx > SWDRx
Stockle 1997	Cold and compression	Cold Rx: ColdPack: changed 4×/day & fixed with elastic dressing Continuous Cryo Rx: 12°C for 8hrs thru cooling cuff (ice Δed 2×/day) AV impulseRx: 130mmHg for 1sec every 20sec continuous thru day	60	AVImpulseRx ContCryoRx ColdRx	Yes	No	No	Edema↓	AVImpulseRx > Continuous CryoRx > ColdRx
Wilkerson 1993	Cold and compression	StrapNormRx: strap with modified air-stirrup-normal temp StrapFrozenRx: strap with modified air-stirrup-frozen All subjects: Cryotherapy for 20-30mins at least 1×/day	34	ElasticTapeRx StrapNormRx StrapFrozenRx	Yes	No	No	Function ↑	StrapNormRx > ElastictapeRx and StrapfrozenRx

(Continued)

Table 7-2. (cont'd)

Article	Modality	Rx Parameters	N	Rx Grps	Random	Control	Blinded	Outcome Measures	Conclusions
Weston 1994	Cold	ColdRx: Sitting for 10mins, prone for 10mins with knee in 15-20° flexion; gel 20°F in damp pillow case for 20mins	15	No Rx ColdRx	NA	Yes	No	Local blood volume↓	ColdRx (during application) > NoRx
Cote 1988	Cold, warm and contrast, bath	Cold Rx: Cold cylinder: 50-60°F for 20 mins for 3 days Warm Rx: Warm whirlpool: 102-106°F for 20mins for 3days ContrastRx: begin with warm for 3mins, 5times; cold for 1min, 4times	30	ColdRx WarmRx ContrastRx	Yes	No	No	Edema↓	ColdRx > HeatRx, ContrastRx
Quillen 1982	Rapid pulsed pneumatic compression and cold	RapidPPCRx: Elasticized stockinet, molded cryoglove, Thera-Nu device with boot, 5mins, 70-90mmHg as tolerated; then removing cryoglove and continuing compression for 15min	19	RapidPPCRx	No	No	No	Pain↓ ROM↑ Edema↓	Rapid pulsed pneumatic compression and cold a safe and therapeutically sound intervention

the clinical trials that have examined the effectiveness of the therapeutic modalities on acute ankle sprains.

Reducing tissue temperature via the application of cryotherapeutic agents during the first 72 hours has been shown in the majority of studies to reduce the amount of ankle swelling after ankle inversion injury (Taber et al. 1992; Hecht et al. 1983). Hypothermia-induced reduction in tissue swelling has in turn been associated with lower pain scores and faster return to full recovery (Basur et al. 1976; Weston et al. 1994). The production of mild tissue hypothermia (5° to 15° C) has the ability to produce beneficial antiinflammatory effect; however, increasing the intensity, frequency, or duration of cryotherapy is not associated with any further improvement in functional recovery post ankle inversion injury (20° to 25° C for 24 hours) (Wilkerson and Horn-Kingery 1993). The ability of cryotherapy to limit edema formation after ankle injury has been compared to other thermal modalities, and cryotherapy has consistently been shown to be superior to the application of local heat or contrast baths (Cote et al. 1988; Hocutt et al. 1982). Cold therapy also has been combined with other modalities as part of a rehabilitation program. The combination of cold therapy with compression and elevation using the rest, elevation, and compression (RICE) principle seems to have an additive effect (Stockle et al. 1997; Garrick and Henz-Schelkun 1997; McClusky et al. 1976). Adding other modalities to cold therapy regime including therapeutic ultrasound (Makuloluwe and Mouzas 1977; Laba and Roestenburg 1989), or high voltage pulsed current (Michlovitz et al. 1988) does not appear to be of additional therapeutic benefit.

Substantial experimental evidence suggests electrical energy delivered using HVPC can reduce edema formation (Bettany et al. 1990a&b; Mendel et al. 1992; Karnes et al. 1992; Fish et al. 1991; and Taylor et al. 1992). Very limited trials using human subjects have been conducted to test the clinical application of these animal studies. The addition of HVPC to a post injury program including cryotherapy was shown by Michlovitz and colleagues in 1988 not to produce any added benefit.

Makuloluwe and Mouzas (1977) reported that the delivery of relatively high intensity of continuous ultrasound at 0.8-1.0 MHz was more effective at reducing ankle swelling and functional outcomes

after ankle injuries than immobilization using a cast. However, a more recent study by Nyanzi et al. (1999) reported no difference between ultrasound and placebo treated groups in the range of motion, perceived pain, ankle swelling, or patient's ability to weight bear on the affected extremity. Although this was an extremely well designed randomized clinical trial that studied more than 50 subjects, the ultrasound treatment regime tested in this clinical trial may not have been optimal. Ultrasound parameters used by Nyanzi and colleagues (1999) included a high frequency (3 MHz) sound head that would have resulted in the absorption of most of the ultrasound energy in superficial structures of the treatment area. A report by Bradnock and colleagues (1995) found that treatment of acute ankle injuries using low frequency (45 KHz) ultrasound was much more effective at improving function post ankle injury than using the traditional high frequency ultrasound waves (3 MHz). Thus this research suggests that relatively high spatial average intensity of pulsed ultrasound that is lower in frequency may be required to obtain beneficial effects of this modality on acute ankle sprains.

De Bie and colleagues (1998) performed a large randomized controlled trial to assess the effectiveness of a high (5 J/cm^2) and low (0.5 J/cm^2) dose of pulsed GalAs (904 nm) laser irradiation on ankle pain and function after an acute inversion sprain. They failed to detect a significant effect of either dose of laser administered. This is in contrast to a previous report by the same group demonstrating that a similar laser therapy regime produced a significant reduction in pain after ankle injury (deBie et al. 1998). Although laser therapy has been shown to reduce pain and improve function after ankle injury, whether laser therapy can produce a significant reduction in ankle swelling following lateral ligament sprain has not been assessed.

Other modalities also suggested to improve recovery after ankle sprain include PEMFs. Wilson (1974) using a Diapulse machine for one hour on three consecutive days post injury showed a reduction in ankle swelling, pain, and general impairment over controls for 20 patients in a matched trial on lateral ligament ankle sprains. Barclay et al. (1983) also found reduced ankle swelling within 36 hours for patients who had received Diapulse treatments twice daily for 30 minutes when compared to placebo treated controls. However, Barker et al. (1985), and McGill (1988) found no difference in any criterion measured between controls and PEMF treated ankles. Although PEMF may be a promising therapy for treatment of ankle injuries, research results to date should be considered inconclusive. Differences in studies examining the effects of PEMF on ankle injuries are likely explained by the variety of diathermy machines used and the lack of knowledge regarding the optimal treatment parameters for pulse frequency and power output.

In summary, based on clinical research evidence available to date, the use of cryotherapy during the first 72 hours after injury is recommended. The application of cold therapy reduces tissue temperature, thereby blocking inflammation and edema formation that in turn reduces pain and ultimately speeds the individual's recovery. Combination with compression and elevation using the RICE principle has been associated with an additive effect. Some evidence exists to support the benefits of low frequency or long-wave ultrasound administered in pulsed mode for the treatment of acute ankle sprains. However, the device used to deliver this low frequency (45 KHz) is not typically used in physical therapy practice. Limited evidence exists that PEMF delivered using a Diapulse machine can reduce swelling post ankle sprain. Whether laser or HVPC can assist with recovery after inversion sprain remains to be investigated.

Periarticular Inflammatory Conditions

Bursitis, Tendonitis, and Epicondylitis

Tendonitis refers to inflammation of tendons and of tendon-muscle attachments (see Chapter 3). Estimates suggest that tendonitis resulting from chronic conditions can account for as much as 48% of reported occupational illnesses. Furthermore, overuse injuries causing tendonitis have been estimated to account for as much as 30% to 50% of sports injuries. Whether the condition is caused by an inflammatory reaction is not settled. The presence of an inflammatory process has not been detected within experimental models of tendonitis involving repetitive overloading of limb muscles (Backman et al. 1990; Zamora and Marini 1988).

Other explanations for the etiology of these common tendon problems are a "tendonosis," which denotes that it is a degenerative process produced by either a single large trauma or several repetitive strains, exceeding the healing capability of the tendon. The result is a progressive degeneration of the connective tissue structure caused by repetitive injuries induced by overuse and deposition of scar tissue. Replacement of normal connective tissue of tendons with scar tissue often results in tendon shortening, a reduction in tendon glide, and the relative loss in tendon strength. Because a lack of agreement exists on the underlying cause of these problems with tendons, these conditions are sometimes generically referred to as "tendonopathy" or tendonosis (Chapter 3).

Rotator cuff tendonitis is thought by many to be the most common cause of shoulder pain with the supraspinatus portion of the cuff most frequently involved. The blood supply to the rotator cuff tendons is partially interrupted by compression between the humeral head and the acromion when the shoulder is flexed or abducted above 90 degrees. In addition, tendons of the supraspinatus muscle are relatively avascular, which reduces the rate of healing of the supraspinatus tendon and makes this structure particularly susceptible to chronic injury. Calcific deposits in the tendon and in the subdeltoid bursae are common, and biceps tendonitis is commonly associated with rotator cuff tendonitis because of the proximity of the rotator cuff to the insertion of the tendon of the long head of biceps. Rotator cuff tendonitis with or without involvement of biceps brachii or subdeltoid bursae is characterized by a painful arc and tenderness to palpation over the affected tendons. Pain often is reported at the end of range or upon resistance to active movements of the shoulder that, if left untreated, will result in loss of both passive and active range of motion as result of soft tissue shortening caused by capsular fibrosis and reduced tendon length.

Epicondylitis of the elbow is also a very common musculoskeletal condition affecting predominantly younger individuals. "Tennis elbow," or lateral epicondylitis, is associated with pain and tenderness on palpation over the lateral epicondylar region with increased discomfort upon wrist extension or forearm supination. This condition is common in individuals who are involved in activities that require excessive, repetitive, quick movements of the wrists such as those performed while playing tennis. Nonsporting activities that require sustained hand gripping, such as gardening or hammering, also can precipitate the development of epicondylitis. A commonly accepted etiology of lateral epicondylitis is an inflammation with or without rupture of the extensor aponeurosis. Most often the tendon of the extensor carpi radialis brevis tendon is involved.

Bursitis results from inflammation within saclike structures lined with endothelial cells, called *bursae*, that are usually present between tendon and bone or skin and serve to facilitate a gliding motion at points of high friction. Bursitis is associated with a variety of clinical symptoms depending on the location of the bursae involved but most often is associated with extreme local tenderness and edema around the joint structures that results in a restriction to both passive and active range of motion. Bursitis has been estimated to be responsible for approximately 0.4 percent of all visits to primary care clinics with the incidence rising to as high as 10% for individuals who do a lot of running. The onset of bursitis may be insidious, resulting from chronic overuse, or acute resulting from a single traumatic event. In most cases bursitis develops as a result of the presence of material not normally present in bursa fluid that stimulates an inflammatory reaction with leukocyte infiltration. The foreign material that most commonly triggers bursitis is the presence of serum proteins and extracellular fluid that are extravagated into the bursa fluid as a result of repetitive subacute injury to the bursae. Blood resulting from a sudden traumatic blow to tissues overlying the bursae also can act a foreign material stimulating an inflammatory response in the bursae. Other foreign materials that can accumulate in the fluid filled cavity of the bursa and stimulate an inflammatory reaction are bacteria and calcium crystals. Calcific bursitis is the result of abnormal deposition of calcium usually in the form of hydroxyapatite in response to chronic inflammation. A bacterial infection of bursae occurs rarely and requires rapid response with appropriate antibiotic therapy. A review of the clinical research studies that have examined the effectiveness of various therapeutic interventions on tendonitis, bursitis and epicondylitis is provided in Table 7-3.

Treatment of Periarticular Inflammatory Conditions

Treatment of shoulder tendonitis, bursitis, and lateral epicondylitis should be directed initially at alleviating pain and reducing the acute inflammatory process by removing the inflammatory stimulus. Rapid resolution of inflammation during the acute stage will in turn lower long-term complications including reduced muscle strength and impaired joint range of motion. If the condition is more chronic or caused by repetitive overloading, degenerative changes are more likely. In these cases of chronic tendonitis, treatment interventions should be directed at optimizing tissue healing. Once pain is resolved and inflammation has been brought under control, subsequent treatment sessions should focus on restoring connective tissue length and returning muscle strength.

Reduction of tissue temperature by the application of cryotherapy agents is known to have potent antiinflammatory effects. Ice massage over the specific affected site is commonly employed clinically. However, a paucity of well-designed clinical research trials have tested the efficacy of cold therapy to effectively manage these chronic inflammatory conditions. Ultrasound, laser, PEMFs and electrical stimulation are known to stimulate many of the cellular processes of inflammation. The application of these proinflammatory agents could serve useful in the treatment of these chronic inflammatory conditions, since these modalities could stimulate the healing processes to move on to later stages of repair involved in new tissue formation. In addition, these modalities are believed to assist with overuse injuries such as shoulder tendonitis and lateral epicondylitis primarily by accelerating the healing process and by supplying more nutrients such as oxygen via increases in local tissue blood flow.

Heating modalities such as continuous ultrasound, hot packs and paraffin wax, may be helpful in the chronic stages of periarticular arthritis when pain and other acute signs of inflammation have subsided. An elevation in tissue temperature could assist healing by improving local blood perfusion and hence tissue oxygenation and by assisting with extensibility of connective tissues to help restore joint range of motion. All of the modalities could indirectly help to restore normal joint range of

Table 7-3. Clinical Research Studies Examining the Effectiveness of Various Therapeutic Interventions on Tendonitis, Bursitis, and Epicondylitis

Article	Modality	Condition	Rx Parameters	N	Rx Grps	Random	Control	Blinded	Outcome Measures	Conclusions
Ebenbichler 1999	Pulsed ultrasound	Calcific tendinitis, bursitis	USRx: 20%P, 0.89 MHz, 2.5W/cm², 15mins, 6wks, 24Rxs	54 (61 shld)	Sham USRx	Yes	Yes	Double	Calcium deposit resolution	USRx > Sham
Perron 1997	Iontophoresis and continuous ultrasound	Calcific tendinitis	Ionto Rx: [-] Electrode, 5mA, 20mins followed by... USRx: 100%C, 1 MHz, 0.8W/cm², 5mins	22	NoRx US/IontoRx	Yes	Yes	Single-evaluator	Area and density of calcium deposits pain↓ Passive ABD↑	NS btwn grps
Ebenbichler 1997	Pulsed ultrasound	Calcific tendinitis	USRx: 20%P, 1 MHz, 2 W/cm², 10mins	3	USRx	No	No	No	Calcium deposit resolution	Successful pulsed US Rx with ↓ deposits on radiograph
Haker 1991	Pulsed ultrasound	Lateral epicondylitis	USRx: 20%P, 1.0MHz, 1.0W/cm², 10min, 3-5wks, 10Rxs	43	Sham USRx	Yes	Yes	Double	Pain↓ ADL↑ grip strength↑	NS btwn grps
Pienimaki 1996	Pulsed ultrasound and exercise	Lateral epicondylitis	USRx: 20%P, 1.0 MHz, 0.3-0.7W/cm², 10-15min, 2-3Rxs/wk, 6-8wks, 12-24Rxs	39	USRx Exerc	Yes	No	No	Pain↓ ADL↑ isokinetic↑ grip strength↑	Exerc > USRx Exerc = USRx Exerc > USRx Exerc > USRx
Lundeberg 1988	Continuous ultrasound	Lateral epicondylitis	USRx: 100%C, 1 MHz, 1 W/cm², 10min, 5-6wks, 10Rxs	99	Sham NoRx USRx	Yes	Yes	Double	Pain↓ Weights ↑ Grip strength↑	USRx = Sham > NoRx
Binder 1985	Pulsed ultrasound	Lateral epicondylitis	USRx: 20%P, 1MHz, 1 - 2W/cm², 5-10mins, 4-6wks, 12Rxs	76	Sham USRx	Yes	Yes	Double	Pain↓ Weights ↑ Grip strength↑	USRx > Sham
Holdsworth 1993	Continous ultrasound and phonophoresis	Lateral epicondylitis	USRx: 3 MHz, 1.5W/cm², 5mins, 12Rxs over 6wks &/or epicondylitis ClaspRx PhonoRx: Gel containing 1% hydrocortisone & 2% dimethicone	36	USRx PhonoRx US/claspRx Phono/claspRx	Yes	No	Double	Pain↓ AROM↑	N.S. btwn grps

Study	Modality	Condition	Parameters	N	Groups				Outcomes	Results
Haker 1991	GaAs and HeNe laser combo	Lateral epicondylitis	LaserRx: 5 GaAs (904nm, 4mm, 10W, 3800Hz, 180nsec, 70mrad) with 1 HeNe (632.8nm, continuous, 5mW, 60mrad)	58	Sham LaserRx	Yes	Yes	Double	Pain↓ grip strength↑ Lifting test↑	NS btwn grps (but the objective outcome indicated favor for the placebo Rx)
Haker 1990	GaAs laser	Lateral epicondylitis	LaserRx: 904nm, 12mW, 8.3W, 70Hz, 0.36J/pt	49	Sham LaserRx	Yes	Yes	Double	Pain↓ Weights↑ Grip strength↓	NS btwn grps
Papadopoulos 1996	GaAlAs laser	Lateral epicondylitis	LaserRx: 820nm, 50mW, 0.4W/cm², 5kHz, 160nsec	29	Sham LaserRx	Yes	Yes	Double	Pain↓	NS btwn grps
Vasseljen 1992	GaAs laser and US and Massage	Lateral epicondylitis	LaserRx: 3.5J/cm², 8Rxs USRx: 0.32W/cm², 8Rxs Massage Rx: 10min, 8Rxs	30	Sham Rx Laser Rx US and Mass Rx	Yes	Yes	Laser Rx -Double USRx -No	Pain Grip strength	Us and Massage Rx> Laser Rx N.S.btwn grps
Lundeberg 1987	GaAs laser and HeNe laser	Lateral epicondylitis	HeNe laser: continuous, 632.8nm, 1.56mW & GaAs laser: pulsed, 904nm, 0.07mW, 73Hz, 10Rxs over 6wks	82	Sham LaserRx -HeNe LaserRx -GaAs	Yes	Yes	Double	N conduct velocity SubQ skin temp Pain↓ Grip strength↑ Weights↑	N.S. btwn grps
Vasseljen 1992	GaAs Laser	Lateral epicondylitis	904nm, 12diodes, 880Hz, 175ns, 10min, 3.5J/cm²	30	Sham LaserRx	Yes	Yes	Double	Pain↓ Grip strength↑	LaserRx > Sham
Demirtas 1998	Iontophoresis	Lateral epicondylitis	[-ve] Electrode, 6-11mA, 20mins, Pads soaked in Na⁺ diclofenac or 2% Na⁺ salicylate, 5x/wk up to 18 days	40	IontoRx -salicylate -diclofenac	Yes	No	NA	Pain↓	IontoRx-diclofenac > IontoRx-salicylate
Stratford 1989	Pulsed and continuous ultrasound and phonophoresis	Lateral epicondylitis	Dosage varied from 1.3 W/cm² continuous output to 0.5 W/cm² pulsed 1:4. Gel had either 10% hydrocortisone or no steroid, 6mins	40	USRx (sham) US&FricRx PhonoRx Phono& FricRx	Yes	Yes	Double	Pain↓ Grip strength↑	N.S. btwn grps

(Continued)

Table 7-3. (cont'd)

Article	Modality	Condition	Rx Parameters	N	Rx Grps	Random	Control	Blinded	Outcome Measures	Conclusions
Halle 1986	Ultrasound, phonophoresis, TENS, injection	Lateral epicondylitis	NA, 5days	48	USRx PhonoRx TENSRx InjectRx	Yes	No	Phono-Double Others-Single evaluator	Pain↓	N.S. btwn grps
Pienimaki 1998	Pulsed ultrasound and exercise	Lateral epicondylitis	NA, 8wks	30	USRx ExercRx	Yes	No	NA	Pain↓ ADL↑ Function↑	ExercRx > USRx
Siebert 1987	HeNe laser and GaAlAs laser and combination	Mixed	HeNe: 632.8nm, GaAlAs: 904nm, pulsed, 30mW, 7.5W/cm², 10Rxs, 15min	64	Sham LaserRx	Yes	Yes	Double	Pain↓ ROM↑	N.S. btwn grps
Klaiman 1998	Continuous Ultrasound and phonophoresis	Mixed	Both grps: 8mins, 1.5 W/cm², 100%. phono grp: 0.05% fluocinonide	49	USRx PhonoRx	Yes	No	Double	Pain↓ Pressure Tolerance↑	N.S. btwn grps
Kleinkort 1975	Ultrasound and phonophoresis	Mixed	1 MHz, 0.0-2.0W/cm², 6mins 1% or 10% hydrocortisone ointment	285	USRx PhonoRx -10% hc -1% hc	NA	No	NA	NA	PhonoRx 10% > PhonoRx 1%
Echternach 1965	Continuous ultrasound	Mixed	1.2W/cm - 1.8W/cm, 5mins - 8mins, 11.8Rxs avg	73	USRx	No	No	No	Pain↓ ROM↑	60% improved; acute > chronic
Inaba 1972	Continuous ultrasound	Painful shoulder syndrome	0.5-2.0 W/cm², 100%, 5mins, 4wks, 15Rxs	33	Sham NoUSRx USRx	Yes	Yes	Double	Pain↓ ROM↑	N.S. btwn grps
Herrera-Lasso 1993	Continuous ultrasound	Painful shoulder syndrome	USRx: 100%C, 0.5-1.0 W/cm², 10mins, 3-6wks, 13Rxs	30	USRx TENSRx	Yes	No	No	Pain↓ ROM↑	N.S. btwn grps
Nykanen 1995	Pulsed ultrasound	Painful shoulder syndrome	USRx: 20%P, 1.0 MHz, 1.0W/cm², 10mins, 3-4wks, 10-12Rxs	72	Sham USRx	Yes	Yes	Double	Pain↓ ROM↑	N.S. btwn grps

(Continued)

Study	Modality	Condition	Treatment	N	Groups			Blinding	Outcomes	Results
Munting 1978	Continuous ultrasound	Painful shoulder syndrome	USRx: 100%C, 1.5 MHz, 0.5 W/cm², 4-5mins, 3wks, 10Rxs	20	Sham USRx	Yes	Yes	Double	Pain↓ A&PROM↑ ADL↑	USRx > Sham
Vecchio 1993	GaAlAs CB Meidco Master III laser	Rotator cuff tendinitis	LaserRx: GaAlAs, 830nm diode laser, continuous, 2x/wk, 8wks, 10min, 30mW, 1.0J, ± 1.5nm	35	Sham LaserRx	Yes	Yes	Double	Pain↓ Function↑ ROM↑	N.S. btwn grps
Chard 1988	Pulsed electro-magnetic field	Rotator cuff tendinitis	PEMFRx: high dose: 8hr/day, low dose: 2hr/day, 8wks	43	PEMFRx -high dose -low dose	Yes	Yes	Double	Pain↓ AROM↑ Weights↑ Painful Arc↓	PEMF highdoseRx > PEMF lowdoseRx
Binder 1984	Pulsed electro-magnetic field	Rotator cuff tendinitis	PEMFRx: 73±2Hz, 5-9 hrs/day,	29	Sham NoRx PEMFRx	Yes	Yes	Double	Pain↓ Weights↑ Painful Arc↓ AROM↑	PEMFRx > Sham
Saunders 1995	GaAlAs laser	Supraspinatus tendinitis	LaserRx: 820nm, 40mW, 5000Hz, 30J/cm²	24	Sham LaserRx	Yes	Yes	Double	Pain↓, Weakness↓	LaserRx > Sham LaserRx > Sham
England 1989	GaAs laser	Shoulder tendinitis	LaserRx: 904nm, 4000Hz, 180nsec, 10W	30	Sham LaserRx	Yes	Yes	Double	Pain↓ Stiffness↓ ROM↑ Function↑	LaserRx > Sham
Bulgen 1984	Injections, mobilizations, cold and exercise	Adhesive capsulitis	Inject: Methyl Prednisolone Acetate 20mg & 1% Li ocaine hydrochloride 0-5mL	42	NoRx InjectRx MobsRx, ColdRx,	Yes	Yes	NA	Pain↓ ROM↑	N.S. btwn grps (Short term: InjectRx > MobsRx ColdRx NoRx)
Berry 1980	Acupuncture, injections, ultrasound	Adhesive capsulitis	AcuRx: Acupuncture 1x/wk InjectRx: 40mg methyl Prednisolone with 2mLof 2% lidocaine with 2 tabs of placebo tolmetin Na+ OR same as above with 1200mg active tolmetin Na+ x3 USRx: Ultrasound:-8 sessions, 10mins	60	AcuRx InjectRx Inject ShamRx USRx USShamRx	Yes		NA	Pain↓ ROM↑	N.S. btwn grps

Table 7-3. (cont'd)

Article	Modality	Condition	Rx Parameters	N	Rx Grps	Random	Control	Blinded	Outcome Measures	Conclusions
Downing 1986	Continuous Ultrasound	Subacromial Bursitis	USRx: 100%C, 1 MHz, 1.2W/cm^2, 6mins, 3x/wk, 4wks, 12Rxs	20	Sham USRx	Yes	Yes	Double	Pain↓ ROM↑ Function↑	N.S. btwn grps
Gudeman 1997	Iontophoresis and ice and exercise	Plantar Fasciitis	IontoRx: Up to 4.0mA, net charge 40mA over 20mins, 0.4% Dexamethasone 6x over 2wks ShamRx: phosphate bulfered saline Trad: includes ice: 20min	40	Sham and Trad Ionto and TradRx	Yes	Yes	Double	Recovery	Ionto and traditionalRx > Sham and traditional (Immediately Post Rx, but NS btwn grps after 1mos)
Basford 1998	GaA1As Laser	Plantar Fasciitis	Laser Rx continuous IR diode laser, 30mW, 0.83um, 3x/wk, 4 wks	32	Sham LaserRx	Yes	Yes	Double	Pain↓ Meds↓ Orthotic Use	NS btwn grps
McKibbin 1989	Laser	Plantar Fasciitis	LaserRx: Low-E, IR laser, pulsed at 904nm, 10 diode head, 4000Hz, 6mW, 20min, 7J/rx	46	LaserRx CortisoneRx	No	No	No	Pain↓	NS btwn grps

motion by reducing pain and permit pain free stretching of noncontractile inert joint structures and strengthening of weakened muscles.

Shoulder Tendonitis

The application of GalAs laser has been shown in two well designed clinical trials to reduce pain and improve joint range of motion in patients with rotator cuff tendonitis (England et al. 1989; Saunders 1995). Another prospective, controlled clinical study that examined the effectiveness of GalAs laser in the treatment of shoulder tendonitis failed to detect a statistically significant difference between the laser treated group compared with individuals randomized to receive treatments from a dummy laser (Vecchio et al. 1993). Pulsed electromagnetic fields applied for a minimum of 2 hours per day were found to significantly improve pain and improve shoulder function in patients with tendonitis of the glenohumeral joint (Chard et al. 1988; Binder et al. 1984). Nykanen (1995) in a well designed clinical trial, failed to demonstrate a benefit of pulsed ultrasound on pain associated with rotator cuff tendonitis.

Initially a brief clinical report that included few details suggested that continuous ultrasound given over a 3-week period reduced pain and improved range of motion of patients (n = 11) with frozen shoulder and adhesive capsulitis (see Chapter 3) to a greater extent than control subjects who did not receive ultrasound treatments (Munting 1978). Echternach (1965) reported that ultrasound treatment produced marked improvement in pain and joint mobility in individuals with shoulder conditions of mixed etiology and that more acute conditions responded better than those individuals with long-standing chronic shoulder problems. However, three subsequent published studies did not find any added benefit of either pulsed or continuous ultrasound treatments over conventional treatment of painful shoulder syndromes that included range of motion exercises (Downing and Weinstein 1986; Griffin et al. 1972; Nykanen 1995). A systematic review of the research literature performed by van der Heijden et al. (1997) concluded that ultrasound was ineffective in the treatment of soft tissue shoulder disorders.

Ultrasound treatment was shown to be as effective at reducing symptoms of adhesive capsulitis as other more invasive forms of therapy including intraarticular injections of steroids (Berry et al. 1980). Other modalities found to be as effective as ultrasound at reducing symptoms of shoulder conditions such as shoulder periarthritis, subdeltoid bursitis, and supraspinatus tendonitis include ice massage (Hamer et al. 1976) and TENS (Herrera-Lasso et al. 1993). However, the effectiveness of cryotherapy for the treatment of adhesive capsulitis was not found to be as effective as steroid injections at reducing pain and improving joint range of motion of individuals with frozen shoulder (see Chapter 3).

Calcific bursitis is the result of abnormal deposition of calcium, usually in the form of hydroxyapatite into bursae in response to chronic inflammation. Calcific deposits in the rotator cuff and biceps tendons and in the subdeltoid bursae are common with chronic shoulder injuries. Calcium deposition also is associated with a condition known as *plantar fasciitis*. This condition develops as a result of prolonged mechanical stress applied to the plantar fascia located between the metatarsal heads and the calcaneus, such as that occuring after a significant increase in body weight. Stretching of plantar fascia causes new tissue formation at the calcaneal tubercules that, if the stress persists, eventually changes to bone. Calcaneal spurs produce microtears in the soft tissues around the anterior and inferior aspect of the calcaneus bone that becomes inflamed and extremely painful upon weight bearing.

Lateral Epicondylitis

Binder et al. (1985), in a well designed randomized controlled clinical study, reported that pulsed ultrasound (1 MHz, 1-2 W/cm^2, 5-10min × 12) enhanced recovery from painful symptoms associated with lateral epicondylagia in twice as many patients than placebo treatments. However two subsequent clinical trials using a similar ultrasound treatment regime found no difference in the outcomes of this patient population between placebo and ultrasound-treated elbows (Haker and Lundeberg 1991b; Lundeberg and Haker 1987). In addition, Lundeberg and Haker (1987) compared the outcomes achieved with patients with lateral epicondylagia after ultrasound treatment and placebo treatment to an additional group of individuals who simply rested and did not receive any treatment. They found that that both placebo and ultrasound-treated groups had better outcomes than those patients who rested. These results, with those of other studies, suggest that a large part of the benefits of ultrasound treatment for inflammatory conditions may be the result of a placebo effect. Pienimaki (1996) and (1998) demonstrated that patients with this condition responded better to a self-administered stretching and progressive strengthening exercise program than those who had received just ultrasound treatments.

A number of laser treatment protocols have been tested for patients with lateral epicondylitis (Lundeberg and Haker 1987; Haker and Lundeberg, 1990, 1991a, b, c). Researchers found that laser treatment using GalAs laser applied locally over the lateral epicondyle was effective in the treatment of this condition. They did not find that laser treatments using GalAs laser applied to distant acupuncture sites had any significant effect on pain and grip strength (Haker and Lundeberg 1990). These results are consistent with two other prospective controlled studies (Vasseljen et al. 1992; Siebert et al. 1987) and one retrospective review of more than 3,000 clinical cases (Simunovic et al. 1998) that showed GalAs laser with or without concomitant HeNe treatment was effective in treating patients with lateral epicondylitis. While the majority of clinical reports suggest that GalAs laser therapy can be effective in the treatment of lateral epicondylitis, some results would not support this suggestion (Haker and Lundeberg 1991c).

Phonophoresis of hydrocortisone using ultrasound has been shown to reduce the symptoms of lateral epicondylitis (Holdsworth and Anderson 1993; Stratford et al. 1989). Transdermal delivery of other antiinflammatory drugs via iontophoresis such as sodium deflonec has also been shown to reduce pain and improve grip strength of individuals with tennis elbow whereas ionotophoretic delivery of sodium salicylate was not as effective at ameliorating the symptoms of lateral epicondylitis (Demirtas et al. 1998).

Halle et al. (1986) compared a number of therapies commonly used for the treatment of lateral epicondylitis including phonophoresis, ultrasound, TENS, and steroid injection and found that all these therapies were associated with improvements in symptoms of lateral epicondylitis. The ability to produce improvements in patient outcomes that were equal to steroid injections could suggest that these conservative treatments that are well tolerated by the patients, are as effective as more invasive techniques involving intra articular steroid injections. Alternatively, these results could suggest that lateral epicondylitis is a self-limiting condition that will resolve spontaneously regardless of the treatment intervention.

Calcific Deposits

For calcific bursitis and tendonitis and plantar fasciitis, treatment must be directed at the removal of the calcium deposits causing inflammation in the soft tissues. Ultrasound has consistently shown to be helpful in the treatment of calcium deposits present in soft tissue lesions, including calcified biceps tendonitis and calcific shoulder and trochanteric bursitis. Ultrasound treatment was reported in 3 case studies to cause resolution of calcium deposits on x-ray exam. These promising results of ultrasound on calcific lesions of periarticular soft tissues were recently confirmed in a well designed, randomized, controlled clinical trial (Ebenbichler et al. 1999).

Another treatment approach that has been used to treat the inflammatory process incited by the calcific deposits is the use of electrical current to deliver antiinflammatory medication such as dexamethasone to the area of calcium deposition. Intraarticular injection of corticosteroids by qualified physicians is a common treatment for these conditions. More recently research found that steroids could be delivered transdermally to the periarticular structure using a less invasive and more comfortable approach using a process called *iontophoresis*. Iontophoresis involves the transdermal delivery of an ionized drug using an electrical field. Gudeman et al. (1997) demonstrated that pain and foot function were significantly improved when dexamethasone delivered ionotophoretically was added to a standard treatment program. Basford et al. (1998) found that transdermal delivery of acetic acid using iontophoresis to calcified shoulder tendons does not however produce a significant resolution of calcium deposits present on x-ray.

McKibbin and Downie (1989) demonstrated that pain associated with plantar fasciitis was significantly reduced below pretreatment levels following administration of GaAs laser (904 nm) daily for 1 week. However, in a more recent prospective, controlled, clinical trial Basford et al. (1998) reported no benefit of infrared laser therapy on any of the outcome measures used to assess pain and function in patients with plantar fasciitis.

Therefore for the purpose of stimulating resolution of calcium deposits of these chronic inflammatory conditions with calcific deposits, ultrasound currently has the most conclusive clinical evidence of effectiveness. The use of iontophoresis of dexamethasone and GaAs laser therapy in these conditions requires further research.

Acute and Chronic Low Back and Neck Pain

Low back and neck pain are some of the most common conditions confronted by orthopedic clinicians. In some clinics, low back pain patients represent up to half of active clientele. In the late 1980s expenditures for low back pain medical care were estimated at $13 billion annually in the United States. A summary of the clinical trials that have examined the effectiveness of therapeutic intervention on acute and chronic neck and back pain has been provided in Table 7-4.

Electrical Stimulation: TENS

The use of TENS for back pain first appeared in the literature in the mid-1970s (Ersek 1976). Initially, electrical currents were delivered to the skin overlying the painful area and stimulus parameters were set to deliver a mild comfortable sensory stimulation. In these studies patients with acute or short-term back pain appeared to have faster and more long-lasting pain relief than those patients with chronic low back pain. However, Ebersold et al. (1975) demonstrated in a large clinical trial involving approximately 200 patients with low back pain that sensory-level TENS treatment also could be effective in the treatment of long-standing conditions with chronic pain. Loeser et al. (1975) also noted that TENS could produce effective analgesia for patients with chronic pain caused by a variety of musculoskeletal disorders. They noted that TENS stimulation did not appear to produce any pain relief if the area where the electrical current was applied was unresponsive to sensory stimulation (denervated). This information strongly suggested that the pain-reducing mechanism underlying sensory level TENS stimulation involved the cutaneous nerve afferents and provides support for TENS induced gate mechanism of analgesia. Not until 1977 did Thorsteinsson and colleagues examine the efficacy of TENS at reducing musculoskeletal pain in a properly designed, randomized, double blind study. They reported effective analgesia in approximately half of the TENS-treated patients, and 47% of these patients had continued pain relief when the TENS stimulator was turned off. They also found that approximately one third of placebo-treated patients reported significant improvement in their pain. This was one of the first studies to suggest that TENS treatments were associated with a significant placebo effect.

Eriksson et al. (1979) was among the first groups to examine the effect of "acupuncture-like TENS" on chronic pain. This form of TENS treatment was fashioned after Chinese electro-acupuncture techniques and involves the delivery of low frequency, high intensity stimuli that produce mild muscle twitch onto acupuncture points that are often located a some distance from the site of pain. Melzack et al. (1983) reported that 85% of subjects with low back pain reported acceptable pain relief after low rate acupuncture like TENS treatments, which was significantly greater than the control group that received local massage. These promising results obtained by Melzack and Wall and Eriksson were later confirmed by work of Cheng and Pomeranz (1986). However, two prospective randomized clinical trials that were published subsequently failed to support the use of TENS for low back pain (Lehmann et al. 1986; Deyo et al. 1990). In particular, the large-scale clinical trial performed by Deyo et al. (1990), which was published in a prominent medical journal, sparked a heated debate that was carried out in the literature challenging the merits of TENS treatment for low back pain. Results reported in a subsequent randomized controlled trial of Marchand et al. (1993) helped to diffuse this skepticism and reaffirm the efficacy of TENS for the treatment of low back pain.

Table 7-4. Clinical Trials that Have Examined the Effectiveness of Therapeutic Intervention on Acute and Chronic Neck and Back Pain

Article	Modality	Condition	Rx Parameters	Rx Grps	N	Random	Control	Blind	Outcome Measures	Conclusions
Falconer et al. 1992	Ultrasound	OA - Knee	USRx: 3 mins, 0.0W/cm²-2.5 W/cm², 2.3×/wk, 4-6wks; Exercise: 30mins, each exercise repeated 10x, 5s repetition, 5s rest and included 5-15mins passive stretch	Sham & ROM Exercises USRx & ROM Exercises	74	Yes	Yes	Yes	Pain↓ ROM↑ Gait↑	NS btwn grps
Nwuga 1983	Ultrasound	Back pain from prolapsed intervertebral disk	USRx: Aquasonic gel, 1-2W/cm², 10mins	NoRx and bed rest and analgesics Sham and bed rest and analgesics USRx and bed rest and analgesics	73	Yes	Yes	Yes	Pain ↓ ROM↑	USRx > NoRx & Sham
Gam et al. 1998	Pulsed ultrasound, massage, exercise	Myofascial trigger points	USRx: 20%P. 100Hz, 3W/cm², 3mins/soundhead -total 15mins/Rx 2×/ wk, 4wks. 8Rxs.	NoRx sham and massage and exercise USRx and massage and exercise	58	Yes	Yes	Yes	Pain↓ Analgesic use↓ Global preference Index of MTrP	NS btwn grps NS btwn grps NS btwn grps USRx = Sham > NoRx
Middlemast & Chatterjee 1978	Pulsed ultrasound, SWD, infrared & wax baths	Soft tissue injuries	USRx: 1.5 MHz, 0.5-2.0 W/cm², 4-10mins; Other Rxs: SWD: 15 mins; Infrared: 15 mins; wax bath; 15mins	USRx OtherRxs -SWD or infrared or wax bath	71	Yes	No	No	Pain↓ Tenderness↓ Erythema↓ AROM↑ Edema↓	USRx > OtherRxs

Study	Modality	Condition	Treatment	Comparison	N				Outcomes	Results
Lewith & Machin 1981	Infrared	OA-Cervical	InfraredRx: 2wks, Infrared: IRS Medtec 100, 240V, 50Hz, output 3.6V, 1.75W, 5-10s/trigger point, 5mins; Sham TENS: 5mins	Sham TENS Infra-RedRx	25	Yes	No	No	Pain↓ Analgesic use↓ Sleep disturbance↓	InfraredRx > ShamTENS
Melzack 1980	Ice massage of hand	Dental pain	Tactils Massage: to web space b/w thumb and index finger on same side as pain, until numb or for 7 mins,	Tactile massage/Rx ice/massage/Rx	40	Yes	No	No	Pain↓	Ice/massageRx > Tactile/massageRx
McCray & Patton 1984	Moist heat and SWD	Myofascial trigger points	SWDRx: Magnothern, 27.12MHz, single layer toweling, inductor 2cm from skin; HeatRx: heated at 68°C for 20mins, each Rx: 20mins	SWDRx heat/Rx	19	Yes	No	No	Pain↓	SWDRx > moist heat
Wagstaff et al. 1986	PEMF & SWD	Low back pain	SWDRx: 27.12MHz, PEMFlowRx: 82Hz and 700W PEMFhighRx 200Hz and 300W All Rxs: 2.4cm space, 15mins, 2×/wk: × 3wks	SWDRx PEMFRx -low -high	23	Yes	No	No	Pain↓	PEMFRxs > SWDRx
Foley-Nolan et al. 1990	PEMF	Chronic neck pain	NA	Sham PEMFRx	20	yes	Yes cross over	No	Pain↓ ROM↑	SWDRx > Sham
Hansen & Thoroe 1991	Laser	Chronic oro-facial pain	LaserRx: 90mm, 30mW, 60 -120s/spot, 4 -9.4J/cm², 200nsec, 78.9mW/cm², 9999Hz	Sham laserRx	40	Yes	Yes	Yes	Pain↓	NS btwn grps
Klein & Eek 1990	GaAs laser	Chronic low back pain	LaserRx: GaAs class I, 1000Hz, 200ns, 904nm, with 10 2W heads in 12cm linear array, 4mins, 1.3J/cm²	Sham laserRx	20	Yes	Yes	Yes	Pain↓	NS btwn grps

(Continued)

Table 7-4. *(cont'd)*

Article	Modality	Condition	Rx Parameters	Rx Grps	N	Random	Control	Blind	Outcome Measures	Conclusions
Ceccherelli et al. 1989	GaAs laser	Cervical myofascial pain	LaserRx: Pulsed IR, 904nm, 200ns, 1000Hz, 25W, 5J, 38/wk, 12Rxs	Sham laserRx	27	Yes	Yes	Yes	Pain↓	LaserRx > Sham
Thorsen et al. 1992	GaAlAs laser	Myofascial pain in neck and shoulder	LaserRx: 830nm, 30mW, 0.9J/pt, max 9J/Rx	Sham laserRx	47	Yes	Yes	Yes	Pain↓ Analgesic use↓	NS btwn grps
Kreczi & Klingler 1986	HeNe laser	Radicular and pseudo-radicular pain	LaserRx: 632.8nm, 100Hz, 2mW, 30secs	Sham laserRx	21	Yes	Yes	Yes	Pain↓	LaserRx > Sham
Walker 1988	HeNe laser	Trigeminal neuralgia	LaserRx: 632 8nm, 1mW, 20Hz, 20secs/site, 3×/wk, 10wks	Sham laserRx	35	Yes	Yes	Yes		LaserRx > Sham
Walker 1983	HeNe laser	Mixed	LaserRx: 632 8nm, 1 mW, 20Hz, 30secs	Sham laserRx	26	Yes	Yes	Yes	Pain↓	Rx grp > placebo and control
Snyder-Mackler et al. 1989	HeNe laser	Trigger points in the neck or back	LaserRx: Dynatron 1120 class II, continuous, 0.95 mW/ trigger pt, 3×20secs	Sham laserRx	24	Yes	Yes	Yes	Pain↓ Skin resistance↓	LaserRx > Sham
Waylonis 1988	HeNe laser	Chronic myofascial pain	LaserRx: Dynatronic 1120, 2×5Rxs	Sham/Sham Sham/laserRx laserRx/Sham laserRx	62	Yes	Yes Cross over	Yes	Pain↓	NS btwn grps
Basford et al. 1999	Laser	Musculoskeletal back pain	LaserRx: Neodymium-Yttrium-Aluminum-Garnet, 1.06um, continuous, 2 simultaneous sites for 90secs × 4 pairs of sites, 542 mW/cm²	Sham laserRx	63	Yes	Yes	Yes	Pain↓ Perceived benefit↑ Function↑	LaserRx > Sham

Study	Modality	Condition	Treatment	Groups	N	Random	Blind	Double	Outcome	Results
Melzack et al. 1980	Ice/massage and TENS	Low back pain	TENSRx: intensity to tolerance, 3 sites × 30mins; IceMassage; 7mins/site with 3min intervals b/w sites to total time of 30mins	Ice/massageRx / TENSRx / TENSRx/Ice-MassageRx / Ice-MassageRx or TENSRx	44	Na	Yes Cross over	Double	Pain↓	Ice massageRx > TENS
Melzack et al. 1983	TENS and massage	Acute or chronic low back pain	TENSRx: electrodes placed center of painful area on back, and on the lateral thigh, 4-8Hz, intensity to tolerance Massage: suction cups with varying pressure changes; both Rxs 2×/wk 30mins	TENSRx MassageRx	41	yes	No	No	Pain↓ ROM↑	TENSRx > massage NS btwn grps
Marchand et al. 1993	TENS	Chronic low back pain	TENSRx: 100Hz, 125μs pulses, low intensity, 30mins	NoRx Sham TENSRx	48	Yes	Yes	No	Pain↓	TENSRx > Sham (short-term) > No Rx
Deyo et al. 1990	TENS and exercise	Chronic low back pain	TENSRx: 80-100Hz, intensity 30 for 2wks then instructed on 2-4Hz intensity 100, (for the last 2wks, pts chose b/w high-rate and APL TENS), 4wks total; Exercise: stretches, 9-12 exercises	Sham Sham and ExerciseRx TENSRx TENSRx and exerciseRx	NA	Yes			Pain↓ Function↑ ROM↑	Sham and exerciseRx = TENSRx and exercise > Sham = TENSRx
Cheng & Pomeranz 1987	Electro-acupuncture and APL TENS	Chronic musculoskeletal pain	Both Rxs: 4Hz & 200Hz, 20mins, 2-12Rxs	Electro-Acupuncture-Rx APL TENSRx	131	Yes	No	No	Pain↓	NS btwn grps (short-term) APL TENSRx > ElectroAcuRx (long-term)

(Continued)

Table 7-4. (cont'd)

Article	Modality	Condition	Rx Parameters	Rx Grps	N	Random	Control	Blind	Outcome Measures	Conclusions
Eriksson et al 1979	APL TENS and conventional TENS	Mixed	APL TENSRx: 100Hz, 1-4burs: $3/sec, intensity 3-5× sensory threshold, 0.2msec; conventional TENS Rx: 10-100Hz, 2.5-3× sensory threshold, Both Rxs 30mins	APL TENSRx Conventional TENSRx		Na	No	No	Pain↓	NS btwn grps
Lehman et al. 1986	TENS	Chronic Low Back Pain	ElectroacupunctureRx: biweekly, 2-4Hz, intensity evoking muscle contraction; TENSRx: 250μsec pulse duration, 60Hz, 5×/wk, subthreshold intensity, All Rxs 3wks	Sham Electro-Acupuncture Rx TENSRx	54	Yes	Yes	Yes	Pain↓ ROM↑ Function↑ Analgesic use↓	ElectroAcupunctureRx > TENSRx & Sham NS btwn grps NS btwn grps NS btwn grps
Ersek 1977	TENS	Chronic & Acute Low Back Pain	TENSRx: conventional	TENSRx	35	No	No	No	Pain↓	50% relief
Ebersold et al. 1975	TENS	Mixed	TENSRx: parameters NA	TENSRx	230	No	No	No	Pain↓	65% LBP pts partial or 100% relief -3.5mos
Loeser et al. 1975	TENS	Mixed	TENSRx: intensity strong (without pain), electrodes local, 10-150Hz, up to 1hr	TENSRx	198	No	No	No	Pain↓	77% LBP pts significant relief
Thorsteinsson et al. 1977	TENS	Mixed	TENSRx: 20mins, 3 days	Sham TENSRx	93	Yes	Yes Cross over	Double	Pain↓	**NS btwn grps**

Ultrasound

Ultrasound treatment has been shown to reduce the pain associated with numerous musculoskeletal conditions, including lateral epicondylitis, shoulder pain, plantar fasciitis, surgical wounds, bursitis, prolapsed intervertebral discs (Nwuga 1983), ankle sprains (Makuloluwe and Mouzas 1977), post herpetic neuralgia (Payne 1984; Jones 1984), postpartum pain (Creates 1987), and myofascial pain dysfunction (Talaat et al. 1986). Continuous ultrasound applied three times a week for 4 weeks at 1.0 to 2.0 W/cm^2 for 10 minutes to the low backs of patients with recent onset of pain caused by prolapsed discs and nerve root compression between L4 and S2 has also been shown to result in significantly faster relief of pain and return of range of motion than placebo ultrasound treatment (Nwuga 1983). The addition of a similar treatment regime using continuous ultrasound to a stretching program also has been found to be more effective than stretching exercises alone in relieving pain and increasing range of motion in patients with shoulder pain. Furthermore, this analgesic effect of ultrasound continued at the time of a 3-month follow-up visit. The authors postulated that heat produced by continuous ultrasound treatments increased patient comfort and improved connective tissue extensibility so that greater gains could be achieved in joint range of motion and functional abilities. Continuous ultrasound (0.5-2.0 W/cm^2) using a low frequency sound head (1.5 MHz) has also been reported to be more effective at relieving the pain from soft tissue injuries than other therapeutic modalities such as superficial heating agents (Middlemast and Chatterjee 1978) or shortwave diathermy (Talaat et al. 1986). Falconer et al. (1992) performed a randomized controlled trial that tested the effect of ultrasound in facilitating exercise in patients with osteoarthritis of the knee. In this study, no differences were found between the two groups treated either with ultrasound or sham ultrasound combined with exercise with respect to range of motion, reduction in pain or gait analysis. Later Gam et al. (1998) also reported no added benefit of the addition of ultrasound treatments to an exercise program for the treatment of patients with myofascial trigger points.

A metaanalysis performed by Falconer et al. (1990) identified 28 research articles that have examined the effects of therapeutic ultrasound treatments on musculoskeletal pain. They concluded that ultrasound appears effective in treatment of pain associated with acute inflammatory conditions such postsurgical or postpartum discomfort. However, no strong effect was reported for the ability of ultrasound to treat chronic conditions such as myofascial pain syndrome or chronic low back pain.

Superficial Hot/Cold

The efficacy of superficial heating agents in producing pain relief in chronic conditions has been tested and shown to produce pain relief in patients with back and cervical pain (Lewith and Machin 1981). Two reports that compared the effects of superficial and deep heating agents on musculoskeletal pain would suggest that deeper heating agents such as continuous ultrasound (Middlemast and Chatterjee 1978) or shortwave diathermy (McCray and Patton 1984) have superior pain-reducing effects. While superficial heating agents may not be as effective for treatment of pain associated with anatomical structures located in deeper layers of the neck and back, cold therapy in the form of ice massage has been shown to be as effective as TENS treatments at reducing low back pain (Melzack et al. 1980). Although both superficial hot and cold agents are known to be able to alter nerve conduction velocities and produce analgesia, the production of pain relief by topical application of cold, rather than heat, may be explained by the ability of cold to penetrate more deeply and produce thermal changes in structures located further beneath the skin surface.

Shortwave Diathermy and PEMFs

Several reports have suggested that PEMFs can reduce pain in both acute and chronic conditions (Foley-Nolan et al. 1990). In addition, Wagstaff et al. (1986) demonstrated that PEMFs, which do not produce a net temperature gain, were superior to shortwave diathermy for treating low back pain. Therefore the analgesic effects of shortwave diathermy may be the result of the electrical currents produced by the electromagnetic field rather than the thermal effects also known to occur with shortwave diathermy. Alternatively changes in local blood flow causing an increase in perfusion of injured tissues that is known to occur after PEMF therapy may reduce pain by washing away pain-inducing chemical mediators.

Laser

Pulsed GalAlAs laser (904 nm) applied to local pain areas and lumbosacral nerves failed to produce significant pain relief (Hansen and Thoroe 1990; Klein and Eek 1990). However Ceccherelli et al. (1989) found the same wavelength of laser (904 nm) applied in the pulsed mode to acupuncture points reduced cervical myofascial pain. Thorsen et al. (1992) found in a double blind crossover study that using a 30 mW GalAs laser that produces infrared light at a wavelength of 830 nm applied in continuous mode to trigger points was not an effective treatment protocol for patients with chronic myofascial pain in the neck and shoulder girdle. Therefore results testing the effectiveness of infrared laser therapy produced by GalAs diodes on chronic pain syndromes such as myofascial pain using properly designed clinical trials have yielded inconclusive results. Furthermore they do not support the beneficial results in previously published papers that analyzed a large number of clinical cases retrospectively and reported a significant improvement of pain symptoms in 40% to 80% of patients with chronic low back pain who were treated locally with 830 nm GalAs laser therapy (Ohshiro and Shirono 1992).

Other types of laser therapy, however, have been associated with beneficial results on musculoskeletal pain. A recent randomized controlled clinical study demonstrated a small but significant analgesic effect of light therapy using a neodymium:yttrium-aluminum garnet laser (Nd:YAG) for the treatment of musculoskeletal pain of mixed etiology (Basford et al. 1999). Several groups have reported a significant benefit of low intensity (1-2 mW) of HeNe laser applied to skin either locally (Synder Mackler et al. 1989; Walker 1983; Walker et al. 1988) or to distant acupuncture points (Kreczi and Klingler 1986), although Waylonis and colleagues (1988) applied HeNe laser therapy to acupuncture points of patients

with chronic myofascial pain and did not find a significant improvement in subjective pain scores between laser sham and control group. Assessing the rationale for the discrepancies in the results of this well designed large-scale clinical trial performed by Waylonis and colleagues is difficult because, unfortunately, they provided only an incomplete laser treatment protocol.

In an attempt to combine information derived from the available research literature on the effects of laser therapy on musculoskeletal pain a meta-analysis was performed by Gam et al. (1993). They combined the results from nine double-blind and four controlled clinical trials that assessed the effects of various types of laser therapy on pain in musculoskeletal syndromes. Their conclusion from the statistical analysis performed was that insufficient clinical research evidence existed to support the use of laser therapy for the treatment of pain associated with musculoskeletal disorders. Beckerman and colleagues also performed a metaanalysis around the same time (Beckerman et al. 1992) and concluded that laser therapy seems to have a substantial beneficial effect on specific musculoskeletal conditions that include myofascial pain syndromes. In 1998, deBie and colleagues reassessed the available research literature examining the effects of laser on musculoskeletal disorders in a systematic review and concurred that some evidence exists for the use of laser in the treatment of myofascial pain syndromes. However, they repeated statements of several previous metaanalyses that further improved research using properly designed clinical trials are needed to determine the effectiveness of laser therapy.

A 1998 survey of therapists working in the United Kingdom revealed that therapeutic modalities commonly used by therapists to treat low back pain include TENS, ultrasound, shortwave diathermy, and PEMFs. Approximately half of the therapists used TENS and 22% of respondents used ultrasound to treat patients with low back pain. Only 5% to 11% of therapists employed the use of PEMFs or shortwave diarthermy on patients with lower back pain. They did not assess whether therapists used superficial hot/cold agents or laser therapy for these conditions.

Sarcova et al. (1988) compared the effectiveness of different modalities for the treatment of pain because of osteoarthritis and found that treatments

Table 7-5. Summary of the Physiologic Effects of Therapeutic Modalities

Modality	Vascular System		Tissue Repair		Neuromuscular System		Connective Tissue	
	Local Blood Flow	Edema	Inflammation	Healing	Pain	Muscle Spasm	ROM	Collagen Plasticity
Superficial heating agents	↑	↑	↑	↑	↓	↓	↑	↑
Cryotherapy	↓	↓	↓	↓	↓	↓	↓	↓
Electrical stimulation	–	↓	↑	↑	↓		↑	
Continuous ultrasound*	–	–	–	↓		↑	↑	
Pulsed ultrasound	–	↓	↑	↑	–			
Electromagnetic fields	↑	↓	↓	↑	↓			
Laser	–		↑	↑	↓			

* – represents a physiological response for which research evidence is inconclusive.

using either ultrasound, TENS and shortwave diathermy therapy all produced rapid reduction of pain reported on a visual analogue scale.

Summary

Table 7-5 provides a summary of the physiologic effects of each of the modalities discussed in previous sections of this chapter. Most of the modalities have the ability to influence neuromuscular, vascular, and connective tissue structures of the body. Apart from cryotherapy, many of these modalities are alleged to produce similar physiologic effects. While cryotherapy tends to produce opposite effects than those induced by other modalities on the vascular system and tissue repair processes, the neuromuscular system seems to be affected similarly by cryotherapy as other modalities. Modalities that produce elevations in tissue temperature such as superficial heat and continuous ultrasound also can improve joint range of motion because of changes in collagen plasticity.

These modalities also can have profound effects on the tissue-repair process initiated after musculoskeletal injury. A schematic diagram that depicts the primary component of the healing process influenced by each of the therapeutic modalities discussed in this chapter is provided in Figure 7-1. Ultrasound is believed to improve healing primarily because of its effects during the inflammatory phase of tissue repair, whereas most research evidence suggests that laser therapy can influence fibroblastic activity. Although PEMFs and superficial heat may directly influence the healing process, both these modalities are more recognized for their ability to improve local blood supply and tissue oxygenation. Extensive examination of the effects of electrical stimulation on the healing process reveals that this modality can aid in the healing process by influencing all of these components of the healing cascade.

Figure 7-4 provides a diagrammatic representation of a relative scale that reflects this author's opinion of the strength of experimental evidence available to suggest the physiologic effects of these therapeutic modalities. For edema management, cold therapy combined with RICE has strong evidence of ability to reduce edema formation following an acute athletic injury. Administration of PEMFs also appears to be effective in the treatment of either acute or chronic edema such as that produced with chronic venous insufficiency. Less research evidence is available to support the use of electrical current (HVPC) for treatment of edema.

Reduction of tissue temperature using cold agents will decrease tissue inflammation and prevent the formation of excessive tissue swelling. Ultrasound has been shown to stimulate the inflammatory process that occurs following an acute injury such as an inversion ankle sprain. Stimulation of the inflammation would be desirable since it would result in a shortening of the inflammatory process and a more rapid resolution of the early phase of tissue healing. Less research evidence exists that laser therapy may also have a similar proinflammatory effect.

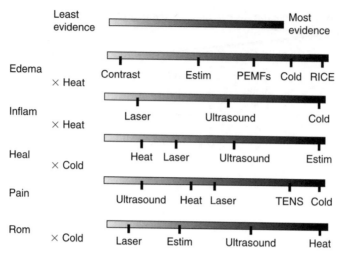

Figure 7-4. Relative strength of research evidence* that supports the ability of the various modalities to reduce edema (EDEMA) and inflammation (INFLAM), accelerate tissue healing (HEAL), resolve pain (PAIN), and increase joint range of motion (ROM). Modalities placed toward the right side of the line are considered to have stronger research evidence than those placed on the left side of the line. X indicates the modality is not indicated for that condition.

*Relative strength of research evidence was based on research articles available to the author at the time of publication.

Numerous research studies have demonstrated the beneficial effects of electrical stimulation on the healing process. Furthermore, clinical trials have consistently shown that impaired healing can be augmented by exogenous application of electrical current. Based on this strong experimental and clinical research evidence this modality is recommended first for the treatment of conditions in which an impaired healing process is believed to underlie the musculoskeletal condition. The experimental research to suggest that ultrasound and laser can influence the healing process is also extensive; however, results from studies investigating this mechanism are less consistent. In particular the effects of the laser therapy on the tissue repair process is dependent on a number of factors for which a complete understanding remains to be determined.

The use of TENS and cryotherapy for the treatment of chronic and acute pain appears to produce analgesic effects most consistently. Both these modalities are used extensively to alleviate such numerous musculoskeletal disorders as acute and chronic neck and back pain. Decreased pain sensation and perception also have been attributed to laser therapy, superficial heating agents, and continuous ultrasound. However, relatively few research studies have been performed to elucidate mechanisms underlying the analgesic properties of these modalities, and clinical research trials have produced inconclusive results.

Joint range of motion can be increased by the application of superficial heat or by using modalities such as continuous ultrasound that produce elevations in tissue temperature. The ability of thermal agents to improve joint movement is attributed to heat-induced changes to collagen plasticity. The application of electrical stimulation and laser therapy has also been associated with moderate improvements in joint range of motion. This is believed to be related secondarily to a reduction in the individual's pain that, in turn, permits more rigorous stretching exercise to be tolerated.

To determine the best modality for the treatment of a particular acute or chronic condition, the clinician must be aware of the cellular and physiologic effects of each modality. The knowledge of the underlying pathophysiology of a particular musculoskeletal condition is critical to formulate a list of possible modalities that would be indicated. To decide between possible modalities that are indicated the clinician must consider the available clinical research evidence. The number of properly designed clinical research trials to test the effectiveness of modalities for the treatment of various musculoskeletal is increasing rapidly. This area of research investigation is very active, and clinicians must continuously refresh their knowledge in this area. Lastly, to make the best decision, the clinician must combine the knowledge of the available research evidence with an appreciation of the relevant contraindications, safety precautions and risks that exist for each different type of modality. These and other practical considerations often factor strongly into the decision-making process.

References

Agaiby AD, Ghali LR, Wilson R, Dyson M. Laser modulation of angiogenic factor production by T-lymphocytes. Lasers Surg Med 2000;26:357-363.

Akai M, Oda H, Shirasaki Y, Tateishi T. Electrical stimulation of ligament healing. Clin Orthopaed Rel Res 1988; 296-301.

Al-Karmi AM et al. Calcium and the effects of ultrasound on frog skin. Ultrasound Med Biol 1994;20:73-81.

Allendorf JDF et al. Helium-neon laser irradiation at fluences of 1, 2 and 4 J/cm2 failed to accelerated wound healing as assessed by both wound contracture rate and tensile strength. Lasers in Surg Med 1997;20:340-345.

Alvarez O et al. The healing of superficial skin wounds is stimulated by external electrical current. J Investigative Derm 1983;81:144-148.

Amano A et al. Histological studies on the rheumatoid synovial membrane irradiated with a low energy laser. Lasers in Surg Med 1994;15:290-294.

Bach S et al. The effect of electrical current on healing skin incision. Eur J Surg 1991;157:171-174.

Backman C et al. Chronic Achilles paratenonitis with tendinosis: an experimental model in the rabbit. J Orthop Res 1990;8:541-547.

Barclay V et al. Treatment of various hand injuries by pulsed electromagnetic energy (Diapulse). Physiotherapy 1983; 69:180-188.

Barker AT et al. A double blind clinical trial of low power pulsed shortwave therapy in the treatment of soft tissue injury. Physiotherapy 1985;71:500-504.

Basford JR et al. Does low intensity helium-neon laser irradiation alter sensory nerve action potentials or distal latencies. Laser Surg Med 1990;10:35-39.

Basford JR et al. A randomized controlled evaluation of low-intensity laser therapy: Plantar Fasciitis. Arch Phys Med Rehabil 1998;79:249-254.

Basford JR et al. Laser therapy: a randomized, controlled trial of the effects of low-intensity Nd: YAG laser irradiation on musculoskeletal back pain. Arch Phys Med Rehabil 1999;80:647-652.

Basford JR. Laser therapy: scientific basis and clinical role. Laser Ther 1993;16:541-547.

Basford JR. Low intensity laser therapy: still not an established clinical tool. Lasers in Surg Med 1995;16: 331-342.

Basur RL et al. A cooling method in the treatment of ankle sprains. Practitioner 1976;216:708-711.

Beckerman H et al. The efficacy of laser therapy for musculoskeletal and skin disorders: a criteria-based meta-analysis of randomized clinical trials. Phys Ther 1992;72:483-491.

Benson TB, Copp EP. The effects of therapeutic forms of heat and ice on the pain threshold of the normal shoulder. Rheumatol and Rehab 1974;13:101-104.

Berry H et al. Clinical study comparing acupuncture, physiotherapy, injection and oral anti-inflammatory therapy in shoulder-cuff lesions. Curr Med Res Opin 1980;7:121-126.

Bettany JA et al. High-voltage pulsed direct current: effect on edema formation after hyperflexion injury. Arch Phys Med Rehabil 1990a;71:667-681.

Bettany JA et al. Influence of high voltage pulsed direct current on edema formation following impact injury. Phys Ther 1990b;70:219-224.

Bierman W, Friedlander M. The penetrative effect of cold. Arch Phys Ther 1940;585-592.

Binder A et al. Is therapeutic ultrasound effective in treating soft tissue lesions? BMJ 1985;290:512-514.

Binder A. Pulsed electromagnetic field therapy or persistent rotator cuff tendinitis: a double-blind controlled assessment. Lancet 1984;695-698.

Bischt D et al. Effect of low intensity laser radiation on healing of open skin wounds in rats. Indian J Med Res 1994;100:43-46.

Bolton PA et al. Macrophage responsiveness to light therapy - a dose response study. Orig Art 1991;101-106.

Bouma MG et al. Low energy laser irradiation fails to modulate the inflammatory function of human monocytes and endothelial cells. Lasers in Surg Med 1996;19:207-215.

Bourguignon GJ et al. Electric stimulation of protein and DNA synthesis in human fibroblasts. FASEB J 1987;1:398-402.

Bradnock B et al. A quantitative comparative assessment of the immediate response to high frequency ultrasound and low frequency ultrasound ('longwave therapy') in the treatment of acute ankle sprains. Physiotherapy 1995;81:78-84.

Braverman B et al. Effect of helium-neon and infrared laser irradiation of wound healing in rabbits. Lasers in Surg Med 1989;9:50-58.

Broadley C et al. Low-energy helium-neon laser irradiation and the tensile strength of incisional wounds in the rat. Wound Rep Reg 1995;3:512-517.

Brown M, Goggia PP. Effects of high voltage stimulation on cutaneous wound healing in rabbits. Phys Ther 1987; 67:662-667.

Brown M et al. Electrical stimulation effects on cutaneous wound healing in rabbits. Phys Ther 1988;68:955-960.

Burgess E et al. Charged beads enhance cutaneous wound healing in Rhesus non-human primates. Plastic Reconstr Surg 1998;102:2395-2403.

Byl NN et al. The effects of phonophoresis with corticosteroids: a controlled pilot study. JOSPT 1993;18:590-600.

Ceccherelli F et al. Diode laser in cervical myofascial pain: a double-blind study versus placebo. Clin J Pain 1989;5:301-304.

Chard MD et al. Controlled study to investigate dose-response patterns to portable pulsed electromagnetic fields in the treatment of rotator cuff tendinitis. J Orthopaed Rheumatol 1988;1:33-40.

Cheng K, Goldman RJ. Electric fields and proliferation in a dermal wound model: cell cycle kinetics. Bioelectromagnetics 1998;19:68-74.

Cheng N et al. The effects of electric currents on ATP generation, protein synthesis, and membrane transport in rat skin. Clin Orthopaed Rel Res 1982;171:264-272.

Cheng RSS, Pomeranz B. Electrotherapy of chronic musculoskeletal pain: comparison of electroacupuncture and acupuncture-like transcutaneous electrical nerve stimulation. Clin J Pain 1986;2:143-149.

Cherry GW, Wilson J. The treatment of ambulatory venous ulcer patients with warming therapy. Ostomy/Wound Manage 1999;45:65-70.

Chu CS et al. Multiple graft harvestings from deep partial-thickness scald wounds healed under the influence of weak direct current. J Trauma 1990;30:1044-1050.

Clemente FR et al. Effect of motor neuromuscular electrical stimulation on microvascular perfusion of stimulated rat skeletal muscle. Phys Ther 1991;71:397-406.

Colver GB, Priestley GC. Failure of a helum-neon laser to affect components of wound healing in vitro. Brit J Dermatol 1989;121:179-186.

Cook HA et al. Effects of electrical stimulation on lymphatic flow and limb volume in the rat. Phys Ther 1994; 74:1040-1046.

Cooper MS, Schilwa M. Electrical and ionic controls of tissue cell locomotion in DC electric fields. J Neurosci Res 1985;13:223-244.

Cote DJ et al. Comparison of three treatment procedures for minimizing ankle sprain swelling. Phys Ther 1988; 68:1072-1076.

Creates VA. A study of ultrasound treatment to the painful perineum after childbirth. Physiotherapy 1987;73: 162-165.

Crowell JA et al. Functional changes in white blood cells after microsonation. Ultrasound Med Biol. 1997;3:185.

Currier DP et al. Effect of graded electrical stimulation on blood flow to healthy muscle. Phys Ther 1986;66: 937-943.

De Bie RA et al. Efficacy of 904 nm laser therapy in the management of musculoskeletal disorders: a systematic review. Phys Ther Rev 1998;3:59-72.

De Deyne P, Kirsch-Volders M. In vitro effects of therapeutic ultrasound on the nucleus of human fibroblasts. Phys Ther 1995;75:629-634.

Demirtas R, Oner C. The treatment of lateral epicondylitis by iontophoresis of sodium salicylate and sodium diclofenac. Clin Rehabil 1998;12:23-29.

Detlavs I et al. Experimental study of the effects of radiofrequency electromagnetic fields on animals with soft tissue wounds. Sci Total Environ 1996;180:35-42.

Deyo RA et al. A controlled trail of transcutaneous electrical nerve stimulation (TENS) and exercise for chronic low back pain. N Engl J Med 1990;322:1627-1634.

Dinno MA et al. The significance of membrane changes in the safe and effective use of therapeutic and diagnostic ultrasound. Phys Med Biol 1989;34:1543-1552.

Downing DS, Weinstein A. Ultrasound therapy of subacromial bursitis. A double blind trial. Phys Ther 1986; 66:194-199.

Dunn MG et al. Wound healing using a collagen matrix: effect of DC electrical stimulation. J Biomed Mater Res: Appl Biomater 1988;22:191-206.

Dyson M, Luke DA. Induction of mast cell degranulation in skin by ultrasound. IEEE Transact UFFC. 1986; 33:194-201.

Dyson M et al. The stimulation of tissue regeneration by means of ultrasound. Clin Sci 1968;35:273-285.

Dyson M, Young S. Effect of laser therapy on wound contraction and cellularity in mice. Lasers Med Sci 1986;1:125-130.

Dyson M. et al. Flow of red blood cells stopped by ultrasound. Nature 1971;232:572-573.

Ebenbichler G et al. Ultrasound therapy for calcific tendinitis of the shoulder. N Engl J Med 1999; 340:1533-1538.

Ebersold MJ et al. Transcutaneous electrical stimulation for treatment of chronic pain: a preliminary report. Surg Neurol 1975;4:96-98.

Ebert DW, Roberts C. In vitro frog sciatic nerve as a peripheral nerve model for studies of the mechanism of action of low energy lasers: part one. Lasers Surg Med 1997; 1:32-41.

Echternach JL. Ultrasound an adjunct treatment for shoulder disabilities. J Amer Phys Ther Assoc 1965;865-869.

El Sayed SO, Dyson M. Comparison of the effect of multiwavelength light produced by a cluster of semiconductor diodes and of each individual diode on mast cell number and degranulation in intact and injured skin. Lasers Surg Med 1990;10:559-568.

El Sayed SO, Dyson M. Effect of laser pulse repetition rate and pulse duration on mast cell number and degranulation. Lasers Surg Med 1996;19:433-437.

El Hag M et al. The anti-inflammatory effects of dexamethasone and therapeutic ultrasound in oral surgery. Br J Oral Maxillofac Surg 1985;23:17-23.

England S et al. Low power laser therapy of shoulder tendonitis. Scand J Rheumatol 1989;18:427-431.

Enwemeka CS et al. The biomechanical effects of low-intensity ultrasound on healing tendons. Ultrasound Med Biol 1990;16:801-807.

Erickson CA, Nuccitelli R. Embryonic fibroblast motility and orientation can be influenced by physiological electric fields. J Cell Biol 1984;98:296-307.

Eriksson MBE et al. Long term results of peripheral conditioning stimulation as an analgesic measure in chronic pain. Pain 1979;6:335-347.

Ersek RA. Low back pain: Prompt relief with transcutaneous neuro-stimulation. A report of 35 consecutive patients. Orthop Rev 1976;5:27-31.

Esclamado RM, Damiano GA, Cummings CW. Effect of local hypothermia on early wound repair. Arch Otolaryngol Head Neck Surg 1990;116:803-808.

Faghri P et al. Venous hemodynamics of the lower extremities in response to electrical stimulation. Arch Phys Med Rehab 1998;79:842-848.

Falanga V et al. Electrical stimulation increases the expression of fibroblast receptors for transforming growth factor-beta. Abstracts 1987;88:488.

Falconer J et al. Effect of ultrasound on mobility in osteoarthritis of the knee. A randomized clinical trial. Arth Care Res 1992;5:29-35.

Falconer J et al. Therapeutic ultrasound in the treatment of musculoskeletal conditions. Arth Care Res 1990; 3:85-91.

Fish DR et al. Effect of anodal high voltage pulsed current on edema formation in frog hind limbs. PhysTher 1991;71:724-733.

Foley-Nolan D et al. Pulsed high frequency (27 MHz) electromagnetic therapy for persistent neck pain. A double blind, placebo-controlled study of 20 patients. Orthopedics 1990;13:445-451.

Foulds IS, Barker AT. Human skin battery potentials and their possible role in wound healing. Br J Dermatol 1983;109:515-522.

Fujita M et al. The effect of constant direct electrical current on intrinsic healing in the flexor tendon in vitro. J Hand Surg (British Volume) 1992;17:94-98.

Fyfe MC, Chahl LA The effect of single or repeated applications of 'therapeutic' ultrasound on plasma extravasation during silver nitrate induced inflammation of the rat hindpaw ankle joint in vivo. Ultrasound Med Biol 1985;11:273-283.

Fyfe MC, Chahl LA. Mast cell degranulation: a possible mechanism of action of therapeutic ultrasound. Ultrasound Med Biol 1982;8(Suppl.1):62.

Gam AN et al. The effect of low-level laser therapy on musculoskeletal pain: a meta-analysis. Pain 1993; 52:63-66.

Gam AN et al. Treatment of myofascial trigger-points with ultrasound combined with massage and exercise: a randomised controlled trial. Pain 1998;77:73-79.

Gan BS et al. The effects of ultrasound treatment on flexor tendon healing in the chicken limb. J Hand Surg 1995; 20B:809-814.

Garrick JG, Henz-Schelkun P. Managing ankle sprains: keys to preserving motion and strength. Physician Sports Med 1997;25:56-68.

Gilcreast D et al. Effect of electrical stimulation on foot skin perfusion in persons with or at risk for diabetic foot ulcers. Wound Rep Reg 1998;6:434-441.

Goddard DH et al. Ultrasound has no anti-inflammatory effect. Ann Rheum Dis. 1983;42:582-584.

Graham DJ, Alexander JJ. The effects of argon laser on bovine aortic endothelial and smooth muscle cell proliferation and collagen production. Cur Surg 1990;27-31.

Greathouse DG et al. Effects of clinical infrared laser on superficial radial nerve conduction. Phys Ther 1985;65:1184-1187.

Griffin JE et al. Patients treated with ultrasonic driven hydrocortisone and with ultrasound alone. Phys Ther 1972; 47:594-601.

Griffin JW et al. Reduction of chronic posttraumatic hand edema: a comparison of high voltage pulsed currnet intermittent pneumatic compression, and placebo treatments. Phys Ther 1990;70:279-286.

Gudeman S et al. Treatment of plantar fasciitis by iontophoresis of 0.4% dexamethasone: a randomized, double-blind, placebo-controlled study. Am J Sports Med 1997;25:312-315.

Haker E, Lundeberg T. Is low-energy laser treatment effective in lateral epicondylalgia? J Pain Symptom Manage 1991a;6:241-246.

Haker E, Lundeberg T. Laser treatment applied to acupuncture points in lateral humeral epicondylalgia. A double-blind study. Pain 1990;43:243-247.

Haker E, Lundeberg T. Pulsed ultrasound treatment in lateral epicondylalgia. Scand J Rehab Med 1991b;23: 115-118.

Haker EHK, Lundeberg TCM. Lateral epicondylalgia: report of noneffective midlaser treatment. Arch Phys Med Rehabil 1991c;72:984-988.

Hall G et al. Effect of low level energy laser irradiation on wound healing. An experimental study in rats. Swed Dent J 1994;18:29-34.

Halle JS et al. Comparison of four treatment approaches for lateral epicondylitis of the elbow. JOSPT 1986;8:62-69.

Hamer J, Kirk JA. Physiotherapy and the frozen shoulder: a comparative trial of ice and ultrasonic therapy. N Z Med J 1976;83:191-192.

Hansen HJ, Thoroe U. Low power laser biostimulation of chronic oro-facial pain. A double-blind placebo controlled cross-over study in 40 patients. Pain 1990;43:169-179.

Harvey W et al. The 'in vitro' stimulation of protein synthesis in human fibroblasts by therapeutic levels of ultrasound. Rheumatol Rehab 1975;14.

Hashish I et al. Anti-inflammatory effects of ultrasound therapy evidence for a major placebo effect. Br J Rheumatol 1986;25:77-81.

Hayashi K et al. The effect of nonablative laser energy on joint capsular properties: An in vitro mechanical study using a rabbit model. Am J Sports Med 1995;23:482-487.

Hecht PJ et al. Effects of thermal therapy on rehabilitation after total knee arthroplasty. Clin Orthopaed Rel Res 1983;178:198-201.

Hecker B et al Pulsed galvanic stimulation: effects of current frequency and polarity on blood flow in healthy subjects. Arch Phys Med Rehabil 1985;66:369-371.

Herrera-Lasso et al. Comparative effectiveness of packages of treatment including ultrasound or transcutaneous electrical nerve stimulation in painful shoulder syndrome. Physiotherapy 1993;79:231-233.

Hinsenkamp M et al. Effects of low frequency pulsed electrical current on keratinocytes in vitro. Bioelectromagnetics 1997;18:250-254.

Hocutt JE et al. Cryotherapy in ankle sprains. Am J Sports Med 1982;10:316-319.

Hogan R et al. The effect of ultrasound on microvascular hemodynamics in skeletal muscle: effects on arterioles. Ultrasound Med Biol 1982;8:45-50.

Holdsworth LK, Anderson DM. Effectiveness of ultrasound used with a hydrocortisone coupling medium or epicondylitis clasp to treat lateral epicondylitis: pilot study. Physiotherapy 1993;79:19-25.

Honmura A et al. Therapeutic effect of ga-al-as diode laser irradiation on experimentally induced inflammation in rats. Lasers Surg Med 1992;12:441-449.

Hoyrup G, Kjorvel L. Comparison of whirlpool and wax treatments for hand therapy. Physiother Canada 1986; 38:79-82.

Hunter J et al. Effects of low energy laser on wound healing in a porcine model. Lasers Surg Med 1984;3:285-290.

Im MJ et al. Effect of electrical stimulation on survival of skin flaps in pigs. Phys Ther 1990;70:37-40.

Indergand HJ, Morgan BJ. Effects of high-frequency transcutaneous electrical nerve stimulation on limb blood flow in healthy humans. Phys Ther 1994;74:361-367.

Jackson BA et al. Effect of ultrasound therapy on the repair of Achilles tendon injuries in rats. Med Sci Sports Exer 1991;23:171-176.

Jones RJ. Treatment of acute herpes zoster using ultrasonic therapy. Physiotherapy 1984; 70:94-96.

Karnes JL et al. Effects of low voltage pulsed current on edema formation in frog hind limbs following impact injury. Phys Ther 1992;72:273-278.

Karu Ti et al. Helium-neon laser induced respiratory burst of phagocytic cells. Lasers Surg Med 1989;9:585-588.

King CE et al. Effect of helium-neon laser auriculotherapy on experimental pain threshold. Phys Ther 1990;70:24-29.

Kjartansson J et al. Transcutaneous electrical nerve stimulation (TENS) increases survival of ischaemic musculocutaneous flaps. Acta Physiol Scand 1988;134:95-99.

Klein RG, Eek BC. Low-energy laser treatment and exercise for chronic low back pain: double-blind controlled trial. Arch Phys Med Rehabil 1990;71:34-37.

Kloth LC et al. Effects of a normothermic dressing on pressure ulcer healing. Adv Skin Wound Care 2000;13:69-74.

Kolarova H et al. Penetration of the laser light into the skin in vitro. Lasers Surg Med 1999;24:231-235.

Kovacs I et al. Laser-induced stimulation of the vascularizaton of the healing wound. An ear chamber experiment. Experientia 1974;15:341-343.

Kowal MA. Review of physiological effects of cryotherapy. J Orthopaed Sports Phys Ther 1983;5:66-73.

Kramer JF, Sandrin M. Effect of low-power laser and white light on sensory conduction rate of the superficial radial nerve. Physiother Canada 1993;45:165-170.

Kramer JF. Ultrasound: evaluation of its mechanical and thermal effects. Arch Phys Med Rehabil 1984;65:223-227.

Kreczi T, Klingler D. A comparison of laser acupuncture versus placebo in radicular and pseudoradicular pain syndromes as recorded by subjective responses of patients. Acupuncture Electro-Therapeut Res Int J 1986;11:207-216.

Laba E, Roestenburg M. Clinical evaluation of ice therapy for acute sprain injuries. New Zealand J Physiother 1989;7-9.

Lamb S, Mani R. Does interferential therapy affect blood flow? Clin Rehab 1994;8:213-218.

Lam TS et al. Laser stimulation of collagen synthesis in human skin fibroblast cultures. Lasers Life Sci 1986; 1:61-77.

Lee JM et al. Effects of ice on nerve conduction velocity. Physiotherapy 1978;64:2.

Lehmann JF et al. Effect of therapeutic temperature on tendon extensibility. Arch Phys Med Rehabil 1970;481-487.

Lehmann TR et al. Efficacy of electroacupuncture and TENS in the rehabilitation of chronic low back pain patients. Pain 1986;26:277-290.

Levine SP et al. Blood flow in the gluteus maximus of seated individuals during electrical muscle stimulation. Arch Phys Med Rehabil 1990;71:682-686.

Lewith GT, Machin D. A randomised trial to evaluate the effect of infra-red stimulation of local trigger points, versus placebo, on the pain caused by cervical osteoarthrosis. Acupuncture Electro-Therapeut Res Int J 1981; 6:277-284.

Litke DS, Dahners LE. Effects of different levels of direct current on early ligament healing in a rat model. J Orthopaed Res 1994;12:683-688.

Liu H-I et al. Circulatory response of digital arteries associated with electrical stimulation of calf muscle in healthy subjects. Phys Ther 1987;67:340-345.

Loeser JD et al. Relief of pain by transcutaneous stimulation. J Neurosurg 1975;42:308-314.

Longo L et al. Effect of diodes-laser silver arsenide-aluminum (Ga-Al-As) 904 nm on healing of experimental wounds. Lasers Surg Med 1987;7:444-447.

Losito JM and O'Neil J. Rehabilitation of foot and ankle injuries. Clin Podiatr Med Surg 1997;14(3):533-557.

Lundeberg T et al. A comparative study of continuous ultrasound, placebo ultrasound and rest in epicondylalgia. Scand J Rehab Med 1988;20:99-101.

Lundeberg T, Haker E, Thomas M. Effect of laser versus placebo in tennis elbow. Scand J Rehab Med 1987; 19:135-138.

Lyons RF, Abergel RP, White RA, Dwyer RM, Castel JC, Uitto J. Biostimulation of wound healing in vivo by a helium-neon laser. Annals of Plastic Surgery 1987;18.

Maeda T. Morphological demonstration of low reactive laser therapeutic pain attenuation effect of the Galium Aluminium Arsenide diode laser. 1988

Makuloluwe RTB, Mouzas GL Ultrasound in the treatment of sprained ankles. Practitioner 1977;218:586-588.

Marchand S, Charest J, Li J, Chenard JR, Lavignolle B, Laurencelle L. Is TENS purely a placebo effect? A controlled study on chronic low back pain. Pain 1993; 54:99-106.

Mardiman S, Wessel J, Fisher B. The effect of ultrasound on the mechanical pain threshold of healthy subjects. Physiotherapy 1995;81:718-723.

Maxwell L. Therapeutic Ultrasound: Its Effects on the Cellular and Molecular Mechanisms of Inflammation and Repair. Physiotherapy 1992;78:421-426.

Mayrovitz H, Larsen P. Effects of pulsed electromagnetic fields on skin microvascular blood perfusion. Wounds 1992;4:197-202.

McCaughan J, Bethel B, Johnston T, Janssen W. Effect of Low-Dose Argon Irradiation on Rate of Wound Closure. Lasers in Surgery and Medicine 1985;5:607-614.

McCray RE, Patton NJ. Pain relief at trigger points: a comparison of moist heat and shortwave diathermy. JOSPT 1984;5:175-178.

McGill SN. The effects of pulsed shortwave therapy on lateral ligament sprain of the ankle. NZ Journal of Physiotherapy 1988;21-24.

McKibbin LS, Downie R. A statistical study on the use of the infared 904-nm low energy laser on calcaneal spurs. n/a 1989;71-77.

McMaster WC. Cryotherapy. The Physician and Sports Medicine 1982;10:112-119.

McMaster WC, Liddle S. Cryotherapy influence on Posttraumatic Limb Edema. Clinical Orthopaedics and Related Research 1980;150:283-287.

McMeeken JM. Magnetic fields: effects on blood flow in human subjects. Physiother Theory Practice 1992; 8:3-9.

Melzack R, Guite S, Gonshor A. Relief of dental pain by ice massage of the hand. CMA Journal 1980a; 122:189-191.

Melzack R, Jeans ME, Stratford JG, Monks RC. Ice massage and transcutaneous electrical stimulation: comparison of treatment for low-back pain. Pain 1980b;9:209-217.

Melzack R, Vetere P, Finch L. Transcutaneous Electrical Nerve Stimulation for low back pain: A Comparison of TENS and Massage for Pain and Range of Motion. Physical Therapy 1983;63:489-493.

Mendel FC, Wylegala JA, Fish DR. Influence of High Voltage Pulsed Current on Edema Formation Following Impact Injury in Rats. Physical Therapy 1992;72:668-673.

Mertz PM, Davis SC, Cazzaniga AL, Cheng K, Reich JD, Eaglstein WH. Electrical Stimulation: Acceleration of Soft Tissue Repair by Varying the Polarity. Wounds 1993;5:153-159.

Mester E, Mester AF, Mester A. The Biomedical Effects of Laser Application. Lasers in Surgery and Medicine 1985;5:31-39.

Michlovitz S, Smith W, Watkins M. Ice and High Voltage Pulsed Stimulation in Treatment of Acute Lateral Ankle Sprains. Journal of Orthopaedic and Sports Physical Therapy 1988;9:301-304.

Middlemast S, Chatterjee DS. Comparison of Ultrasound and Thermotherapy for Soft Tissue Injuries. Physiotherapy 1978;64:331-333.

Miller CR, Webers RL. The Effects of Ice Massage on an Individual's Pain Tolerance Level to Electrical Stimulation. JOSPT 1990;12:105

Mohr T, Akers TK, Wessman HC. Effect of High Voltage Stimulation on Blood Flow in the Rat Hind Limb. Physical Therapy 1987;67:526-533.

Mortimer AJ, Dyson M. The effect of therapeutic ultrasound on calcium uptake in fibroblasts. Ultrasound in Med and Biol 1988;14:499-506.

Munting E. Ultrasonic therapy for painful shoulders. Physiotherapy 1978;64:180-181.

Nessler JP, Mass DP. Direct-current electrical stimulation of tendon healing in vitro. Clinical Orthopaedics and Related Research 1987;303-312.

Noble PB, Shields ED, Blecher PDM, Bentley KC. Locomotory characteristics of fibroblasts within a three-dimensional collagen lattice: modulation by a helium/neon soft laser. Lasers in Surgery and Medicine 1992;12:669-674.

Nussbaum E, Rush P, Disenhaus L. The Effects of Interferential Therapy on Peripheral Blood Flow. Physiotherapy 1990;76:803-807.

Nwuga VCB. Ultrasound in treatment of back pain resulting from prolapsed intervertebral disc. Arch Phys Med Rehabil 1983;64:88-89.

Nyanzi C, Langridge J, Heyworth J, Mani R. Randomized controlled study of ultrasound therapy in the management of acute lateral ligament sprains of the ankle joint. Clinical Rehabilitation 1999;13:16-22.

Nykanen M. Pulsed Ultrasound treatment of the painful shoulder: a randomized, double-blind, placebo-controlled study. Scand J Rehab Med 1995;27:105-108.

Ohshiro T, Shirono Y. Retroactive study in 524 patients on the application of the 830nm GaAIAs diode laser in low reactive-level laser therapy (LLLT) for lumbago. Laser Therapy 1992;4:121-126.

Ohta A, Abergel RP, Uitto J. Laser modulation of human immune system: inhibition of lymphocyte proliferation by a gallium-arsenide laser at low energy. Lasers in Surgery and Medicine 1987;7:199-201.

Olson SL, Perez JV, Stacks LN, Walsh MH. The effects of TENS and interferential current on cutaneous blood flow in healthy subjects. Physiotherapy Canada 1999; Winter:27-31.

Orida N, Feldman JD. Directional protrusive pseudopodial activity and motility in macrophages induced by extra-cellular electric fields. Cell Motility 1982;2:243-255.

Ottani V, DePasquale V, Govoni P, Franchi M, Zaniol P, Ruggeri A. Effects of pulsed extremely-low frequency magnetic fields on skin wounds in the rat. Bio-electromagnetics 1988;9:53-62.

Owoeye I, Spielholz NI, Nelson AJ. Low-intensity Pulsed Galvanic Current and the Healing of Tenotomized Rat Achilles Tendons: Preliminary report using Load-to-break Measurements. Arch Phys Med Rehabil. 1987; 68:415-418.

Oztas O, Turan B, Bora I, Karakaya MK. Ultrasound thera-py effect in carpal tunnel syndrome. Arch Phys Med Rehabil 1998;79:1540-1545.

Patino O, Grana D, Bolgiani A, Prezzavento G, Mino J, Merlo A, et al. Pulsed electromagnetic fields in experi-mental cutaneous wound healing in rats. J Burn Care Rehab 1996;17:528-531.

Passarella S, Casamassima E, Quagliariello E, Caretto G, Jirillo E. Quantitative Analysis of Lymmphocytes-Salmonella interaction and Effect of Lymphocyte Irradiation by Helium-Neon Laser. Biochemical And Biophysical Research Communications 1985;130: 546-552.

Payne C. Ultrasound for post-herpetic neuralgia. Physiotherapy 1984;70:96-97.

Pienimaki T, Karinen P, Kemila T, Koivukangas P, Vanharanta H. Long-Term Follow-Up of Conservatively Treated Chronic Tennis Elbow Patients. A Prospective and Retrospective Analysis. Scand J Rehab Med 1998;30:159-166.

Pienimaki TT, Tarvainen TK, Siira PT, Vanharanta H. Progressive strengthening and stretching exercises and ultrasound for chronic lateral epicondylitis. Physio-therapy 1996;82:522-529.

Pourreau-Schneider N, Ahmed A, Soudry M, Jacquemier J, Kopp F, Franquin JC, et al. Helium-neon laser treatment transforms fibroblasts into myofibroblasts. American Journal Of Pathology 1990;137:171-178.

Rabkin JM, Hunt TK. Local Heat Increases Blood Flow and Oxygen Tension in Wounds. Arch Surg 1987;122:221-225.

Reddy GK, Stehno-Bittel L, Enwemeka CS. Laser photo-stimulation of collagen production in healing rabbit achilles tendons. Lasers in Surgery and Medicine 1998;22:281-287.

Reed BV. Effect of High Voltage Pulsed Electrical Stimulation on Microvascular Permeability to Plasma Proteins. Physical Therapy 1988;4:491-495.

Reich JD, Cazzaniga AL, Mertz PM, Kerdel FA, Eaglstein WH. The effect of electrical stimulation on the number of mast cells in healing wounds. J Am Acad Dermatol 1991;25:40-46.

Rennie GA, Michlovitz SL. Biophysical Principles of Healing and Superficial Heating Agents. In: Thermal Agents in Rehabilitation. Ed. SL Michlovitz. 3rd Edition FA Davis Co. Philadelphia 1996.

Roberts M, Rutherford JH, Harris D. The effect of ultra-sound on flexor tendon repairs in the rabbit. Hand 1982;14:17-21.

Robinson SE, Buono MJ Effect of continuous-wave ultra-sound on blood flow in skeletal muscle. Phys Ther 1995;75:145-150.

Rochkind S, Rousso M, Nissan M, Villarreal M, Barr-Nea L, Rees DG Systemic effects of low-power laser irradiation on the peripheral and central nervous system, cutaneous wounds, and burns. Lasers in Surgery and Medicine 1989; 9:174-182.

Rodemann HP, Bayreuther K, Pfleiderer G. The differentia-tion of normal and transformed human fibroblasts in vitro influenced by electromagnetic fileds. Exp Cell Res 1989;182:610-621.

Rood PA, Haas AF, Graves PJ, Wheeland RG, Isseroff RR. Low-energy helium neon laser irradiation does not alter human keratinocyte differentiation. J Invest Dermatol 1992;99:445-448.

Rubin MJ, Etchison MR, Condra KA, Franklin TD, Snoddy AM. Acute effects of ultrasound on skeletal muscle oxy-gen tension, blood flow and capillary density. J Med Biol 1990;16:271-277.

Santilli SM, Valusek PA, Robinson C. Use of a Noncontact Radiant Heat Bandage for the Treatment of Chronic Venous Stasis Ulcers. Adv Wound Care 1999;12:89-93.

Santoro D, Ostrander L, Lee BY, Cagir B. Inductive 27.12 MHz diathermy in arterial peripheral vascular disease. J Rehab Res Dev 1992;25:19-24.

Saperia D, Glassberg E, Lyons RF, Abergel P, Baneux P, Castel JC, et al. Demonstration of elevated type I and type III procollagen mRNA levels in cutaneous wounds treated with helium-neon laser. Biochemical and Biophysical Research Communications 1986;138:1123-1128.

Saunders L. The efficacy of low-level laser therapy in supraspinatus tendinitis. Clin Rehab 1995;9:126-134.

Sarcova J, Trnavsky K, Zvarova J. The influence of ultra-sound, galvanic currents and shortwave diathermy on pain intensity in patients with osteoarthritis. Scand J Rheumatology 1988;67:83-85.

Schultz RJ, Krishnamurthy S, Thelmo W, Rodriquez JE, Harvey G. Effects of varying intensities of laser energy on articular cartilage. Lasers in Surgery and Medicine 1985;5:577-588.

Shamberger R, Talbot T, Tipton H, Thibault L, Brennan M. The Effect of Ultrasonic and Thermal Treatment on Wounds. Plastic Reconstr Surg 1981;68:860-870.

Shiroto C, Ono K, Ohshiro T. Retrospective study of diode laser therapy for pain attentuation in 3635 patients: detailed analysis by questionnaire. Laser Therapy 1989;41-47.

Siebert W, Seichert N, Siebart B, Wirth CJ. What is the efficacy of "soft" and "mid" lasers in therapy of tendinopathies? Arch Orthopaed Traum Surg 1987; 106:358-363.

Simunovic Z., Trobonjaca T., Trobonjaca Z. Treatment of medial and lateral epicondylitis – tennis and golfer's elbow – with low level laser therapy: a multicenter double blind, placebo-controlled clinical study on 324 patients. J Clin Laser Med Surg 1998;16:145-151.

Skinner S, Gage J, Wilce P, Shaw R. A Preliminary Study of the Effects of Laser Radiation on Collagen Metabolism in Cell Culture. Australian Dental Journal 1996;41: 188-192.

Sluka KA, Christy MR, Peterson WL, Rudd SL, Troy SM. Reduction of Pain-Related Behaviors with either Cold or Heat Treatment in an Animal Model of Acute Arthritis. Arch Phys Med Rehabil 1999;80:313-317.

Smith J, Romansky N, Vomero J, Davis R. The effect of electrical stimulation on wound healing in diabetic mice. J Am Pod Assoc 1984;74:71-75.

Snow CJ, Johnson KA. Effect of therapeutic ultrasound on acute inflammation. Physiother Can 1988;40:162-167.

Snyder-Mackler L, Barry AJ, Perkins AI, Soucek MD. Effectsof helium-neon laser irradiation on skin resistance and pain in patients with trigger points in the neck or back. Phys Ther 1989; 69:336-341.

Sroka R et al. Effects on the mitosis of normal and tumor cells induced by light treatment of different wavelengths. Lasers Surg Med 1999;25:263-271.

Stamford B. Giving injuries the cold treatment. Phys Sports Med 1996;24(3):15-16.

Steckel RR et al. Electrical stimulation on skin wound healing in the horse: Preliminary studies. Am J Vet Res 1984;45:800-803.

Stevenson JH et al. Functional, mechanical and biochemical assessment of ultrasound therapy on tendon healing in the chicken toe. Plastic Recon Surg 1986;77:965-970.

Stockle U et al. Fastest reduction of posttraumatic edema: continuous cryotherapy or intermittent impulse compression? Foot Ankle Inter 1997;18:432-438.

Stratford PW, Levy DR, Gauldie S, Miseferi D, Levy K. The evaluation of phonophoresis and friction massage as treatment for extensor carpi radialis tendinitis: a randomized controlled trial. Physiotherapy Canada 1989; 41:93-99.

Strickler T et al. The effects of passive warming on muscle injury. Am J Sports Med 1990;18:141-145.

Surinchak JS et al. Effects of low-level energy lasers on the healing of full-thickness skin defects. Lasers Surg Med 1983;2:267-274.

Taber C et al. Measurement of reactive vasodilation during cold gel pack application to Nontraumatized ankles. Phys Ther 1992;72:294-299.

Talaat AM et al. Physical therapy in the management of myofacial pain dysfunction syndrome. Ann Otol Rhino Laryngol 1986;95:225-228.

Taylor K et al. Effect of a single 30-minute treatment of high voltage pulsed current on edema formation in frog hind limbs. Phys Ther 1992;72:63-68.

ter Haar GR, Hopewell JW. Ultrasound heating of mammalian tissues in vivo. Br J Cancer 1982;45:65-67.

Thorsen H. et al. Low level laser therapy for myofascial pain in the neck and shoulder girdle: a double-blind cross-over study. Scan J Rheumatol 1992;21:139-141.

Thorsteinsson G et al. Transcutaneous electrical stimulation: A double blind trial of its efficacy for pain. Arch Phys Med Rehabil 1977;58:8-13.

Tracy JE et al. Comparison of selected pulse frequencies from two different electrical stimulators on blood flow in healthy subjects. Phys Ther 1988;68:1526-1532.

Trelles MA et al. The action of low reactive level laser therapy (LLLT) on mast cells: a possible pain relief mechanism examined. J Orthopaed Sports Phys Ther 1989;27-30.

Turner SM et al. The effect of ultrasound on the healing of repaired cockerel tendon: is collagen cross-linkage a factor? J Hand Surg 1989;14B:428-433.

Utsunomiya T. A histopathological study of the effects of low-power laser irradiation on wound healing of exposed dental pulp tissues in dogs, with special reference to lectins and collagens. 1998;24:187-193.

Van der Heijden GJ et al. Physiotherapy for patients with soft tissue shoulder disorders: a systematic review of randomised clinical trails. BMJ 1997;315:25-30.

Vasseljen O et al. Low level laser versus placebo in the treatment of tennis elbow. Scan J Rehabil Med 1992;24: 37-42.

Vecchio P et al. A double-blind study of the effectiveness of low level laser treatment of rotator cuff tendinitis. Br J Rheum 1993;32:740-742.

Wagstaff P et al. A pilot study to compare the efficacy of continous and pulsed magnetic energy (short-wave diathermy) on the relief of low back pain. Physiotherapy 1986;72:563-566.

Walker DC et al. Effects of high voltage pulsed electrical stimulation on blood flow. Phys Ther 1988;68:481-485.

Walker J. Relief from chronic pain by low power laser irradiation. Neurosci Lett 1983;43:339-344.

Walker JB et al. Laser therapy for pain of Trigeminal Neuralgia. Clin J Pain 1988; 3:183-187.

Ward RS et al. Evaluation of topical therapeutic ultrasound to improve response to physical therapy and lessen scar contracture after burn injury. J Burn Care Rehab 1994; 15:74-79.

Waylonis GW. The physiologic effects of ice massage. Arch Phys Med Rehabil 1967;37-42.

Waylonis GW et al. Chronic myofascial pain: management by low-output helium-neon laser therapy. Arch Phys Med Rehabil 1988;69:1017-1020.

Webb C, Dyson M, Lewis WHP. Stimulatory effect of 660 nm low level laser energy on hypertrophic scar-derived fibroblasts: possible mechanisms for increase in cell counts. Lasers Surg Med 1998;2:294-301.

Wessling KC et al. Effects of static stretch versus static stretch and ultrasound combined on triceps surae muscle extensibility in healthy women. Phys Ther 1987;67:674-679.

Weston M, Taber C, Casagranda L, Cornwall M. Changes in Local Blood Volume during Gel Pack Application to Traumatized Ankles. JOSPT 1994; 19:197-199.

Wilkerson GB, Horn-Kingery H.M. Treatment of the inversion ankle sprain: comparison of different modes of compression and cryotherapy. JOSPT 1993; 17:240-246.

Williams AR et al. Effects of MHz ultrasound on electrical pain threshold perception in humans. Ultrasound Med Biol 1987;13:249-258.

Williams AR et al. Haemolysis in vivo by therapeutic intensities of ultrasound. Ultrasound Med Biol 1986;12: 501-509.

Wilson DH. Comparison of short wave diathermy and pulsed electromagnetic energy in treatment of soft tissue injuries. Physiotherapy 1974;60:309-310.

Young S et al. Macrophage responsiveness to light therapy. Lasers Surg Med 1989;9:497-505.

Young SR, Dyson M. Effect of therapeutic ultrasound on the healing of full-thickness excised skin lesions. Ultrasonics 1990a;28:175-179.

Young SR, Dyson M. Macrophage responsiveness to therapeutic ultrasound. Ultrasound Med Biol 1990b;16: 809-816.

Young SR, Dyson M. The effect of therapeutic ultrasound on angiogenesis. Ultrasound Med Biol 1990c;16: 261-269.

Yu H-S et al. Low-energy helium-neon laser irradiation stimulates interleukin-1 alpha and interleukin-8 release from cultured human keratinocytes. J Invest Dermatol 1996;107:593-596.

Yu W et al. Effects of photostimulation on wound healing in diabetic mice. Lasers Surg Med 1997;20:56-63.

Zamora AJ, Marini JF. Tendon and myo-tendinous junction in an overloaded skeletal muscle of the rat. Anat Embryol 1988;179:89-96.

Zarkovic N et al. Effect of semiconductor GaAs laser irradiation on pain perception in mice. Lasers Surg Med 1989;9:63-66.

Zhao M et al. Electric field-directed cell motility involves up-regulated expression and asymmetric redistribution of the epidermal growth factor receptors and is enhanced by fibronectin and laminin. Mol Biol Cell 1999a; 10:1259-1276.

Zhao M et al. A small, physiological electric field orients cell division. Proc Natl Acad Sci 1999b;96:4942-4946.

Zhao M et al. Human corneal epithelial cells reorient and migrate cathodally in a small applied electric field. Curr Eye Res 1997;16:973-984.

Zhuang H et al. Electrical stimulation induces the level of TGF-β1 mRNA in osteoblastic cells by a mechanism involving calcium/calmodulin pathway. Biochem Biophys Res Comm 1997;237:225-229.

Index

Note: Page numbers followed by *f* indicate figures; *t* indicates tables; *b* indicates boxes.

A

Abrasion arthroplasty, for cartilage repair, 79
Acetic acid, transdermal delivery of, 166
Achilles tendon, 35, 38
  attachment of, 36*f*
  overuse injury of, 42
  surgical repair of, 47
Acupuncture
  clinical studies on effectiveness of, 163*t*
  laser therapy combined with, 174
  with TENS, 173
Adhesive capsulitis, 57
Adipocytes, of connective tissue, 6, 7
Aggrecans, 5, 35
  in articular cartilage, 64, 64*t*
  in tendons, 36
Aging process
  articular cartilage and, 71
  and cartilage repair, 78
  collagen in, 26
  and disc herniation, 108
  and disease process, 28, 29
  effect on IVD of, 97, 104-105, 106
  and interstitial collagens, 28*t*
  and ligament growth, 51-52
  musculoskeletal function and, 25, 26, 27, 27*f*
  vs. osteoarthritis, 74
  and overuse injury, 41
Allografts
  in ligamentous injury, 55
  in meniscal repair, 84-85
Amino acids
  in collagen, 11
  in polypeptide chain, 14-15
Analgesia. *See also* Pain
  cryotherapy-induced, 141
  heat-induced, 141
Anchorin CII, in articular cartilage, 66, 66*t*
Animal models
  cartilage repair, 81
  collagen organization in, 152
  of CPM, 123
  for electrical stimulation, 145
  of healing ligaments, 55
  immobilization studies, 51, 130, 130*f*, 131
  laser therapy, 149
  of ligament growth, 51, 52
  mechanical stress in, 51

Animal models—cont'd
  of meniscal apoptosis, 84
  meniscal repair, 85
Animal models—cont'd
  osteoarthritis, 73-74
  Rhesus macaque, 75
Ankle sprains, 139
  prevalence of, 153
  therapeutic modalities for, 153, 157-158
Ankylosis, intraarticular, 128
Annulus fibrosus, 100-101
  of cervical IVD, 99
  composition of, 112
  in disc degeneration, 109
  effect of aging on, 105, 106, 107
  mechanical stimulation of, 111
  ultrastructure of, 102*t*
Anterior cruciate ligament (ACL)
  effect of aging on, 52
  exercised *vs.* nonexercised, 131*f*
  healing response of, 53
  and hormone levels, 52
  repair of, 52
  rupture of, 53
  strains in, 50
Antifibrotic therapy, 25
Antiinflammatory medication
  clinical trials of, 167
  NSAIDS, 134-135
Apoptosis, in meniscus, 84
Areolar (small space) tissue, 3
Arthrogenic restriction, of contractures, 133
Arthrography, limitations of, 74
Arthropathies, joint, 74
Arthroplasty
  abrasion, 79
  CPM following, 123-124
Arthroscopy, 76
Articular cartilage, 1, 3
  age-related changes in, 71
  biochemistry of, 64-67
  biomechanics of, 68-69, 70, 73, 86
  collagen in, 11, 65, 65*t*
  compartmentalizaiton of, 68
  defined, 63
  degradation of, 71, 86
  ECM of, 5
  effect of CPM on, 123

Articular cartilage—cont'd
formation of, 69-70
functional integrity of, 68-69, 86
heterogeneity of, 67-68
laminae of, 67-68, 86
non-collagenous proteins in, 66, 66*t*
normal, 67*f*
in osteoarthritis, 72, 72*f*
proteoglycans in, 64, 64*t*, 86
remodeling of, 70
type II collagen in, 14
visualization of, 74-77, 75*f*-77*f*
Articular cartilage repair, 80-81
biologic agents for, 79
bone marrow stimulation in, 78
cell-seeded approach to, 79-80
current treatment method, 77-78
lavage and debridement, 78
microfracture technique, 79
noncell-seeded/biosynthetic approach to, 80
Athlete, ligamentous injury in female, 52
Augmented soft tissue mobilization (ASTM), 124-125
Autografts, in ligamentous injury, 55
Autologous chondrocyte implantation (ACI)
in cartilage repair, 80
of knee, 75
Axonotmesis, 141

B

Back pain, 97, 139
clinical trials for, 168*t*-172*t*
cold therapy for, 173
electrical stimulation for, 167, 173
electromagnetic fields for, 173-174
etiology of, 97*f*
heat therapy for, 173
and IVD changes, 106
laser therapy for, 174
lumbar disc degeneration in, 107
manipulation of spine for, 127
therapeutic modalities for, 175
ultrasound therapy for, 173
Basement membranes, collagen in, 29
Beighton scale, 135
Biglycan, in articular cartilage, 66, 66*t*
Biomechanical studies, of tendon, 40
Blood, in connective tissue, 2
Blood flow
effects of electrical stimulation on, 144
effects of hot and cold agents on, 140-141
effects of PEMFs on, 147
effects of ultrasound on, 150-151
and tissue repair, 146
Blood viscosity, in cold therapies, 140
Bone
connective tissue in, 2
and ligament development, 51
Bone-ligament-bone complex model, 51
Bone marrow, cellular components of, 7
Bone marrow stimulation, in cartilage repair, 78
Bone morphogenetic proteins (BMPs), in articular
cartilage repair, 79
Bone patella-tendon bone autograft procedure, 55
Bracing, *vs.* accelerated rehabilitation, 55-56
Bulging, IVD, 111

Bursae
associated with tendons, 38
calcific deposits in, 159
Bursitis
calcific, 159, 166-167
clinical studies of, 160*t*-164*t*
etiology of, 159
prevalence of, 158-159
treatment of, 159, 165

C

Calcific deposits, clinical research on, 166-167
Calcium levels, in tendinopathy, 38
Capsules, collagen in, 11
Cartilage. *See also* Articular cartilage
dynamic loading of, 69
hyaline, 63
mechanical properties of, 1
tissue-engineered, 81
viscoelastic properties of, 73
Cartilage canals, 63, 86
Cartilage diseases, clinical diagnosis of, 71
Cartilage matrix, 9
Cartilage matrix glycoprotein (CMP), 66, 66*t*
Cartilage oligomeric matrix protein (COMP), 66, 66*t*
Cartilage repair, 77-78. *See also* Articular cartilage repair
cell-seeded approach to, 79-80
with chondrocyte transplantation, 81
Casting
functional ankle, 47
joint motion restricted by, 128
Cataphoresis, 145
Cell biology, 6-7
Cells
in annulus fibrosus of IVD, 102*t*-103*t*
of connective tissue, 5-6
smooth-muscle, 6, 8, 12
synovial, 38
Cell-to-matrix ratio, of tendon, 36
Chondral lesions, in knee arthroscopies, 76
Chondrocytes
in articular cartilage, 63
in articular cartilage repair, 77
collagens produced by, 12
in embryonic development, 70
in nucleus pulposus, 100
in vitro studies of, 69
Chondrogenesis, 5
Chondroitin sulphate
in articular cartilage, 64, 64*t*
from damaged tendon, 42
Chondromalacia, of patella, 12
Chondronecrosis, 70
Chondronectin, in articular cartilage, 66, 66*t*
Chondrons, in articular cartilage, 63
Clinical studies, on effectiveness of therapeutic modalities,
160*t*-164*t*
Clinical trials
of calcific deposits, 166-167
on effectiveness of therapeutic intervention, 168*t*-172*t*
of lateral epicondylitis, 166
on musculoskeletal injuries of shoulder, 165-166
of therapeutic modalities, 154*t*-156*t*
Cold therapy, 139. *See also* Cryotherapy
for ankle injury, 157

Cold therapy—cont'd
  for back pain, 90
  clinical studies on effectiveness of, 163*t, 164t*
  clinical trials of, 154*t*-156*t, 171t, 174t*
  for edema, 141-142, 173-174
  effects on blood flow of, 140
  effects on pain of, 141
  for increased ROM, 143
  for neck pain, 90
  physiologic effects of, 140*t*
  research on, 176*f*
Collagen. *See also* Fibrillar collagens
  age-related loss of, 26
  in annulus fibrosus of IVD, 102*t*-103*t*
  in articular cartilage, 64-65
  biosynthesis of, 10-11, 17-21, 19*f*
  in chondromalacia of patella, 12
  in connective tissue, 1
  defined, 11
  effects of electrical stimulation on, 146
  excessive formation of, 25
  fiber-forming, 13-15
  fibrillar, 11
  function of, 7, 10-11
  interstitial, 14-15, 29
  in lamina of articular cartilage, 67
  molecular structure of, 12
  mutations of, 22
  in OA cartilage, 73
  response to mechanical elongation, 119
  in scar tissue formation, 44, 45*f*, 46
  structural organization of, 10-11, 11*f*
  in tendons, 13, 13*f*, 34, 35
  in therapeutic ultrasound, 152
  types of, 12-13
Collagen, type I, 13, 14-15
  in annulus fibrosus, 112
  formation of, 15, 16*f*
  in hypermobility syndrome, 134
  in ligamentous injury and repair, 52, 54
  in ligaments, 57
  mutations in, 23
  in nucleus pulposus, 100
  occurrence of, 29
  in severe OA, 73
  in tendon, 34
Collagen, type II, 14-15
  in articular cartilage, 65
  in ECM, 63
  in lamina of articular cartilage, 68
  mutations in, 23
  in nucleus pulposus, 100, 112
  occurrence of, 29
  in severe OA, 73
  in vertebral end-plate, 101
Collagen, type III, 14-15
  in hypermobility syndrome, 134
  in ligaments, 57
  mutations in, 23
  occurrence of, 29
Collagen, type IV, occurrence of, 29
Collagen, type VI, in articular cartilage, 65
Collagen, type IX
  in articular cartilage, 65
  in vertebral end-plate, 101

Collagen, type X, in articular cartilage, 65
Collagen, type XI, in articular cartilage, 65
Collagenase, in articular cartilage, 63
Collagen biosynthesis
  ECM components of, 26
  extracellular events in, 18-21
  posttranslational modifications of, 18
Collagen cross links, in articular cartilage, 65
Collagen disease, genetic, 29
Collagen fibers, 13, 13*f*
  crimp of, 40
  fibroblast assembly of, 20*f*
  idealized weave pattern of, 130*f*
  of meniscus, 82, 83
  and proteoglycan granules, 59*f*
  in tendinopathy, 42
  within tendons, 33, 56
  ultrastructure of, 34, 35*f*
Collagen fibrils, 12, 37, 37*f*
  and age, 48
  of articular cartilage, 64
  connective tissue mechanics and, 118-119
  formation of, 15, 16*f*
  forms of, 6, 6*b*
  imaging of, 15
  after immobilization, 130
  of joint capsules, 56, 56*f*, 57
  and ligament development, 51, 52
  radial growth of, 16
  structure of, 16
Collagen synthesis inhibitors, for joint contractures, 134
Colony-forming units, of bone marrow, 7
Compressive loading, role of articular cartilage in, 69
Condylar flattening, in meniscectomized knees, 84
Connective tissue
  across lifespan, 25-26
  adaptation to mechanical stress of, 40
  aging and, 26
  biomechanical properties of, 11, 117
    elastic range, 120
    mechanisms underlying extensibility,
      117-118
    plastic range, 120-121
    response to physical stress, 119
    role of collagen fiber, 118-119
  components of, 5-8
  dense nonmineralized, 3
  disorders of, 21-22
  in distraction osteogenesis, 134
  diversity of, 1
  functions of, 2*t*, 29
  hard *vs.* soft, 3*b*
  loose *vs.* dense, 3, 6
  manipulation of, 124-125
  mechanical properties of, 135
  mobilization of, 124-125
  nonmineralized, 7-8
  postinjury, 142-143
  regular dense, 8-11
  remodeling of, 128, 136
  response to immobility of, 127-132, 129*f*-131*f*
  response to injury of, 2-3
  "soft," 2
  structure of, 1
  viscoelastic characteristics of, 132-133

Continuous passive motion (CPM)
  in cartilage repair, 79
  clinical use of, 123
  dose-response curve for, 47
  of synovial joints, 123
  in total knee replacement, 123
Contractures
  in elderly, 128
  after immobilization, 129
  of ligaments, 51
  management of, 132-133
  prevention of, 133, 134
Contractures, joint
  conservative approach to, 133
  pathogenesis of, 132
  stretching exercises to prevent, 142-143
  treatment techniques for, 133-134
  uncomplicated, 133
Controlled motion, for ligament injury, 55. *See also* Continous
      passive motion
Corticosteroids
  clinical trials of, 167
  for soft tissue injuries, 135 (*See also* Steroids)
C-proteinase, procollagen, 24
Creep
  in aged discs, 107
  mechanical, 117
  resistance to, 54
  in viscoelastic tissue, 117
Crimp
  defined, 40, 57
  and stress-strain curve, 120
Cross-linking defect, in connective tissue diseases, 22
Cryotherapy, 139-140. *See also* Cold therapy
  analgesia produced by, 141
  for ankle injury, 157
  for ankle therapy, 158
  benefits of, 141
  effectiveness of, 176
  physiologic effects of, 157*t*, 175, 176*f*
Cryotherapy agents, 143. *See also* Ice
Crystal deposits, in joint disorders, 74
CT scans
  IVD morphological changes on, 111
  limitations of, 74
C-type fibrils, 6, 6*b*

D

Debridement
  in cartilage repair, 78
  in ultrasound therapy, 151
Decorin
  in articular cartilage, 66, 66*t*
  in ECM, 9
Degenerative changes
  age-related, 48
  IVD, 107, 108-109
Degenerative disorders, and musculoskeletal system, 25
Degenerative joint disease (DJD)
  cartilage degradation associated with, 71
  of knees, 84
Deoxypyridinoline, in articular cartilage, 65
Desmosine, 25
Development
  embryonic, 69

Development—cont'd
  and interstitial collagens, 28*t*
  and ligament growth, 51-52
Diabetes, and IVD changes, 107
Diapulse machine, for ankle injury, 158
Digital extensors, 40
Digital flexors, 40
Disc. *See* Intervertebral disc
Disc osteophyte complex, 106
Diseases
  and aging process, 28, 29
  cartilage, 71
  collagen in, 29
  fibrotic, 25
  fracture, 127
  genetic, 24
  joint, 5
  vascular, 107
Dose-response curve, for controlled passive motion,
      47
Duchenne muscular dystrophy, 133

E

Edema
  effects of electrical stimulation on, 144-145
  effects of hot and cold agents on, 141-142
  management of, 175
Education
  in hypermobility syndrome, 134
  proprioceptive training, 134
Ehlers-Danlos syndrome (EDS), 21, 29
  collagen mutation in, 23
  and physical rehabilitation, 24
Elasticity
  of connective tissue, 8
  fibers contributing to, 6
Elastin
  in annulus fibrosus, 102*t*-103*t*
  in ECM, 25
  in tendons, 34, 35, 36
Elbow
  epicondylitis of, 159
  tennis, 125, 156
  ultrasound-treated, 166
Elderly, immobilization of extremities in, 128
Electrical stimulation. *See also* Transcutaneous electrical
      nerve stimulation
  for ankle injury, 157
  for back pain, 166, 173, 168
  beneficial effects of, 176
  clinical trials of, 176
  in edema, 144, 175
  effect on pain of, 144
  effects on blood flow of, 144
  effects on fibroblastic activity of, 146*f*
  and inflammation, 144, 145*f*
  mechanism of action of, 143*f*
  physiologic effects of, 157*t*, 175, 176*f*
  physiologic responses to, 146
  research on, 176*f*
Electroacupuncture, clinical trials of, 171*t*
Electromagnetic fields
  for back pain, 174
  clinical studies on effectiveness of, 163*t*
  clinical trials of, 155*t*

Electromagnetic fields—cont'd
  physiologic effects of, 157*t*
  pulsed, 147
Embryonic development, apical ectodermal ridge in, 69
Endoplasmic reticulum (ER), collagen formation in, 21
Endotenon
  defined, 38, 39*f*
  fibroblasts from, 44
Endothelial cells
  in connective tissue, 6, 8
  in electrical stimulation, 143*f*
Entactin, 9
Entheses, 35, 36*f*
Epicondylitis
  clinical research trials of, 166
  clinical studies of, 160*t*-164*t*
  of elbow, 159
  treatment of, 159, 165
Epiligamentous repair phase, of ACL, 53
Epitenon
  defined, 38, 39*f*
  fibroblasts from, 44
  on surface of tendon, 37*f*
Epithelial cells
  collagens secreted by, 12
  effects of electrical stimulation on, 145, 146
Exercise. *See also* Physical activity
  clinical studies on effectiveness of, 163*t*, 164*t*
  clinical trials of, 168*t*
  in hypermobility syndrome, 134
Extensibility, tissue, 33
  of connective tissues, 117
  effect of hot and cold agents on, 142-143
  effect of US on, 153
Extracellular matrix (ECM)
  of cartilage, 63
  in chondromalacia of patella, 12
  components of, 5, 6-7
  of connective tissue, 2
  defined, 8*b*
  degeneration of, 71
  fibrous component of, 10
  and meniscal strength, 83
  meniscus, 82
  metabolism of, 36
  noncollagenous components of, 25
  nonfibrous component of, 8
  synthesis and degradation of, 63
  of tendons, 33, 35

F

Femur-ACL-tibia complex (FATC), tensile testing of, 51
Fibril-associated collagens with interrupted triple helices
       (FACIT), 12
Fibril-forming collagens
  in tendon structure, 13, 13*f*
  types of, 13
Fibrillar collagens
  biosynthesis of, 17*b*
  overview of, 14-15, 29
  pathophysiology of, 21
  stabilization of, 15-16; 17*b*
Fibrilogenesis, extracellular events in, 18
Fibroblast growth factor, in articular cartilage repair, 79. *See
       also* Growth factors

Fibroblasts
  and aging process, 47, 48
  of bone marrow, 7
  collagens secreted by, 12
  in connective tissue, 2, 5-6, 7, 7
  effect of electrical stimulation on, 143*f*, 145, 146, 146*f*
  effect of ultrasound on, 152
  effects of laser therapy on, 150
  in ligamentous repair, 52
  from ligaments, 52
  in scar tissue formation, 43
  stress responses of, 41
  in tendons, 36*f*
Fibrocartilage
  enthesial, 36*f*
  periosteal, 35
  sesamoid, 35
  of tendon, 35
Fibrochondrocytes, meniscal, 84, 85
Fibrocytes, 33
Fibromodulin, in articular cartilage, 66, 66*t*
Fibronectins
  in articular cartilage, 66, 66*t*
  functions of, 9
Fibroplasia, in scar formation, 43, 44
Fibrosis, 22, 41
Fibrotic diseases, 25
Fixed (resident) cells, in connective tissue, 7
Fracture, disuse-induced changes after, 128
Fracture disease, 127
Friction massage, 124, 125

G

Gene therapy, 56
Genetic diseases, involving collagen, 24
Glycine, in collagen, 11
Glycoproteins, in articular cartilage, 65-67, 66*t*
Glycosamines, from damaged tendon, 42
Glycosaminoglycan (GAG) chains, 9
  in articular cartilage, 35, 64
  dermatan sulphate, 65
Glycosaminoglycans (GAGs), 9
  of adult meniscus, 82
  immobilization in, 131
  movement and, 124
  in tendinous tissue, 35-36
Gly-X-Y triplets, repeating, 11
Golfer's elbow, 125
Gout, 74
Grafts
  allografts, 55, 84-85
  tendon, 55
Ground substance, of ECM, 8
Growth, and interstitial collagens, 28*t*. *See also* Development
Growth factor injection, 43
Growth factors, 56
  effects of electrical stimulation on, 145, 146
  in laser therapy, 149
Growth regulatory factors, 44

H

Haluronic acid, of ECM, 8
Healing process. *See also* Tissue repair
  maturation of, 128
  for MCL, 56*b*

Healing process—cont'd
  mechanical loading during, 47
Heart-valve lesions, 29
Heating agents
  examples of, 139
  physiologic effects of, 157*t*
Heat therapy, 139, 140
  for back pain, 90
  clinical trials of, 154*t*, 156*t*, 169*t*
  effects on blood flow of, 140
  effects on pain of, 141
  for extensibility, 143
  for inflammation, 142
  for neck pain, 90
  for periarticular arthritis, 165
  physiologic effects of, 140*t*, 175, 176*f*
  research on, 176*f*
  and ROM, 175
  and stretching exercises, 153
  and tissue repair, 142
HeNe laser, 148
Hepatocyte growth factor (HGF), in articular cartilage repair,
      79. *See also* Growth factors
Herniation, IVD, 107-108, 108*f*, 109*f*
  aging and, 106
  clinical presentation of, 111*t*
High voltage pulsed current (HVPC)
  for ankle injury, 157
  clinical trials of, 155*t*
  for edema, 175
  treatment with, 144
Histamine, effect of electrical stimulation on, 145
Hormonal replacement, and musculoskeletal system, 27
Hormones, and ligament metabolism, 52
Hunting response, 140
Hyaline cartilage, 63. *See also* Articular cartilage
Hyaluronan (HA), 5
  hydrated, 10
  role of, 10
Hyaluronate, 10
Hyaluronic acid, in articular cartilage, 64, 64*t*
Hydrocortisone, phonophoresis of, 166
Hydroxyapatite crystals, 2
Hydroxylysine, 11, 19*f*
Hydroxyproline, 11
Hydroxypyridinium cross links
  in articular cartilage, 65
  in ligamentous injury, 54
Hypermobility syndrome, 134
  diagnosis of, 135
  management of, 134
Hypoesthesia, 141
Hysteresis, 126*f*

I

Ice bath, 139
Ice massage, 139, 159, 169*t*
Imaging techniques, to assess AC lesions, 74-77, 75*f*-77*f*
Immobilization
  vs. accelerated rehabilitation, 55-56
  of connective tissue, 135
  connective tissue response to, 127-132, 129*f*-131*f*
  effect on tendons of, 34
  effects of, 119
  and joint immobility, 132

Immobilization—cont'd
  after knee surgery, 85
  periarticular tissues response to, 129
  of uninjured ligament, 51
Infant, IVD development in, 104
Inflammation
  effects of electrical stimulation on, 144-145
  effects of hot and cold agents on, 141-142
  general principles of, 43*b*
  NSAIDS for, 135
Inflammatory mediators
  in edema, 142
  in heat therapy, 141
  in therapeutic ultrasound, 152-153
Infrared therapy, clinical trials of, 175*t*
Injuries. *See also* Tissue repair
  and advancing age, 25-26
  overuse, 41, 42, 48, 165
  tendon, 41, 43
Insulin-like growth factors (IGFs), 79. *See also* Growth factors
Integrins, 9, 119
Interterritorial matrix, 68
Intervertebral disc (IVD), 1, 3, 97
  alterations in structure of, 112
  biomechanics of, 101-107
  bulging of, 109, 110*f*
  cervical, 99, 99*f*
  collagen in, 11
  common pathologies of, 107-109
  degeneration of, 108-109
  ECM of, 5
  effect of age changes in, 104-105, 106-107
  effects of loading on, 100
  function of, 111
  general morphology of, 100-101
  herniation of, 107-108, 108*f*, 109*f*
  lesions of, 109-111, 111*t*
  lumbar, 98, 98*f*, 99*f*, 111
  manipulation of, 127
  nature of loading on, 104
  nonimpaired, 97-98
  protrusion of, 109, 110*f*
  structure of, 98, 98*f*
  tears in, 109
  thoracic, 98-99
  ultrastructure of, 102*t*-103*t*, 105
Intracartilagenous morphology, qualitative assessment of, 76
Intradiscal pressure, measurement of, 105
In vitro studies
  of electrical stimulation, 144, 145, 146
  laser therapy, 148-150
  of macromolecular biosynthesis, 69
  of therapeutic ultrasound, 151-152
In vivo studies, of therapeutic ultrasound, 151-152
Iontophoresis
  clinical studies of effectiveness of, 160*t*, 161*t*, 164*t*
  clinical trials of, 167
  for lateral epicondylitis, 165
Isodesmosine, 25

J

Joint capsule, 1, 3
  collagen fibrils of, 57
  ECM of, 5
  histology, 56, 56*f*

Joint contracture, 51. *See also* Contractures
Joint disease, and skeletal development, 5
Joint loading, in youth, 70
Joint motion, effect of, 124. *See also* Range of motion
Joint pain, of cartilage degeneration, 77
Joints. *See also* Elbow; Knee
  hypermobility of, 134-135
  hypomobility of, 132-134
  immobilization of, 130-132
  manipulation of, 127
  mobilization of, 124, 126
  synovial, 123, 130-132

K

Keloid scar tissue, 46
Keratan sulphate, in articular cartilage, 64, 64*t*
Keratinocyte migration, effects of electrical stimulation on, 146
Knee. *See also* Meniscus
  ACI of, 75
  articular defects of, 81
  immobilization of, 129, 131
  mechanics of, 84
  and role of menisci, 86
  shock-absorbing capacity of, 84
Knee ligament, effects of immobilization on, 130

L

Lamina, articular cartilage, 67-68, 86
Laminins, 8-9
  in articular cartilage, 66
  function of, 7
Laser therapy, 147
  acupuncture combined with, 174
  for ankle injury, 158
  antiinflammatory effects of, 149
  for back pain, 174
  for calcium deposits, 167
  clinical studies of effectiveness of, 161*t*-164*t*
  clinical trials of, 154*t*, 165, 169*t*, 170*t*
  effect on tissue repair of, 148-150
  effects on fibroblastic activity of, 146*f*
  for lateral epicondylitis, 166
  for pain, 148
  physiologic effects of, 157*t*
  research on, 176*f*
Lavage, in cartilage repair, 78
Ligament, 1, 3
  biomechanical properties of, 49-51, 50*f*
  characteristics of, 48
  collagen in, 11
  ECM of, 5
  effect of aging on, 48
  effect of immobilization on, 129, 130
  effects of immobilization on, 51, 128
  healing and repair of, 52
    allografts *vs.* autografts, 55-56
    histological changes, 53
    promotion of, 55
    research in, 56
    response to microdamage in, 53
    role of other joint structures in, 54-55
    staging for, 54*b*
    structural limitations after, 53-54, 54*f*
  mechanical behavior of, 119
Ligament—cont'd

mechanical properties of, 41
  and mechanical stress, 51
  multiple injuries to, 55
  normal growth of, 51-52
  one year postinjury, 55*t*
  strain values for, 40
  stress-strain curve for, 50*f*
  ultrastructure of, 49, 50*t*
Ligament-bone complexes, mechnical properties of, 52
Ligamentomuscular reflex loop, 49
Ligamentous injury, and hormone levels, 52
Ligamentum flava, 25
Load-deformation curve, for tendon, 117, 118*f*
Longitudinal bucket-handle lesion, 85
Lumbar spine, IVDs of, 111
Lymphocytes, in connective tissue, 6, 7
Lysyl hydroxylase, in collagen synthesis, 24
Lysyl oxidase, in collagen synthesis, 24

M

Macrofailure, of connective tissue structure, 127
Macromolecules, of ECM, 6
Macrophages
  in connective tissue, 2, 6, 8
  effect of electrical stimulation on, 145
Maitland grades, 126, 127
Manual therapy, effect on connective tissues, 125-127, 126*f*
Marfan syndrome, collagen mutation in, 23, 29
Marrow stromal cells, 7
Massage
  clinical studies of effectiveness of, 161*t*
  clinical trials of, 168*t*, 171*t*
  defined, 125
  friction, 124, 125
  ice, 139, 165
Mast cells, in connective tissue, 2, 6, 7-8
Matrix gla protein (MGP), in articular cartilage, 66, 66*t*
Matrix metalloproteinases, 44
Maturation, and ligament growth, 51-52. *See also* Aging process
Mechanical distraction, and ligament growth, 51
Mechanical loading
  effect on connective tissue of, 121, 122*f*
  effects on tendon of, 41
  during healing process, 47
  in scar tissue repair, 46
Mechanical stimulation, of uninjured ligament, 51
Mechanical stress
  and articular cartilage, 68
  connective tissue adaptation to, 40
  effect on tendons of, 34
  essential, 52-53
Mechanotransduction processes, 125
Medial collateral ligament (MCL)
  stages of healing of, 54*b*
  strains in, 50
  tissue flaws in healing of, 54, 54*f*
Meniscal repair, 84
Meniscectomy
  experimental models of, 84
  mechanical effects of, 84
Meniscoid structures, repositioning of, 127
Meniscus
  anatomy of, 81-82, 82*f*, 86
  biomechanics of, 83-84, 86
  degradation of, 84, 86

Meniscus—cont'd
    functions of, 83
    infant *vs.* adult, 81
    structure of, 82
    traumatic injury of, 84
Mesenchymal stem cells
    of bone marrow, 7
    in senescent process, 26
Mesenchyme
    connective tissue formed in, 2
    origin of, 5
Metalloproteinases
    in articular cartilage, 63
    matrix, 44
Microfailure, of internal mechanisms, 126-127
Microfibrils, 15-16, 17*f*
Microfracture technique, of cartilage repair, 79
Middle-aged population, musculoskeletal impairment in, 1
Mobilization. *See also* Range of motion
    graded, 126
    after knee surgery, 85
    response of connective tissue to, 121, 122*f*
Monocytes, in connective tissue, 8
MRI (magnetic resonance imaging)
    of AC lesions, 75-76, 77*f*
    degenerative disc changes in, 107
    of disc height, 100
    IVD morphological changes on, 111
Musculoskeletal injury, spontaneous rupture, 48
Musculoskeletal pain
    laser therapy for, 174-175
    ultrasound therapy for, 173-174
Musculoskeletal system
    and aging process, 26, 27, 27*f*
    connective tissue in, 1
    impairment of, 1, 27
    and physical activity, 28
Mutations, of collagen genes, 22, 23
Myofascial pain syndromes, laser therapy for, 174, 175
Myofibroblasts, 45
Myogenic restriction, of contractures, 133
Myotendinous junction, 33, 33*f*

N

Neck pain
    clinical trials for, 168*t*-172*t*
    cold therapy for, 174
    electrical stimulation for, 167, 173
    heat therapy for, 174
    and IVD changes, 106
    laser therapy for, 174, 175
Neuromuscular disease, progressive, 133
Neuropraxia, 141
Newborn, tendons of, 36
Nonsteroidal antiinflammatory drugs (NSAIDS)
    in hypermobility syndrome, 134
    for soft tissue injuries, 134-135
N-proteinase, procollagen, 24
Nuclear medicine scans, limitations of, 74
Nucleus pulposus, 98, 98*f*, 100, 107
    composition of, 112
    defined, 111
    degradation of, 108
    effect of aging on, 104, 105-106, 107
    and loading of IVD, 104

Nucleus pulposus—cont'd
    pathology of, 110
    ultrastructure of, 102*t*

O

Office workers, loading of IVD in, 100
Older population, musculoskeletal impairment in, 1
Osteoarthritis, 29
    vs. aging, 74
    animal models, 73-74
    articular cartilage in, 5
    biochemistry of, 72-73
    biomechanics of, 73
    clinical manifestation of, 71
    ECM degeneration in, 71
    histology of, 72, 72*f*
    pain due to, 174
    pathogenesis of, 72
Osteoblasts, collagens produced by, 12
Osteogenesis, distraction, 134
Osteogenesis imperfecta, collagen mutation in, 23, 29
Osteophyte formation, in meniscectomized knees, 84
Overuse injury
    aging and, 41
    musculoskeletal pain in, 48
    of tendon, 42
    therapeutic modalities for, 165
Oxygen partial pressure (PO2), of IVD, 97-98

P

Pain
    in adhesive capsulitis, 57
    back, 97, 97*f*, 106, 107 (see also Back pain)
    effect of electrical stimulation on, 144
    effect of laser therapy on, 148
    effects of hot and cold agents on, 141
    effects of ultrasound on, 151
    IVD pathology associated with, 111
    joint, 77
    of osteoarthritis, 175
    spinal, 112
    in tendinopathy, 42
Paratenon, defined, 38, 39*f*
Paresthesia, 141
Patella, chondromalacia of, 12
Pathobiology, of connective tissue, 3
Pentosidine level, of arthritic patients, 73
Peptidases, procollagen, 29
Periarticular inflammatory conditions
    identification of, 158-159
    treatment of, 159, 165
Periocytes, in connective tissue, 6, 8
Pharmacological intervention, for joint contractures, 134
Phonophoresis
    clinical studies of effectiveness of, 160*t*, 162*t*
    for lateral epicondylitis, 166
Physical activity. *See also* Exercise
    and cartilage thickness, 70
    extreme levels of, 34
    lifelong, 48
    response of connective tissue to, 121, 122*f*
Physical therapy, orthopedic, 1. *See also* Rehabilitation
Plantar fasciitis, 166-167
Plasma cells, in connective tissue, 6, 7
Poly(vinyl alcohol)-hydrogel (PVA-H), 80

Posttranslational events, in collagen biosynthesis, 17*b*, 18
Procollagen molecule, 18
Prolapse, clinical presentation of disc, 111*t*
Prolyl hydroxylase, in collagen synthesis, 24
Proprioception, joint, 48
Proprioceptive training, in hypermobility syndrome, 134
    prostaglandins, in laser therapy, 149
Prostheses, for meniscal repair, 85
Proteins
    in articular cartilage, 65-67, 66*t*
    multiadhesive matrix, 8-9
    structural, 10
Proteoglycan granules, and collagen fibers, 50*f*
Proteoglycans (PGs)
    aggregating, 9
    in annulus fibrosus of IVD, 102*t*-103*t*
    in articular cartilage, 64, 64*t*
    of ECM, 6, 8, 9-10, 63
    in nucleus pulposus, 100, 106
    of tendon, 35, 36
Protrusion, disc
    anterior and lateral, 110-111
    clinical presentation of, 111*t*
    posterior, 109-110
Pseudogout, 74
Pulsed electromagnetic fields (PEMFs), 147
Pulsed electromagnetic fields (PEMF) therapy
    for ankle injury, 158
    for back pain, 174
    clinical trials of, 169*t*
    for edema, 175
    physiologic effects of, 175, 176*f*
    research on, 176*f*
Pyridinoline, in articular cartilage, 65
Pyridinoline cross links, in disc aging, 107

Q

Quadriceps tendon, 34

R

Radiography, limitations of, 74, 75*f*
Range of motion (ROM)
    in adhesive capsulitis, 57
    after CPM intervention, 124
    effect of hot and cold agents on, 142-143, 175
    effect of US on, 153
    effect on articular cartilage, 124
    for joint contractures, 132
    in tendon injury, 43
    therapeutic approaches to, 176
Rapid pulsed pneumatic compression, clinical trials of, 156*t*
Recovery. *See also* Tissue repair
    principles of, 121
    and prolonged immobilization, 127
Regeneration, of articular cartilage, 77
Rehabilitation
    and advancing age, 25-26
    in Ehlers-Danlos syndrome, 24
    after ligament injury, 55-56
Repair, disuse-induced changes after, 128. *See also* Tissue repair
Reticulin, in ECM, 25
Retinacula, 38
Rhesus Macaque model, 75
Rheumatoid arthritis, 29
    articular cartilage in, 5

Rheumatoid arthritis—cont'd
    ECM degeneration in, 71
    joints involved in, 74
RICE (rest, ice, compression, elevation) principle, 157, 158
    for edema, 175
    research on, 176*f*
Rotator cuff tendonitis, 125
"Russian current," 144

S

Scar tissue
    breaking strength of, 46
    creep behavior of, 54
    in ligamentous repair, 52, 53
Scar tissue formation
    contraction and shrinkage, 45-46
    and friction massage, 125
    inflammation, 43
    maturation phase, 46
    mechanism of, 43
    proliferation/fibroplasia, 44-46
    remodelling/consolidation, 46
    after surgery, 55
    in therapeutic ultrasound, 152
Scar tissue repair, effect of loading on, 46-47
Schmorl's nodes, 110
Semilunar cartilage, 81
Shear properties, of meniscus, 83
Shear stress, and cartilage destruction, 70
Shivering, stimulation of, 140
Shortwave diathermy (SWD), 147
    for back pain, 174
    clinical trials of, 155*t*, 168*t*, 169*t*
Shoulder
    adhesive capsulitis of, 57
    periarticular inflammatory conditions of, 159, 160, 165
Shoulder capsule, internal composition of, 56
Shoulder injuries, clinical trials of, 165
Skeletal development, articular cartilage in, 70
Skin, connective tissue in, 2
Skin temperature, elevating, 140-141
Smoking, and IVD changes, 107
Smooth-muscle cells
    collagens produced by, 12
    in connective tissue, 6, 8
Soft tissue injuries, pharmacological management of, 134-135
Space narrowing, in meniscectomized knees, 84
Spalteholz technique, 39*f*
Spinal column, ligaments of, 49. *See also* Intervertebral disc
Spinal deformity, and IVD changes, 107
Spine, manipulaiton of, 127
Splinting, joint motion restricted by, 128
Steroids
    clinical trials of, 167
    for joint contractures, 134
    for lateral epicondylitis, 165-166
Stiffness, in adhesive capsulitis, 57
Strain, defined, 119*b*
Strain values, for tendons, 41
Stress
    and cartilage destruction, 70
    defined, 119*b*
    as physical stimulus, 119

Stress relaxation
  for connective tissue, 135
  in viscoelastic tissue, 117, 118
Stress-relaxation tests, 51
Stress-strain curves, 119, 120*f*
  for ligament, 50*f*
  linear region of, 120
  for tendon, 117, 118*f*
  toe-linear region, 120
Stretches, for connective tissue, 133
Stretching, in hypermobility syndrome, 134
Stromelysin, in articular cartilage, 63
Surgery
  of Achilles tendon, 47
  for joint contractures, 134
  meniscus, 84
Syndecan, 9
Synovial cells, in tendons, 38
Synovial fluid, 63
Synovial joints
  and CPM, 123
  immobilizaiton of, 131
  response to immobilization of, 130-132
Synovial sheaths, around tendons, 38

T

Telopeptides, 14
Temperature, therapeutic range for, 133
Temperature elevation
  and tissue repair, 142, 143*f*
  vascular changes induced by, 141
Tenascin, in articular cartilage, 66, 66*t*
Tenascin-C, 40, 41
Tendinopathy
  Achilles, 42
  calcifying, 38
Tendinosis, chronic Achilles, 42
Tendon
  biochemical properties of, 39-41
  calcific deposits in, 159
  cellular component of, 36-37, 37*f*
  collagen in, 11
  composition of, 33, 34*f*, 56
  ECM of, 5
  effects of aging on, 48
  effects of mechanical loading on, 41
  effects of physical strain on, 121
  gross structure of, 34
  healing and repair of, 37
  healing process in, 125
  human flexor, 36, 37*f*, 38*f*
  immobilized, 34
  inorganic composition of, 37-38
  mechanical behavior of, 119
  mechanical properties of, 41
  organization of, 38-41
  overuse injury of, 41
  primary function of, 40
  properties of, 35
  strain values for, 40, 41
  structural organization of, 1, 13*f*, 37*f*
  ultrastructure of, 34-36
Tendon grafts, 55
Tendon injury, healing and repair in,
  41, 43

Tendonitis
  Achilles, 125
  clinical studies of, 160*t*-164*t*
  defined, 158
  epicondylar, 139
  management of, 124
  rotator cuff, 125, 158-159
  shoulder, 139
  treatment of, 159, 165
  "Tendonosis," 158
Tennis elbow, 125, 159
Tenoblasts, 36
Tenocytes, 36
Tenotomies, 47
Tensile strength, 6
  for articular cartilage, 69
  of cartilage matrix, 64
  of collagen fibrils, 118
  of collagens, 10
  of tendon, 40, 56
Tensile testing, of FATC, 51
TENS (transcutaneous electrical nerve stimulation). *See also*
    Electrical stimulation "acupuncture-like," 173-174
  for back pain, 167, 173
  clinical trials of, 171*t, 172t*
  effectiveness of, 176
  for lateral epicondylitis, 166
  research on, 176*f*
Thawing phase, in adhesive capsulitis, 57
Therapeutic damage, 127
Therapeutic modalities
  for ankle injuries, 153, 157-158
  for back pain, 168*t*-172*t*
  choosing, 176-177
  clinical studies of effectiveness of, 160*t*-164*t*
  clinical trials of effectiveness of, 154*t*-156*t*
  electrical stimulation, 143-147
  electromagnetic fields, 147
  laser therapy, 147-150
  for neck pain, 168*t*-172*t*
  for periarticular inflammatory conditions, 158-159
  physiologic effects of, 157*t, 175, 168t*-172*t*
  superficial hot and cold, 139-143
  ultrasound, 150-153
Therapeutic pressure, 125
Thermal energy, 139
Thermoregulatory reflex, 141
Tissue repair
  effects of electrical stimulation on, 145-147
  effects of electromagnetic fields on, 147
  effects of hot and cold agents on, 142
  effects of laser on, 148-150
  effects of ultrasound on, 143, 151-153
Total knee joint replacement (TKR), and CPM intervention,
  123
Transcription, in collagen biosynthesis, 17*b*
Transcutaneous electrical nerve stimulation. *See* TENS
Transforming growth factor-beta (TGF-ß). *See also* Growth
    factors
  in articular cartilage, 66
  in articular cartilage repair, 79
Translation, in collagen biosynthesis, 17*b*
Transplantation, meniscal, 84-85
Trapeziometacarpal joint, 49*f*, 56*f*
Tri-joint complex, of IVD, 97

Triple helical region, of collagens, 14-15
T-type fibrils, 6, 6*b*

U

Ultrasonic imaging, 74-75, 76*f*
Ultrasound therapy
  administration of, 150
  for ankle injury, 157-158
  for back pain, 173
  clinical studies of effectiveness of, 160*t*, 161*t*, 162*t*, 163*t*,
      164*t*, 173-174
  clinical trials of, 154*t*, 165, 168*t*
  effect on inflammation of, 175
  effect on ROM of, 153
  effects on blood flow of, 150-151
  effects on tissue repair of, 151-153
  and fibroblastic activity, 146*f*
  for lateral epicondylitis, 166
  for pain, 151
  physiologic effects of, 157*t*, 175, 176*f*
  research on, 176*f*
  for resolution of calcium deposits, 167
  timing of, 152-153

V

Van Hoff's law, 142
Vapocoolant sprays, 143

Vascular disease, and IVD changes, 107
Vasculature
  of ligaments, 49
  of tendon, 38, 39*f*
Vasoconstriction, stimulation of, 140
Vasodilation
  in electrical stimulation, 143*f*, 146
  mechanisms underlying, 140
Vertebral body, effect of age changes in, 104-105
Vertebral end-plate, 101
  composition of, 111
  congenital defects at, 108
  effect of aging on, 106-107
Viscoelastic properties, of connective tissue, 118

W

Wandering (nonresident) cells, in connective tissue, 7
Wax baths, clinical trials of, 168*t*
Weight bearing, and GAG content, 124
Wound healing, scar tissue formation in, 44. *See also* Scar
      tissue formation
Wound repair, 22. *See also* Tissue repair

Z

Zygoapophyseal joints, 104
  and IVD health, 107
  manipulation of, 127